Praise For Dr. Michael Galitzer

"It's no secret why people from six continents seek out Dr. Galitzer as their doctor. The work he does is truly cutting-edge and transformational, resulting not only in better health, but also greater energy, restored youthfulness, and a renewed passion for life. With *Outstanding Health* he is sharing his knowledge with the world so that you, too, can experience the same healthy transformations as his patients. I highly recommend you read this book and put what he shares to action."
   ~ Tony Robbins, Bestselling author

Dr. Galitzer is the best kind of doctor, cutting edge and thoughtful. He has kept me well for over a decade. I lead an active and stressful life, traveling constantly for work, which wears down the body. Before and after every trip I go to his office and utilize protocols that protect and build up. As a result, I never get sick. We work together, rarely resort to drugs, and his approach allows me to enjoy superb health. He keeps my insides healthy, which manifests on the outside, making me look young and feel young. He is a true healer and a dear friend.
   ~ Suzanne Somers, Actress and bestselling author

You can reach a new level of amazing at any age. In *Outstanding Health*, Dr. Michael Galitzer shows you how to turn back the clock for increased energy, improved sex drive, renewed vigor and stamina, and an enviable body at any decade. In this book you'll learn simple, effective strategies to never settle for anything less than your leanest, healthiest, most fabulous self. Can't recommend this one enough!
   ~ JJ Virgin, CNS, CHFS, bestselling author of *The Virgin Diet, The Virgin Diet Cookbook*, and *The Sugar Impact Diet*

How do we stay focused, sane and balanced in this crazy world we live in? How do we balance our hormones? What about our organs? Why does everyone seem to be existing rather than living full and enriching lives? We are living on fumes disguised as energy! How do we achieve great and sustaining energy, vitality, restoring sleep so that we can live long, healthy sexy lives far beyond where we originally thought? Consciousness is changing and Dr. Galitzer is the pied piper of this change. This book should be a reference book for everyone looking to become educated in finding a heathier, richer, fuller life. I want to dance my way to 120,feeling as energetic as possible. How about you?

~ Linda Gray, Actress

Dr. Galitzer is an outstanding physician with an approach that goes far beyond the typical scope of anti-aging medicine, detoxification and hormone replacement. His Energy Medicine addresses the deepest level of disease and is as preventative as it is curative. This is the medicine of the future and Dr. Galitzer is one of its pioneering experts.

~ Hans Gruenn, M.D., Anti-Aging Physician, Longevity Medical Center, Los Angeles, CA

Dr. Michael Galitzer uses homeopathic and naturopathic medicines in conjunction with bioidentical hormone replacement. There's no better specialist in this area in the world, and he's given many women a new lease on life.

~ Melanie Simon, cofounder, Circ-Cell Skin Care

Five minutes after being treated by Dr. Galitzer I knew I was in the right place. At that point I couldn't even walk around the block. After my first visit, I felt a huge difference, and within a week I was running! He saved my life. Since then he keeps me healthy and totally energized. I adore you, Dr. Galitzer. I'd be lost without you!

~ Cornelia Guest, Socialite, author, businesswoman, and philanthropist

Dr. Galitzer has been my physician since 1990, and I have been in excellent health ever since then. I look about 10 years younger than just about all of my friends. In addition to having mastery of alternative and anti-aging medicine, he is a very caring and empathic human being. I am truly grateful that I have Dr. Galitzer in my life.

~ Dave Davis, M.D., Psychiatrist, Orange County, CA

Dr. Galitzer has been a tremendous force in making a smooth transition into my middle years as a woman. His technique, supplements and guidance have helped to steer me clear of the unknown symptoms of going through menopause. His methods not only work for me, but also for my adolescent child, and for aging men. Be open to new technology and lend an ear to a refreshing approach to health.

~ Vanessa Williams, Actress and singer

I have known Dr. Michael Galitzer for over 20 years. He is an eminent physician who cares for his patients in a way that is unique and powerful. He is very up-to-date with technological changes in both alternative and allopathic healthcare. He continues to get patients well from diseases which other doctors say are impossible to see even slight improvement. In all he is a wonderfully talented physician and human being, and it's a pleasure to see him write this meaningful book.

~ Barry Morguelan, M.D., Gastroenterologist, Los Angeles, CA

I've known Dr. Michael Galitzer and Larry Trivieri Jr for many years. Their knowledge, passion and commitment to helping others is exemplary. Their book *Outstanding Health* is exactly that—an outstanding book about what you must do to stay healthy in today's toxic world. I highly recommend it.

~ Burton Goldberg, the Voice of Alternative Medicine and creator of *Alternative Medicine: The Definitive Guide*

As an elected official and the father of two teenagers, I recognize the importance of being energetic and maintaining good health. Thanks to my friend and physician, Dr. Michael Galitzer, I have all of that and more. Read *Outstanding Health* and try out his recommendations. You will be glad you did.

~ Michael D. Antonovich, the most senior serving member of the Los Angeles County Board of Supervisors.

Outstanding Health

THE 6 ESSENTIAL KEYS TO MAXIMIZE YOUR ENERGY AND WELL BEING

HOW TO STAY YOUNG, HEALTHY AND SEXY FOR THE REST OF YOUR LIFE

Michael Galitzer, MD
Larry Trivieri Jr

AHI PUBLISHING–LOS ANGELES, CA

Disclaimer

The information in this book is not to be used to treat or diagnose any particular disease or any particular patient. Neither the authors nor the publisher is
engaged in rendering professional advice or services to the individual reader.
The ideas and recommendations in this book are not intended as a substitute
for professional health care advice or a consultation with a professional health
care provider. The publisher and authors are not responsible nor liable for
any adverse effects, losses, damages, or other consequences arising from any
information or recommendations in this book. All matters pertaining to your
personal health should be supervised by a healthcare professional.

AHI Publishing

Library of Congress Control Number: 2015900964

ISBN 978-0-9863947-0-6

Cover design by Damon Za.
Cover photo by William Werts.

Table of Contents

Foreword by Suzanne Somers xi

Introduction xv

Part One: A New Standard For Health 1

Chapter 1. Committing to Outstanding Health 3

Chapter 2. Your Body Is A Dynamic Energy System 29

Chapter 3. The ABCs of Optimal Energy 59

Part Two: Knowing The 6 Essential Keys To Outstanding Health 77

Chapter 4. The Breakthrough Action Plan 79

Chapter 5. Essential #1: Cleanse and Fortify the Mind 91

Chapter 6. Essential #2: Cleanse and Renew Your Body 131

Chapter 7. Essential #3: Super Nutrition 171

Chapter 8. Essential #4: Ignite Your Energy 207

Chapter 9. Essential #5: Regenerate With Energy Medicine 249

Chapter 10. Essential #6: Hormonal Happiness 273

Chapter 11. Awaken Your Brain 325

Chapter 12. Heal Your Heart; Hold the Sugar 353

Chapter 13. Radiant Skin 383

Chapter 14. Medicine's Exciting Future 399

Conclusion: Dancing Your Way to 120 and Beyond 427

Resources and Recommended Reading 433

Acknowledgments 447

About the Authors 449

Dedication

To every person who desires outstanding health, and to their doctors who need to understand this new medical paradigm.

Foreword by Suzanne Somers

I have been a patient of Dr. Galitzer's for longer than a decade. He is my doctor and one of my teachers. We have a unique relationship and friendship. I work *with* him; 'with,' being the operative word. His is the *new* medicine, quite different from the old version, and this is how he works with all his patients. He works *with* them.

I grew up being told the doctor was god and you never questioned anything he or she told you to do. *They* knew it all. But in today's world it's imperative that you take responsibility for your health, and make a plan for aging that includes a longevity doctor such as Dr. Galitzer.

For most of us, aging is something far down the line (we think); something we really don't have to deal with right now. That's not true. Every day, by the choices we make, we are either maintaining and improving our health, or we are not. Aging well requires a plan. If you fail to plan, then you are planning to fail. It's as simple as that.

At present, aging for most people in our society is not an attractive scenario: decrepit, frail, sick, memory-less, brain fog, heart disease, cancer and/or Alzheimer's, with the final destination: the nursing home. What a horrible end. I often think about all those people I've seen when visiting nursing homes for my research, tied to their wheel chairs, with sagging heads from being over-medicated to shut them up, and wonder how many of these people EVER thought that this was how they would end up.

Thanks to Dr. Galitzer, I now know that it doesn't have to be that way. In fact, I not only know this, I daily experience what Dr. Galitzer calls *Outstanding Health.* I'm enjoying aging. I'm 68 and feel I still have my 'juice'. I enjoy robust health. I sleep eight hours nightly, my hormones are perfect, my sex life is rockin', and my overall appearance is youthful, which is enjoyable because I know what manifests on the outside comes from good health on the inside.

I attribute much of my good health to the 6 Essential Keys that Dr. Galitzer has identified and uses as the foundation of his approach to medicine with me and all of his other patients. Putting all that he has taught me into practice, I do all I can to daily cleanse and fortify my mind and regularly detoxify my body. I also am conscientious about what I eat and drink, follow a naturally energizing lifestyle, and, to keep myself on track, I use Energy Medicine to diagnose my health status and then treat any imbalances before they become problematic. And, as you know if you have read my books, I also work with Dr. Galitzer to ensure that my hormones and the organs that manufacture them remain in a vibrantly youthful state.

In all these years that I've been Dr. Galitzer's patient, I can't recall a time when he wrote me a prescription. Instead, I go to him to stay well. I travel a lot for my work and before a trip I go to his office to load up on IV nutrients, and upon my return I go to him again to detoxify from the contamination I could not control on the trip. I unload my toxic burden regularly. Longevity experts such as Dr. Galitzer understand that no one person has the same biochemical and bio-energetic makeup as the next. Therefore, treating patients most effectively requires critical thinking about each individual patient. This is more of a hands-on type of medicine; a doctor working *with* you to eliminate the things and substances in your life that are bringing you down, and providing what you need to reverse illness and, yes, even aging.

In my books about hormones, many of which Dr. Galitzer has so eloquently written the forewords to, I tell my readers that, for example, having a chronic 'itch' on your leg or elsewhere on your body is reason to call your new thinking doctor. The itch is the *language;* it's your body communicating with you that something is amiss. To go to an orthodox doctor for an itch would appear frivolous and the remedy will most likely be some type of cortisone cream, a Band-Aid that will never address why and where the itch came from and what is behind it. Longevity doctors look for the source; a simple itch can be symptomatic of so many possibilities: a highly toxic body causing eczema from a GI tract that is out of balance from a lack of healthy flora? Or your 'itch' might be from declining hormones. This is just a simple example of the detective work longevity doctors practice by paying attention to the 'language'. Dr. Galitzer understands this 'language', and has done a marvelous job of communicating it to you in this book.

Because I follow the approaches you are about to learn, I truly do expect to live a very long life well into my 100's. I can't imagine the life I would be living had I not met Dr. Galitzer and embraced this new way to health and aging that he has shown me. Because of it, I am a productive member of society, not a drain on society. Because of my great health I require (at this time) no pharmaceutical drugs so my brain is clear and has allowed for my wisdom to manifest; I have perspective so my thinking feels clear and has order. Wisdom is a gift to the next generations; important for the evolution of humanity.

Knowledge is power. Understanding the role we each play in our own health puts the responsibility on us to educate ourselves in order to stay well and avoid declining health as we get older. Your education about how best to do so begins now. Let Dr. Galitzer teach *you* what *you* need to do to prepare for this new way to age. It's *your* life, it's *your* health. Embrace *Outstanding Health* and start creating it for yourself and your loved ones now. Read Dr. Galitzer's book. Apply the information he shares, and get ready for a whole new life you never thought possible.

I am and always will be extremely grateful for having Dr. Galitzer in my life and that gratitude manifests and trickles over as happiness with who I am and the life I am living. It's a win, win, win. And I am thrilled to be able to introduce Dr. Galitzer and this book so that you, too, can create your own win-win lifestyle for outstanding health.

~ Suzanne Somers

Introduction

In 2003, I got a phone call from actress and best-selling author Suzanne Somers. Suzanne was writing a book on hormones and menopause, and as I am a medical doctor and an acknowledged expert in bio-identical hormone therapy and anti-aging medicine, she wanted to interview me. Within a few months of that first interview, Suzanne came to my clinic in Santa Monica, California. While she had no symptoms or complaints, she was curious about what I did and how it differed from the other doctors she had interviewed. She was so impressed that she elected to become my patient. A decade later, Suzanne still comes to my clinic for treatments, and I have been a featured contributor in eight of her bestselling books.

In a city full of doctors offering every kind of anti-aging treatment, why have stars like Suzanne Somers and Vanessa Williams, as well as the "movers and shakers" in the entertainment industry, successful business people, doctors, psychiatrists, and psychologists, made the journey to my clinic in Santa Monica for over 25 years? Why do they, like Cornelia Guest, tell me, "You saved my life ... I'd be lost without you"? Why am I considered the "best-kept secret" in youth-centric Hollywood? And why do I have people calling me from every continent except Antarctica to ask for my help?

Simple: I have developed a program that consistently helps people look and feel years younger than their actual age. And now I want to share it with you so that you, too, can quickly start to improve your health and feel better than you may not have felt in years.

The sad truth is that poor health is something that most people in this country are struggling with. They may not necessarily be suffering from specific illnesses, but they certainly lack the energy they had when they were younger to do the things they most enjoy. In fact, lack of energy is the number one complaint among my patients, just as it is among patients of most other physicians. Add to that chronic stress, low libido, memory problems and "foggy" thinking, joint pain and lack of flexibility, and you have the potpourri of symptoms that the majority of Americans experience each and every day.

I am here to tell you that it doesn't have to be that way. Your body is designed to be healthy and to retain its youthful vigor well beyond what most people today expect and think of as normal. My patients and I are living proof of this, and I wrote this book so that you can be too.

The reason my program is both unique and so effective is because it combines the best of leading edge discoveries from both conventional and complementary, or alternative, medicine, and in particular, because of its focus on *Energy Medicine*, which addresses health at the cellular or energetic level. In this book, you will discover how and why both aging and disease are created energetically by such factors as environmental toxins, nutrient deficiencies, and excess stress. More importantly, you will learn what you can do to prevent and reverse this process in order to regain and maintain lasting good health, abundant energy, and a true buoyant enjoyment of your daily life or, as the French say, *joie de vivre.*

While conventional medicine views the body mostly from a physical and chemical perspective—using tools such as x-rays, CT scans, biopsies, MRIs, and mammograms to look inside the body, and blood, urine, stool, and lymph tests to do chemical analyses of bodily fluids—Energy Medicine sees the physical body as an energetic system. Any imbalance or disease is a result of disturbances in the energy field of a particular organ or system. If left untreated, these disturbances eventually produce biochemical abnormalities, and then alterations to tissues and organs. Therefore, *Energy Medicine has the capability of diagnosing and treating problems at the energetic level before they ever manifest as specific symptoms.*

This is important because millions of people in the U.S. today aren't really sick—but they aren't really well either. Many patients come to my practice complaining of fatigue, lack of focus, diminished productivity and enjoyment of life. They've been to their primary care physicians and had batteries of tests that show nothing wrong. But these people *know* they're not healthy, and they are seeking solutions that will restore their missing vitality, energy, and zest for life.

When they walk into my office, their experience is very different. Yes, I run the usual blood and urine tests to confirm that their readings are in the normal range. But then I use tests such as bio-impedance analysis, heart rate variability, applied kinesiology, and electro-dermal screening, to assess the energetic health of their cells. I ask about their lifestyle, how well they eat, how much they exercise. I ask whether they have amalgam dental fillings (which leak mercury, a toxic metal, into the body), and how many hours they spend exposed to electromagnetic radiation from their cell phones and computers. I ask about their work and relationships, and how much stress they've been under. (You will learn more about the testing methods I employ, and find the same questionnaire that I use with my patients, in the pages that follow.)

It quickly becomes clear where the patient's energetic weaknesses are located—typically, depleted adrenals in combination with overtaxed elimination systems (kidneys, liver, and lymph). Once I determine where the weaknesses are, I then can prescribe specific lifestyle changes, nutritional support, and other treatments to bring the body gently back to electrical, chemical, and physical balance. The information I am sharing here in *Outstanding Health* has been designed to create the same changes for you.

By making use of the precepts of Energy Medicine to treat the causes of ill-health rather than symptoms, and to increase well-being by increasing energy, *Outstanding Health* will guide you towards renewing and revitalizing yourself at every level of your body, mind, and spirit, so they you can enjoy greater health and vitality no matter your age or current health status.

Here is what you will discover in the pages ahead:

- What being healthy really means
- Why you are so tired and what you can do about
- How to determine your current health and overall energy status
- The "energy factories" in your cells that are the key to turning your health around
- How to supercharge your sex drive
- What your specific metabolic type is and what that means in terms of your diet and hormones.

Then you will learn the six essentials for achieving new levels of health and vitality and how to implement them in your daily life. And I will also show you how you can protect yourself from our nation's most serious health issues—Alzheimer's and dementia, heart disease, and obesity and diabetes. Additionally, you will discover cutting edge medical treatments to further help you along your journey to optimal wellness, along with where you can find physicians who offer such services and how to best create a health partnership with them.

You may be wondering how I came to develop my approach to health care. My journey began in 1986, when I went from being a burnt-out emergency room physician to practicing at a holistic clinic in Westwood, California. One of my best friends, Bill, came to see me complaining of fatigue, and I diagnosed mercury toxicity from the amalgam fillings in his teeth. I advised him to have his fillings removed and ran a blood test (similar to a food allergy test) to determine which metals would be compatible with his body to use in the replacement fillings.

But when Bill came back from the dentist, he had a list of recommendations the dentist had produced by using an energy screening device that measured skin resistance changes when various metals were introduced into the circuit. I compared the results from the blood test and the results from the device, and they were identical. I said, "If measuring skin resistance (a noninvasive test) could produce the same results as a blood test, I want to know more."

Thus began my comprehensive education in Energy Medicine, which has included trainings in Germany, certifications in medical acupuncture, homeopathic medicine (including creating my own line of homeopathic remedies), nutritional and supplement studies, as well as studying the sub-clinical effects of stress and lifestyle on health.

In the years since then, I have applied the precepts and principles of Energy Medicine to both my extensive conventional medical knowledge and my work with bio-identical hormones to create a comprehensive program that has helped thousands of people live more healthy, vital lives. My patients range from ages 1 to 95 and come from every continent except Antarctica. I also have trained, consulted with, and recommended doctors who practice Energy Medicine all over the world. And I believe that anyone, armed with an understanding of Energy Medicine and following the program in this book, can re-ignite their spark of energy and health.

Because most of the six essential keys (lifestyle changes, nutrition, and so on) are easily accomplished, and any of the suggested treatments are available from practitioners throughout the U.S., I believe that the information you are about to learn can make vibrant health possible for anyone, regardless of location or economic circumstances. So, if you are ready to reclaim your health and youthful vigor, turn the page and read on.

PART ONE

A New Standard For Health

CHAPTER 1

Committing to Outstanding Health

Imagine a day in the distant future. See yourself at 90 or even 100 years old. What state of health is your future self in? It is a sad fact of life in our society today that most people, when they visualize such a future, see themselves in a state of worsening health at that age, fully expecting that their vitality and physical and mental health will decline, and that they will be frailer and riddled with more aches and pains. And they explain this by saying that such a reality is simply a natural consequence of getting older. Some people, in fact, so dread the thought of such a consequence that they actually prefer dying before they reach such an age in order to be spared from the suffering that they imagine inevitably accompanies reaching it. In my own practice, when I ask patients how long they'd like to live they always say 90, "but not if I'm in a walker."

Are you such a person? Do you believe that getting older means an ongoing experience of diminishing health? If so, chances are that you do so because your current state of health is no longer what it once was when you were younger.

Now imagine this potential future:

You've been an active participant in your own health for many years, partnering with your doctor, who, like me, is well-versed in the field of anti-aging and energy medicine. Under your physician's guidance, you continue to make all of the necessary lifestyle and mindset changes to stay young and healthy. You've eliminated most sources of external toxins, and you're using every means necessary to keep your internal biological environment clean and functioning at optimal levels.

You sit down in the doctor's office and look at the results of your last set of tests. Your muscle mass is strong and indicative of your daily exercise regimen. Your body fat is in the ideal range, and all of your other indicators (blood levels, sugar metabolism, and so on) are extremely healthy. Your adrenal health—indicative of your stress level—shows your stress is way down. Your hormone levels are those of a thriving 25-year-old. Your sex drive, mental clarity, respiratory efficiency, energy production, immunity and anabolic activity (the phase of your body's metabolism that is concerned with repair, rebuilding, and regeneration) are all superb. All of your neurotransmitters show that you are healthy, happy, and younger than you were last year. You walk out of the doctor's office feeling great. You call your spouse or partner to say you'll meet up at the gym later. "I can't think of a better way to celebrate my 100th birthday!" you remark.

Impossible, you say?

Not at all! And over the course of this book, I will prove it to you.

As a society, our beliefs about aging have to change. That's where I and my fellow doctors who specialize in anti-aging medicine come in. A lot of people ask what's more important, the patient's belief in the doctor or the doctor's belief in the patient. I know it's the doctor's belief in the patient. That's because when the doctor believes in the patient, the patient gets it immediately. And once the patient gets it, all things are possible.

As you read this book, I want you to consider yourself as my patient. My greatest value as a doctor is in providing people like you the information to allow you to feel, look, and be more energetic with every passing year, and to believe in your own well-being. As we make this journey together through this book, I'd like you to remember this: It's not hard to get out of balance. *Yet it's also not hard to get back into balance.* That is what the information I'm sharing with you, will help you do.

What if you could dance your way to 100, 120, and even 150 and beyond? What if each year you could feel the same or greater levels of energy and vitality, no matter what the age on your birth certificate? I'm here to tell you that not only is such a future possible for you, it is becoming increasingly probable. That's why I wrote this book—to give you the tools and information you need to live long, feel well, and look well. And to address the number one complaint that I hear from my patients when they first come to see me:

"Why Am I So Tired?"

Several years ago Sarah walked into my office and sat down. At 49 years old, she had a range of symptoms—total body pain, chronic stress, insomnia, and always feeling cold, among others. She also told me that her energy level had decreased. "Dr. Galitzer, I'm too young to feel this old and tired," she protested.

I hear a variation on those words from the majority of my patients. Most of them come not because they have a specific disease, but because they "just don't feel well." The problem is that most Western-based modern medicine looks at health and disease as two ends of a spectrum—and it rarely addresses the range of symptoms in between. The tests you get through most doctors' offices (CAT scans, MRIs, biopsies, mammograms, x-rays, blood tests, and so on) are designed to tell you if your body has become sick enough to qualify as having a "disease." If not, then the doctor will do little for you other than prescribing something to help with whatever symptoms you may have. If you complain of low energy, they may tell you to sleep more. If you have digestive problems, you may get a prescription for Prilosec. Skin issues? Cortisone or other creams. Trouble sleeping? Ambien or some other sleeping pill.

But to me, it's not enough that a patient isn't sick; I want to help them in whatever ways I can to feel completely, abundantly healthy. And that takes more than looking at their cholesterol levels and prescribing medications; it takes assessing their health at the energetic, cellular level.

In my practice, we evaluate a patient's health in six specific areas: toxicity level, ability to regenerate, terrain status, metabolic status, endocrine balance, and flow of bio-energy throughout the body. In Sarah's case I ordered blood, saliva, urine, and stool tests. But I also used Energy Medicine tests that a typical Western-trained physician knows nothing about, but which are key to assessing the fundamental functioning of the body. And I look at all of these tests from a different perspective: I want to see how far off the patient is from *optimal* functioning.

Sarah's Energy Medicine tests included a *bio-impedance test*, which measures the percentage of water inside and outside of the cell—the more water in the cell, the healthier you are. It also measures the amount of fat in your body, and how quickly you are creating new cells. (Bio-impedance shows what I call the Vitality Index, which represents a patient's ability to respond to treatment.) I also did a *biological terrain assessment* (BTA), which measures the level of digestive enzymes, the health of the lymphatic system and the kidneys, how much energy the cells are making, and whether the patient needs antioxidants or oxidants. (This test, developed by the Germans in the early 1970's, was used by NASA to monitor Apollo series astronauts on flights to our moon.) Then I ran a *heart rate variability test* (HRV), which measures the responsiveness of the autonomic nervous system, the level of stress or tension in the nervous system, and the health of the adrenal glands. I also tested Sarah using *electro-dermal screening*, which measures the energy flowing through the body. All of these non-invasive tests took no more than an hour. (You will learn more about each of the above tests and how to find doctors who provide them later on in this book.)

I then asked Sarah about her lifestyle. Did she drink coffee, alcohol, soda, or commercial, non-herbal tea? Did she smoke cigarettes? What medications was she on? Did she use artificial sweeteners like Sweet 'N Low, Equal, or Splenda? Did she eat a lot of sugar, or crave salt? Did she eat pork, bacon, ham, or breakfast sausage? How many fruits and vegetables did she eat in a typical day? Did she have PMS, did she exercise, did she drink enough water, and was it filtered or straight from the tap? What supplements was she taking? Had she ever had a root canal, and did she currently have silver amalgam fillings or dental implants?

Then I asked Sarah about her emotional life. Did she meditate? How were her relationships with others? Did she like her work? Did she feel she had a purpose in life? Did she feel connected to God or a higher power? Did she have a healthy support system of family and friends? Hardly the questions asked by most doctors, I know, yet each of them provided me with further clues for accurately assessing and addressing the root causes of Sarah's health complaints.

Sarah's tests indicated an autoimmune condition, a weak thyroid, and deficiencies in estrogen, progesterone, and testosterone. I also diagnosed a sluggish liver with high levels of toxicity, and severe adrenal fatigue. Would a conventional Western-trained endocrinologist have come to the same conclusions? Probably not. But many of Sarah's results were not extreme enough to cause other doctors concern. Instead, they might write the results off as an indication of a natural decrease in hormonal functioning due to her age and/or perimenopausal status. But to my eyes, the results indicated clearly why Sarah was feeling so ill—and I knew that I had a range of treatments that could help restore her to health and vitality.

I explained my program to Sarah and showed her exactly why she was feeling so exhausted. I directed her to avoid peanuts, dairy, and corn, and to get at least 30 minutes of exercise each day, preferably outdoors. To accelerate her healing, I prescribed bioidentical hormones, vitamin and mineral supplements, proteolytic enzymes, intravenous vitamin C and glutathione, herbal and homeopathic formulas, and photon light therapy. (You will learn more about these approaches later on in this book.)

Within one month Sarah was back in my office, beaming. She was completely pain free for the first time in years. Her hormone levels were optimal, and all of her tests indicated that her cells and metabolic processes were functioning exactly as they should. She reported that she felt better than she had when she was in her 20s. You could see from the glow of her skin, the light in her eyes, and the bounce in her step that she had returned to vibrant health. "On a scale of 1 to 10, I'm a 20!" she said happily.

Sarah's dramatic turnaround is typical of the results I see in my patients. We are in the midst of an era where it is possible to reverse physical damage caused by our environment and poor lifestyle choices, and return ourselves to vibrant health. Equally important, we can catch that damage long before it creates real havoc with our bodies, and we can *heal ourselves at the cellular and energetic level.*

As a medical doctor specializing in Energy Medicine, for the past 30 years I have used cutting-edge conventional and alternative treatments to help people of all ages and from six of the seven continents. My patients tell me that my program has helped them reverse the debilitating effects of conditions like chronic fatigue, depression, diabetes, impotence, stroke, MS, even cancer. And every one of them reports that they feel younger and healthier, with more energy, passion, and zest for life than they've had in a long, long time.

Now I want to help you achieve the same results for yourself and for your loved ones. To begin, let's explore what it means to be truly healthy.

What Is Health?

Health is commonly mistaken to mean the absence of disease. In reality, it is so much more than that. From a medical point of view, health is ultimately based upon the level of *energy* you experience on a daily basis. The more energy you have, the healthier you are and the more you are able to enjoy your life.

Energy allows us to regenerate the cells and tissues of the body. Ill health is caused by a loss of energy at the level of our cells. When there isn't enough energy for the body to accomplish its basic physiological processes efficiently, we don't feel well. It's harder for the body to absorb nutrients from food and to eliminate toxic wastes. The immune system is less effective in fighting off bacteria, viruses, parasites, and other invaders. Cell turnover decreases, and it takes far longer for the body to recover from illnesses, or just to get through the day.

Most people's health complaints today can be attributed to functional disturbances in their bodies' ability to produce and utilize energy. Such disturbances occur well before specific tissue or organ damage can be identified by conventional medical tests, which is why so many patients today continue to experience symptoms of poor health even when their doctors can't find anything wrong with them. The use of the energy medicine techniques I will be introducing you to can help detect and identify these disturbances very early on. Doing so makes it easier to effectively reestablish balance to the energetic pathways that run through all of your body's organs, glands and tissues, thereby restoring and maintaining optimal health.

When we are young, the processes of optimal energy production, regeneration, and a host of other physiological functions within the body chug along very happily, doing exactly what they're supposed to—keeping the body healthy, clean, and vibrant. But over the years we bombard our bodies with internal and external stressors. *Lack of energy is created by the slow accumulation of damage due to toxicity, hormone depletion, lifestyle choices, and mindset.* Addressing each of these factors is the key to reclaiming the energy of your youth.

Toxins: When I was an ER doctor, the only times we talked about toxicity were when we saw an overdose of sleeping pills or other drugs, carbon monoxide poisoning, or a chemical or oil spill—the acute care/disease approach. However, in Energy Medicine we see toxins as substances that produce energetic imbalances in the body, resulting in physical, emotional and mental symptoms. (Most symptoms are actually the body's way of trying to get rid of toxins and to regain homeostasis and balance.) Toxicity can produce both specific illnesses (like migraine, arthritis, psoriasis, influenza, sinusitis, immune deficiencies, and tumors), and nonspecific illnesses (clusters of symptoms that are identified as fatigue, headaches, insomnia, bad breath, muscle stiffness, depression, hypoglycemia, candidiasis, allergies, and stress).

We are constantly exposed to toxins every day. Toxins can come from the outside environment or be produced as a result of imbalances in our metabolism. *Environmental* toxins can come from tap water, smog and petrochemicals, coffee, tobacco, alcohol, sugar, food preservatives, pesticides, heavy metals (mercury, aluminum, lead, cadmium), viruses such as Epstein-Barr, influenza, cytomegalovirus, herpes, and HIV, bacteria (streptococcus, staphylococcus, salmonella, and so on), parasites, even prescription or over-the-counter medication. *Internally-generated* toxins are produced as a result of compromised digestion, inefficient metabolism, pancreatic digestive enzyme deficiency, poor eating habits, and wrong food combinations.

Both internally-generated and environmental toxins need to be cleared out by the body's elimination organs (liver, kidneys, lymph, colon, lungs, and skin) for us to feel healthy. However, if there are too many toxins for these organs to handle, these toxins start to accumulate—first in the connective tissues of the body, and then in the organs. The body tries to compensate by having the endocrine system secrete more hormones to help stimulate detoxification, but over time these glands also become inefficient and "tired."

As the cells and tissues of your body become more toxic, you feel less well, your energy drops, and an ideal environment that allows yeast and viruses to grow is created. An inefficient elimination system with toxin accumulation, coupled with depleted hormones and reduced organ function, equals autointoxication and ill health.

While the tests offered by most Western medical doctors aren't sensitive enough to diagnose the kinds of toxicity that contribute to so many diseases, Energy Medicine (which can track the impact of toxins and other stressors on a cellular level) is designed specifically to assess toxin damage in the body. Based on the levels of toxicity I have seen in almost every single one of my patients, I believe that proper and thorough detoxification is just as important as good nutrition in creating health.

Hormone Depletion: Researchers have long known that a decline in hormone levels in the body contributes to many different diseases and symptoms. Since hormones affect virtually every bodily process, low levels of hormones and impaired communication within the endocrine system, which oversees and balances hormone production, create havoc with all other body systems, including the immune, cardiovascular, detoxification, and gastrointestinal. Chronic illness is frequently associated with the body's decline in hormone production.

Nutritional deficiencies, lack of exercise, and exposure to toxins, can all result in diminished hormone production that ultimately leads to diminished biological functioning. Chronic stress can seriously impact hormone production. Other factors include malnutrition, sleep disorders, exposure to electromagnetic fields (EMFs), lack of sunlight, and the long-term use of over-the-counter and prescription medications.

There are seven key "players" on your hormonal "team": testosterone, estrogen, progesterone, insulin, thyroid, human growth hormone (HGH), and adrenal hormones. For you to be healthy, each player has to perform well, while also playing well with the rest of the team. There are a variety of ways to help restore energy and promote hormone regeneration and balance, which you will learn more about in Chapter 10.

Lifestyle Choices: In the 1960s and 1970s, we all heard the phrase that "life was all about sex, drugs, and rock and roll." Well, nowadays for many people the pleasure of sex has been replaced by the pleasure of food, drugs have been replaced by alcohol or prescription medication, and rock and roll has been replaced by TV, the Internet, or anything that keeps us sedentary, on the couch, not exercising, and passively entertained.

But food, alcohol, and TV are not the only elements of our toxic modern lifestyle. Exposure to almost constant electromagnetic radiation through our smart phones, cell towers, microwave ovens, and computer screens, also contribute to our declining health. And when you throw into the mix the heightened levels of stress created by a culture where we're expected to be accessible to work and our families 24/7, and the lack of sleep caused by our overscheduled, overstressed lives, it's no wonder we feel so exhausted.

The good news is that making changes to lifestyle can be fairly simple and extraordinarily effective. In fact, studies done by the Harvard School of Public Health show that simple changes in diet and exercise, combined with basic preventive medical care, can add 20 more years of healthy and productive life to the average individual. Lifestyle changes are some of the easiest ways for anyone to feel more energized.

Mindset: Our general state of health is directly tied to our feelings, thoughts, beliefs, attitudes, and intentions—our consciousness, if you will. Our bodies are constantly renewing themselves, and our consciousness can affect the regeneration of cells and organs positively or negatively. *A change in our health, either better or worse, involves a change in our consciousness.*

Your mind has the power and ability to cure any disease in the body. However, many people unknowingly use the mind to create illness. Because the mind plays a dominant role in health and disease, emotions such as fear, worry, tension, frustration, hate, aggression, and other negative emotions can render us more susceptible to illness.

At least sixty percent of all illness involves a psychosomatic (mental/emotional) contributing factor. The most debilitating emotion I see in my patients is fear. We are afraid of poverty, criticism, and ill health. We fear old age; we fear death; and most important, we fear the "big four" diseases: diabetes, heart disease, Alzheimer's, and cancer. Negative, fearful thinking creates disharmony in the body, literally acting like harmful frequencies. So eliminating fear is crucial for us to be able to move out of the survival mode and into the growth mode required for vibrant health.

Replacing fear-based thoughts with positive thoughts of love, gratitude and joy is one of the most effective ways that you can proactively start to take better control over your health. Such thoughts are to your body like sunlight is to plants and produce healing frequencies that resonate with every cell in your body. As I tell my patients, *Thoughts that make you happy make you well!*

Mindset also includes elements like our level of happiness, sense of purpose, our connections with friends and family, our belief and connection to a higher power. Since health is the balanced functioning of body, emotions, and mind, rejuvenation must always include mind, body, and spirit. Mindset and emotions are part of the six essential elements of an energetic life that you will discover in Part Two of this book.

How Healthy Are You?

The following test will help you assess your current health and energy. Check the applicable box for each question. Please answer as honestly and completely as you can.

Section 1: Overall Health and Energy

1. How would you rate your current level of health?

Poor (1)	Average (2)	Good (3)	Very good (4)	Excellent (5)

2. Compared to *five years ago*, how would you rate your level of health?

A lot worse (1)	A little worse (2)	The same (3)	A little better (4)	A lot better (5)

3. Compared to *ten years ago*, how would you rate your level of health?

A lot worse (1)	A little worse (2)	The same (3)	A little better (4)	A lot better (5)

4. How long has it been since you felt your health was at an optimum level?

Six months or less (5)	1 year (4)	2 years (3)	5 years (2)	More than 5 years (1)

5. How would you rate your current levels of energy?

Poor (1)	Average (2)	Good (3)	Very good (4)	Excellent (5)

6. Compared to *five years ago,* how would you rate your levels of energy?

A lot worse (1)	A little worse (2)	The same (3)	A little better (4)	A lot better (5)

7. Compared to *ten years ago,* how would you rate your levels of energy?

A lot worse (1)	A little worse (2)	The same (3)	A little better (4)	A lot better (5)

Scoring: Add up the numbers that correspond to each of you answers above. The closer your total score is to 35, the greater your overall health and energy is. Conversely, the lower your score is, the greater your need to improve your health and energy.

Section 2: Emotional Health and Wellness

8. How do you feel about your life in general?

Terrible (1)	Mediocre (2)	Good (3)	Very good (4)	Excellent (5)

9. Describe how you feel about these issues:

	Great	Okay	Problem	Comments: Why did you give this ranking?
Spouse	(5)	(3)	(1)	
Significant other	(5)	(3)	(1)	
Children	(5)	(3)	(1)	
Work	(5)	(3)	(1)	
Sex Life	(5)	(3)	(1)	
Finances	(5)	(3)	(1)	

10. How would you describe your current stress level?

Low (5)	Moderate (4)	High (2)	Very high (1)

11. What emotional or stress-related factors are of concern to you currently?

_____

12. What do you do to reduce stress in your life?

_____

Scoring: Add up the numbers that correspond to each of you answers above. The closer your total score is to 35, the greater your overall health and energy is. Conversely, the lower your score is, the greater your need to improve your emotional health and how you deal with stress. Pay attention to the written answers you gave for this section, too, because they provide clues to what you most need to do to make improvements in this area of your well-being.

Section 3: Your Current Lifestyle

13. Rank your enjoyment of your work:

Low (1)	Moderate (2)	High (4)	Very high (5)

14. How much of your work day is spent sitting?

Less than 1 hour (5)	1 to 2 hours (4)	2 to 4 hours (3)	4 to 6 hours (2)	More than 6 hours (1)

15. How much time daily do you spend on a cell/mobile phone?

Less than 1 hour (5)	1 to 2 hours (4)	2 to 4 hours (3)	4 to 6 hours (2)	More than 6 hours (1)

16. Do you have a headset or Bluetooth? _____ Yes (1) _____ No (5)

17. How many hours do you spend in front of a computer screen each day?

Less than 1 hour (5)	1 to 2 hours (4)	2 to 4 hours (3)	4 to 6 hours (2)	More than 6 hours (1)

18. How much time do you spend each day online?

Less than 1 hour (5)	1 to 2 hours (4)	2 to 4 hours (3)	4 to 6 hours (2)	More than 6 hours (1)

19. How much time do you spend watching television each day?

Less than 1 hour (5)	1 to 2 hours (4)	2 to 4 hours (3)	4 to 6 hours (2)	More than 6 hours (1)

20. How often do you exercise each week?

I don't exercise (1)	Once or twice a week (2)	3 times a week (3)	4 times a week (4)	More than 4 times a week (5)

21. Do you do exercise both aerobically and anaerobically?
_____ Yes (5) _____ No (3)

22. How long is a typical exercise session?

Less than 15 minutes (1)	15 to 30 minutes (2)	30 to 45 minutes (3)	45 minutes to 1 hour (4)	More than 1 hour (5)

23. How long have you been exercising regularly?

I don't exercise (1)	Less than 6 months (2)	6 months to a year (3)	1 to 3 years (4)	More than 3 years (5)

24. Do you enjoy exercising? _____ Yes (5) _____ No (1)

25. How often do you have bowel movements?

My bowel movements are every third day (1)	Every other day (2)	Once a day (3)	Twice a day (4)	Three times a day (5)

26. How much water do you drink per day? (Do not include other beverages.)

I don't drink water (1)	Less than 1 liter (2)	1 liter (3)	2 liters (4)	3 or more liters (5)

27. What kind of water do you drink?

Fluoridated tap water (1)	Unfluoridated tap water (2)	Bottled water (3)	Filtered water (4)	Filtered, Ionized, Alkaline Water (5)

28. Do you have a water purifier? _____ Yes (5) _____ No (1)

29. If so, what kind (reverse osmosis, charcoal filter, distilled, etc.)?

_____

30. Do you use an electric blanket? _____ Yes (1) _____ No (5)

31. Do you have any allergies or sensitivities to drugs, supplements, herbs, foods, pollens, animals, or chemicals

32. _____ Yes (1) _____ No (5)

33. If so, what are you allergic to?

_____

Scoring: Add up the numbers that correspond to each of your answers above. The closer your total score is to 90, the healthier your overall lifestyle is. Conversely, the lower your score is, the greater your need to improve your lifestyle choices. Pay attention to the written answers you gave for this section because they provide clues to what you most need to do to make improvements in this area.

34. FOR WOMEN ONLY: What percentage of time in a 24-hour day do you wear a bra?

I don't wear a bra. (5)	Less than 25 percent (4)	25 to 50 percent (3)	50 to 75 percent (2)	More than 75 percent (1)

Scoring: A growing body of research indicates that bras, especially those that contain metal in them, can negatively impact health because of how they block the flow of circulation within the lymphatic system. Bra-wearing has been linked to an increased risk of breast cancer, as well as a greater and prolonged incidence of back and shoulder pain, as well as headache and migraine because of the way bras constrict and put pressure on the back and shoulders. The lower percentage of time that you wear a bra each day, the better.

Section 4: Hormonal and Other Symptoms

(Please check any that apply.)

35. Symptoms of estrogen deficiency:

hot flashes	depression
warm rushes	headaches & migraines
temperature swings	heart palpitations
night sweats	vaginal dryness
kicking covers off at night	weight gain
trouble falling asleep	intestinal bloating
racing mind at night	back & joint pain
mental fogginess	diminished sexuality & sensuality

36. Symptoms of estrogen excess:

breast tenderness [especially central]	breast swelling or enlarging
water retention & swelling	impatient & snappy thought with clear mind
pelvic cramps	nausea

37. <u>Symptoms of progesterone deficiency</u>:

difficulty sleeping	anxiety & nervousness
no period	cystic breasts
infrequent period	painful breasts
shorter cycle	endometriosis
frequent & heavy periods	fibroids
spotting before period	PMS

38. <u>Symptoms of testosterone deficiency</u>:

diminished sex drive	flabbiness
diminished energy & stamina	diminished sense of security
diminished coordination & balance	Indecisiveness
diminished armpit, pubic & body hair	facial hair loss
diminished love of your body image	muscle weakness

39. <u>Symptoms of adrenal fatigue</u>:

trouble adapting to stress	unexplained anxiety
fatigue/exhaustion unrelieved by sleep	loss of sex drive
confused thinking	restless hands or legs
drop in productivity	increased allergies/allergic reactions
nervous under pressure	headache
nervous stomach/indigestion	low blood pressure
decreased tolerance for cold	suddenly run out of energy
difficulty sleeping	tired when you don't eat regularly
increased irritability	frequent/recurring colds or other illnesses
unexplained nausea	bruise more easily
difficulty getting up in the morning	crave sweets, caffeine

40. <u>Symptoms of thyroid deficiency</u>:

weight gain	vertical ridges on nails
fatigue	fingernails weak, breaking, splitting, or peeling
hands and feet often cold	hair falling out or thinning
energy drop in the morning	memory problems
constipation	loss of sex drive
muscles weak or prone to cramping	outside portion of eyebrows thinning or gone

41. <u>Symptoms of insulin resistance</u>:

extra weight in the abdominal area	put on weight easily and have difficulty losing it
fluid retention	sleepy after eating
food cravings	mental confusion
mood swings	hypertension
frequent urination	food allergies
irregular menstrual periods	

42. <u>Symptoms of low HGH</u>:

low energy	decreased tissue healing
decreased strength	comprehension challenges
decreased exercise tolerance	increased emotionality
decreased muscle or bone mass	lack of focus
anxiety/depression	lack of follow-through on tasks
thin, dry skin	decreased libido and sexual function
impaired concentration/memory	increased body fat and weight (around waist)

43. <u>Symptoms of acidosis and body toxicity:</u>

cardiovascular damage	free radical damage
weight gain/obesity	hormone concerns
diabetes	premature aging
yeast/fungal overgrowth	osteoporosis
immune deficiency	joint pain
low energy	aching muscles
chronic fatigue	slow digestion and elimination
bladder and kidney conditions, including kidney stones	

Scoring: Count up the number of symptoms you have in each of the above categories, then note which categories you have the most symptoms within. Those categories are where your greatest health problems lie. Take note of them so that you will know which areas of your health to focus on first with regard to the self-care techniques I share in the rest of this book.

Section 5: Past and Current Medications

44. Please list any medications that you are currently taking (include birth control pills and nonprescription drugs, including vitamins/supplements). Indicate the dosage, length of time taking the medication, and frequency of use.

Medication name & type	Dosage	Length of time taking it	Frequency of use

45. Have you ever had a frequent or prolonged use of the following drugs? If so, provide your age at the time and for how long you took them.

Medication name & type	Dosage	Length of time taking it	Frequency of use
Antibiotics			
Antihistamines			
Cortisone			
Prednisone			
Steroids			

Section 6: Current State of Health and Beliefs about Healing

46. How old do you feel in relation to your contemporaries?

Significantly younger than people my age (5)	Somewhat younger than people my age (4)	About the same as people my age (3)	Somewhat older than people my age (2)	Significantly older than people my age (1)

47. How long since you've felt really well?

Six months (5)	1 year (4)	2 years (3)	5 years (2)	More than 5 years (1)

48. What percentage of your body's healing power do you feel you are using now?

100% (5)	75% (4)	50% (3)	25% (2)	Less than 25% (1)

49. How long do you think it will take for you to regain your health?

3 months (5)	6 months (4)	1 year (3)	2 years (2)	More than 2 years (1)

Scoring: Add up the numbers that correspond to each of you answers above. The closer your total score is to 20, the greater your health and your beliefs about health and healing are. Conversely, the lower your score is, the greater your need to improve your health and examine your beliefs.

50. What lifestyle/dietary changes do you think you need to regain your health?

_____

51. How will your life be different when you reach a state of optimal health?

_____

Answering these questions should give you a clear sense of where you stand as far as your health, energy, and youthfulness are concerned. Hopefully, it will galvanize you to read the rest this book and to put its principles and suggestions into practice.

Optimum, Energetic Health Is Possible

To recap what I pointed out earlier in this chapter, optimal health occurs when a patient is physically, emotionally, mentally, and spiritually in flow, and when the organs and glands of the body are functioning at maximum capacity. Conversely, disease is a condition precipitated by a toxin-filled, nutritionally deficient and stress-dominated system, which will ultimately result in changes in energy and hormone production.

Conventional medicine tends to suppress these symptoms through the use of drugs, allowing them to smolder quietly until they erupt with increased intensity later on. In anti-aging medicine, we want to remove the underlying cause and allow the embers of an illness to never get an opportunity to smolder; we want patients to have lots of energy.

Again, your body is like an orchestra and your organs and glands are the instruments in that orchestra; some are in tune and some are out of tune. Some organs age faster than others; for instance some people have hearts and brains that are working fine, yet they fall and break a bone, and that is when they find that their bones are aging faster than their heart and brain. Other people may have heart and bones that are in good order, but they can't think or remember. so in this orchestra, if you can get everything in tune, and get the music "right," meaning getting all your organs and body systems in good working order, you will feel better.

To help the body rejuvenate requires a specific program designed to (1) cleanse the body of toxins, (2) reestablish balance within the electrical or energetic pathways that run throughout the body, and (3) provide the kind of optimum physical, mental, and emotional support that will allow the body to "re-set" itself to its state of youthful vitality and vigor.

As you'll discover in the second half of this book, there are six essential elements that are needed to re-ignite your spark and feel the kind of energy and enthusiasm you desire. My patients have used this rejuvenation program successfully for over 20 years. My wife and I follow these principles as well, and we plan to keep doing so for many years to come. No matter what your current level of health and youthfulness, know that rejuvenation *is* possible. But *you must start now, today, to take charge of your health and energy.*

An excellent example of someone who has done this is a Japanese doctor, Shigeaki Hinohara. Dr. Hinohara is over 100 years old and still practicing medicine, and serves as chairman of the board of trustees at St. Luke's International Hospital in Tokyo. He's written and published 150 books since his 75th birthday, including one called *Living Long, Living Well*, which is also the theme of this book.

Dr. Hinohara attributes his excellent health to the fact that he has taken full responsibility for his well-being and lifestyle choices. He still weighs what he weighed when he was in his 30s, and points out that one of the things that all people who live long share in common is that none of them are overweight. Every day, he makes a point of walking at least 2,000 to 2,500 steps and also engages in daily stretching exercises. According to Dr. Hinohara, his breakfast consists of a glass of fruit juice mixed with a tablespoon of olive oil, a glass of milk containing three teaspoons of lentil powder, and a banana. Because of his busy medical practice, he typically has a very light lunch, and for dinner, he eats 90 grams of beef filet two days of the week and fish on the other five. He also eats fresh vegetables, such as broccoli and lettuce, after pouring olive oil on them.

I think when we see more people like Dr. Hinohara still living full and active lives past 100 that more and more people will be inspired to learn what they need to do in order to accomplish the same thing. My wish is that, by reading this book, you will become one of them.

By following the principles outlined in this book, you are a pioneer, part of the forefront of the next wave of healthy living. The code of the pioneers always includes personal responsibility—and you, too, must take responsibility for your health. Over the past few years it's become somewhat fashionable for people to look for someone to blame for their disease or disability or plain lack of health. "It's the fault of health insurers and the cost of health care." "It's the fault of the pharmaceutical industry, whose drugs are too expensive with too many side effects." "It's the fault of our genes, or our lack of self-discipline, or our addictive personality, or the doctor who failed to catch our condition in time." Some of those factors certainly may have contributed to your current state of health, but I believe that we've been trained to give away our power over our health, and that our doing so starts at a very early age.

Here's a story to illustrate what I mean. A woman—let's call her "Mary"—is pregnant with a baby she calls Johnny. Johnny goes through nine months in Mary's belly, and then is delivered by a doctor. The first day after Johnny is born a pediatrician comes to see him and does a well baby check-up. For his first two years Johnny goes to the pediatrician every few months for check-ups and vaccinations. Every time Johnny gets sick his mom takes him to the doctor, to get the treatments to make him feel better. Eventually Johnny gets the idea: the *doctor* is the one responsible for Johnny's health, not Johnny! So we grow up giving most of the power for our health decisions into our doctors' hands—never realizing that *it's the choices we make each and every day that are the real foundation of our health or illness, youthfulness or old age.*

Author and cancer surgeon Bernie Siegel reminds us that the Latin root for the word *patient* means "submissive sufferer." All too often going to the doctor involves the patient relinquishing power over his or her health. A smart doctor will try to empower patients, but *you*, as a *smart patient*, must be willing to take responsibility for your health choices. As a doctor, I am your partner in your journey back to health, youth, and energy. *You* have the power to get and stay healthy, year after year, decade after decade. You alone have the power to experience the vital, vibrant health of your youth. Here are some key steps you can take to do so:

- Know that your health is in your control and that you have the power to improve it.
- Find your purpose in life and stay passionate and grateful.
- Make your relationship with your family a top priority in your life and stay in touch with your friends.
- Reduce the toxic load in your body through detoxification and drainage.
- Eat a healthy diet that reduces cell tissue acidity and promotes healthy, pH balance.
- Improve your nutrition with appropriate nutritional supplements.
- Develop an effective and enjoyable exercise program.
- Get sufficient exposure to sunlight each day.

- Optimize your hormone levels.
- Improve your ability to handle stress.
- Associate with like-minded health-oriented friends.
- Make time to regularly engage in hobbies and other pleasurable activities.

I will be sharing a variety of proven and effective tips and techniques that you can use to accomplish all of the above goals in the remainder of this book.

I know that you are ready to take charge of your rejuvenation! So please keep reading, and let's make this fun!

Key Points To Remember

Living a long, healthy and fulfilling life is not only possible, it's very likely once you educate yourself on the steps you need to take to do so.

Your health is your responsibility. By taking action now to improve your health you lay the foundation for optimally good health for many years to come.

True health depends on a vibrant level of energy production by the body.

Disease begins to occur long before conventional medical techniques can diagnose it, and is always due to depleted energy production.

Ongoing fatigue is a sure sign that your health is out of balance even when your doctor can't find anything wrong with you.

The primary causes of energy depletion and, thus, disease are toxic buildup in your cells, organs and glands; hormonal imbalances and diminished hormone production; unhealthy lifestyle choices; and limited and/or negative thoughts and beliefs (a poor mindset).

Doctors of anti-aging and energy medicine are trained to look for the underlying causes of diminished energy and disease in ways that conventional physicians ignore or are not trained in.

Just as it is not hard to get out of balance in today's hectic, fast-paced world, it is also not hard to get back into balance.

The power to achieve and maintain optimal health lies in your hands.

CHAPTER 2

Your Body Is A Dynamic Energy System

"Energy medicine is the future of all medicine. We're beginning now to understand things that we know in our hearts are true but we could never measure. As we get better at understanding how little we know about the body, we begin to realize that the next big frontier in medicine is energy medicine. It's not the mechanistic part of the joints moving. It's not the chemistry in our body - it's the understanding for the first time how energy influences how we feel."

~ Dr. Mehmet Oz

The underlying basis and foundation of my approach to healing lies in what has been termed Energy Medicine. From this perspective, I recognize that all of us are beings of energy, that our bodies are first and foremost energy systems, and that health and disease are first and foremost the outcomes of energy flow or disruption.

Such concepts may be foreign to you and even, at first, difficult to grasp. Indeed, that is the case for many doctors who practice conventional Western medicine. Their education in medical school primarily taught them to view the human body from a physical and biochemical perspective, and, for those who went on to become medical specialists, to focus solely on the organ systems that they treat. This is why today we have medical specialties such as cardiology (the heart), urology (the urinary tract), gastroenterology (the GI tract), and so forth. Doctors in these areas are typically well-versed in recognizing and treating conditions related to the organ systems they specialize in, yet, for the most part *they overlook the interrelationship said systems have with the entirety of their patients' bodies.*

This state of affairs of conventional medicine increasingly becoming a field of specialization ignores the patient as a whole person. And it reminds me of the following quote by Leonardo da Vinci, who wrote, "Learn how to see. Realize that everything connects to everything else."

Going beyond specialization and recognizing how everything in the body is connected is a hallmark of the art and science of Energy Medicine, and reflects the approach I take with all of my patients. In this chapter, I want to share that approach with you, so that you have a better understanding of the basics of Energy Medicine, and how an energetic disturbance in one organ or organ system can produce a seemingly unrelated symptom in a different area of your body. You will also learn how toxic emotions can disrupt your body's energetic systems, and discover revolutionary techniques that can read the energy in any organ, and how treating the energetic imbalances in your body is often more effective than many common drugs utilized in conventional medicine. Let's begin by exploring what Energy Medicine actually is, as well as its roots.

Energy Medicine Is Not New

It may surprise you to learn that Energy Medicine is not a new development when it comes to health and healing. In actuality, it is the basis of the world's two oldest and most complete systems of medicine—traditional Chinese medicine (TCM) and the Ayurvedic system of healing that originated in India. Both TCM and Ayurveda originated more than 3,500 years ago, and in both systems it was well-established even back then that health is a condition of harmony, or balance, within all of the body's organ systems, and also in "body, mind and spirit," whereas disease is the result of disharmony, or imbalances, within the patients' overall being. As these imbalances take hold, the flow of vital life force energy becomes disrupted, setting the stage for disease to occur.

In TCM, this vital life force energy is known as *qi* (pronounced as "Chee"), while Ayurvedic medicine refers to it as *prana*. Both systems of medicine seek to restore and maintain the balance and proper flow of that energy via a variety of integrated approaches, such as meditation, diet, herbs, movement exercises (yoga, Tai chi, etc), detoxification therapies, and breathwork. In addition, both TCM and Ayurveda recognize the existence of energy pathways in the body that can be regulated via specific points along these pathways, called acupoints in TCM and *marmas* in Ayurveda. Such regulation is achieved via acupuncture and marma therapy, respectively.

TCM and Ayurveda are far from the only systems of medicine that recognize the importance of the healthy flow of vital life force energy to good health. In ancient Greece, the mystic scientist Pythagoras named this subtle energy *pneuma*. A century later, Hippocrates, the Father of Western Medicine, taught his students that good health depended on the unimpeded flow of *pneuma*.

In the Judeo-Christian tradition, this same life force is commonly referred to as *spirit*, and throughout European history many healers and scientists also taught that an invisible life force was at the heart of good health. Among them were the famed Roman physician Galen, the Renaissance physician and scholar Paracelsus, Sir Isaac Newton, and Samuel Hahnemann, the developer of homeopathy, which today is widely used as a primary form of medicine around the world, including by England's Royal Family.

Despite such widespread acceptance of the existence of this vital life force and its importance of life and health, it was not until the 20th century that modern Western medicine began to become open to such concepts. In part, this occurred because of the discoveries of quantum physicists in the early 20th century. They discovered that, at the sub-atomic level, solid matter is not composed of any material substance, but, rather, is made up of packets of light energy known as quanta. But even then, the concept of energy medicine was largely ignored by conventional physicians until the early 1970s.

This change occurred due in part to an article in the *New York Times* written by James Reston. A highly respected journalist, Reston had been assigned to cover President Nixon's historic visit to China. While there, Reston underwent an emergency removal of his appendix. Following his surgery, he was amazed by the pain relief he experienced as a result of an acupuncture treatment he received, and wrote about it in the Times.

Reston's report garnered the interest of a number of influential leaders in the American medical community, resulting in a number of them traveling to China to confirm for themselves the healing benefits that acupuncture can provide. What they discovered, and then reported back to their colleagues, is that acupuncture not only relieves pain, but can also be used to effectively treat a variety of other conditions. By the end of the 1970s, interest in acupuncture grew to the point that acupuncture schools appeared throughout the US, supported by dozens of professional associations. Today, because of its proven effectiveness, acupuncture is covered by a growing number of health insurance companies and more and more doctors now refer their patients to acupuncturists or, to physicians like me, that have trained to become certified practitioners of medical acupuncture.

As a result of ongoing studies which continue to prove the effectiveness of acupuncture and other types of energy-based healing therapies, Energy Medicine is now officially recognized by the US Government as a subspecialty within the overall field of integrative, complementary and alternative medicine. The National Center for Complementary and Alternative Medicine (NCCAM), a part of the National Institutes of Health (NIH), is the federal government's primary agency for researching alternative medical therapies. The NCCAM has determined that there are five primary categories, or domains, that comprise the alternative medicine field, one of which is Energy Medicine. Such recognition by the NCCAM has provided further credibility to Energy Medicine approaches to health and has at last reopened the door to the acceptance of concepts of energetic healing that originated thousands of years ago.

Using Energy Medicine To Diagnose Illness

Even though the term Energy Medicine may not be familiar to you, chances are that you've already been a beneficiary of it in your past. Have you ever had an X-ray, CT scan, an EKG (electrocardiogram), EEG (electroencephalogram), EMG (electromyelogram), or MRI (magnetic resonance imaging)? All of these sophisticated diagnostic techniques are commonly used by conventional medical doctors, hospitals, and clinics, and they all work by employing the principles of Energy Medicine. And they are all very useful for determining various types of disease conditions and structural imbalances in the body.

However, there are also a variety of other Energy Medicine devices that are far less common, yet which can be even more effective in detecting illness and its underlying causes, in many cases months, and even years before conventional medical testing can do so. The use of such devices has dramatically improved my ability to help my patients, keeping them younger and healthier than they previously thought imaginable.

The advent of such devices occurred in the early to mid-20ᵗʰ century. They are primarily based on the 12 major energy pathways of acupuncture and TCM, also known as meridians, which traverse the entire body. One of the most important pioneers in this field was Reinhold Voll, MD, of Germany. Dr. Voll had an extensive background in acupuncture. Beginning in the 1940s, Dr. Voll recognized that meridian acupoints emit and conduct electrical current. He was able to measure skin resistance along these different meridians, which allowed him to correlate these meridian channels to different organ systems. For example, the large intestine meridian starts on the index finger and ends up at the nose. The different points along this large intestine meridian correlate to different areas of the large intestine. Dr. Voll was able to demonstrate that when an acupoint had a change in skin resistance, there existed a weakness in the large intestine that was associated with the symptoms that the patient was experiencing.

As his research progressed, Dr. Voll trained other German physicians in his methods. They soon determined that, compared to other areas of the body's skin, acupoints on the skin have a significantly less electrical resistance. Dr. Voll and his colleagues also discovered that when people are in a state of good health, each acupoint exhibited a standard measurement, but that this measurement changed when illness manifested.

Since meridian acupoints correspond to specific organs and organ systems within the body, Dr. Voll realized that measuring the electrical resistance of such points could provide an accurate and noninvasive way to quickly determine which areas of the body were out of balance and verging towards disease, as well as the degree to which that was occurring. He went on to develop the first generation of Energy Medicine devices to make such diagnoses, with the first such device known as the Dermatron. The Dermatron (so called because it measured acupoints on the skin, or *derma*) enabled Dr. Voll to precisely measure the electrical resistance of acupoints and thus determine which organs or organ systems were out of balance in the body. Because of his research in this field, this method of assessment initially became known as electroacupuncture according to Voll, or EAV, but today is more commonly referred to as electrodermal screening, or EDS.

Dr. Voll's work has resulted in a variety of EDS devices. Practitioners like me who use EDS devices do so in order to quickly and accurately determine energetic imbalances in the body that conventional diagnostic methods cannot. For example, when an acupoint reading is higher than the standard measurement, I know that its corresponding organ is in a state of inflammation or irritation even when conventional testing shows it to be normal. Similarly, when acupoint readings test lower than their standard measurements, I know that their corresponding organs are fatigued. Detecting such imbalances early on makes it much easier to restore them back to healthy harmony, and also makes it possible for me to detect contributing factors, such as toxins or allergens (substances that cause an allergic reaction) that very often escape detection when conventional testing methods are used.

The benefits of using nonconventional Energy Medicine devices do not end with diagnoses, either. Electrodermal screening not only allows me to determine what areas of the body are in need of attention, and which factors are causing those areas of imbalance, but can also help me to decide upon the most effective remedy or remedies to prescribe for my patients. This ability of EDS also originally came about because of Dr. Voll's work. His great discovery was that he was able to show that when he added a natural substance to return the skin resistance to normal, that substance helped the patient feel better.

The real value of this type of medicine is to discern what substances work for people, and at the same time do no harm. For instance, a great example of something that may be effective but is not well tolerated is chemotherapy. It kills cancer but also harms the body. By employing Energy Medicine, I am able to make sure I provide my patients everything they may require, be it antibiotics, herbs, vitamins or minerals, or homeopathic remedies, while also knowing in advance that it will be effective and well tolerated. This is why I regard EDS testing as one of the great advances in the overall field of medicine. I actually feel that if you're not testing at this level you're not as complete as you could be as a physician.

When necessary, of course, I also make use of conventional medical tests, including blood, urine, saliva and stool analyses, as well as other diagnostic methods such as X-rays, CT scans, or MRI, to confirm my EDS findings. This integrative approach enables me to provide truly comprehensive care for my patients.

Understanding Physical, Chemical and Energetic Health

As I pointed out above, while conventional medicine continues to develop at a rapid rate, as it does so it is becoming ever more technical and specialized. For example, consider the conventional medical approach to headaches. Depending on what type of headache you have, you may visit an internist, who may in turn refer you to a neurologist, an ophthalmologist, or even a psychiatrist. In this conventional form of medicine, the different symptoms are viewed as different body parts being ill.

But what if all of these symptoms are interrelated? What if your headache, skin rash, constipation, insomnia, and muscle spasms are all symptoms of the same underlying problem? What if the medicines that suppress your pain also suppress your immune system and possibly compromise your health over the long term? These are questions that most physicians today never stop to consider, in large part because their area of specialization never trained them to do so.

Conventional medicine primarily looks at the body from two levels: physically (structural) and chemically. Conventional doctors look at the body from a structural point of view by doing x-rays, CT scans, biopsies, MRI's, mammograms, and so forth. They also look at the body from a chemical level when they analyze blood, saliva, urine and stool tests. If these physical and chemical tests are found to be normal, then the patient is considered healthy. In other words, if you have no discernible sign of a disease on a physical or chemical level, then your doctor will most likely tell you that you are healthy.

As we discussed in Chapter 1, however, the absence of disease does *not* always mean that you are healthy. Optimal health only exists when a patient is physically, emotionally, mentally, and spiritually in flow, and when the organs and glands of the body are functioning at maximum capacity. Disease is a condition precipitated by a toxin-filled, nutritionally deficient and stress-dominated system which will ultimately result in changes in enzyme production and hormone production.

Many of the patients that I see have normal blood tests and X-rays and so forth, yet their major complaint to me is, "I don't feel well." They complain about a wide range of symptoms, such as fatigue, insomnia, arthritis, poor memory and concentration, and gastrointestinal issues such as bloating and constipation. These patients are not healthy.

So we need to go a little deeper – to the electrical or energetic level – to help these people feel better. As I observed above, conventional medicine does utilize energy medicine. Cardiologists take EKG's to analyze the electrical heart. Neurologists do EEG's and EMG's to evaluate the electrical brain and peripheral nerves. And just as there is electricity in the heart, brain, and nervous system, there are also electrical connections in all of the other organs and tissues of the body.

To repeat, think of your body as an orchestra, with all of its organs and glands as the instruments in that orchestra. Some organs age faster than others; for instance, some people have hearts and brains that are working fine, yet they fall and break a bone and that is when they find that their bones are aging faster than their heart and brain. For other people they may have heart and bones that are in good order, but they have cognitive or memory problems.

If all of the instruments in an orchestra are in tune and playing in harmony with each other, the music sounds great. In the same way, when all of the body's organs and organ systems are balanced and harmoniously interacting with each other, vibrant health exists and people feel great, too. That is my goal for you as you read this book.

Most symptoms that you may find yourself experiencing are your body's way of trying to get rid of toxins and to regain homeostasis and balance. Therefore, most diseases should be treated not by suppressing the body's defense mechanisms, *but by cooperating with these systems.* Modern physics has determined that matter and energy are interrelated, and that matter can be seen as a denser form of energy. That's why it is so vital to understand that your physical body is an energy system, composed of wave forms or oscillations at various frequencies. Consequently, imbalances and diseases of the physical body are a result of disturbances in the energy field of a particular organ or system. This is why Energy Medicine in all of its forms is so important, and why it will increasingly become the primary approach for treating illness and maintaining health in the future. With the knowledge that I am sharing with you, you can be in the vanguard of that future, *so long as you apply it.*

Why a Migraine May Mean An Issue With Your Liver

When I was an emergency doctor we were concerned about life-threatening toxins: an overdose of sleeping pills, carbon monoxide inhalation, an oil spill, or chemical spill. Anti-aging and Energy Medicine regard toxins as cumulative exposures. There are toxins in the air, water, and food and then there are pesticides and heavy metals and they all add up and stack up on one another. Consequently the organs get overloaded and then symptoms start. The end result is that that majority of people today feel lousy even when their doctors are unable to find anything wrong with them.

The type of medicine I practice looks at the electrical, or energetic, status of the liver, kidneys, pancreas, adrenals, thyroid, and other organs and glands. In an electrocardiogram, the electrical impulse of the heart precedes the physical heartbeat. The same thing is true for all of your body's other organs. In every case, electrical changes in the organs precede physical symptoms, often months or more before the physical symptoms themselves arise. So when the electrical status of the liver becomes abnormal, people will often have symptoms such as migraine or insomnia, and this is something you can't see on a liver function blood test or an ultrasound of the liver.

Energy Medicine reveals that most people's livers today are sluggish due to toxic overload, tissue acidity, and various other factors. Part of what I do as a physician is to help increase toxin elimination from the liver, thus reducing tissue acidity and restoring the liver to an optimal state of energetic, physical and chemical balance.

Here is a point I often tell my patients, and one which I want to emphasize with you, as well: *If you looked at nothing else in your body and only went about cleaning up your liver and improving its energetic and overall functioning, you would go a very long way toward improving your health and feeling better.* Don't forget, the first four letters in *liver* are L-I-V-E. (By the way, most people don't even know the location of the liver in the body. It sits right behind the right breast.)

Improving Liver Function and Energy: There are a variety of methods for restoring optimal liver function, many of which you can do on your own. For example, you can start your day by drinking a glass of pure, filtered water to which you add the juice of a fresh-squeezed, organic lemon. Doing so will help reduce acidity in your body and help your liver to eliminate toxins. Eating liver-cleansing foods on a regular basis will also help. In this category, some of the best foods are cruciferous vegetables, such as broccoli, Brussels sprouts, cabbage, cauliflower, kale, and radishes. These foods help boost the production of enzymes in the liver that flush out toxins. As an added and very important bonus, cruciferous vegetables have also been shown to reduce the risk of cancer. Various nutritional supplements, such as vitamin C, alpha lipoic acid, and N-acetyl-cysteine (NAC), can also help, as can various herbal remedies, such as dandelion root, milk thistle, peppermint, and turmeric. (You will learn a lot more about diet and nutrition in Chapter 7.)

Here is a juice recipe you can also use to nourish your liver if you have a juicer or a blender or food processor capable of making vegetable juice. It is very simple to make. All you need is one medium-sized, organic carrot, one medium, organic cucumber, two medium-sized, organic beets (including the beet tops), and one whole, peeled, organic clove of garlic. (It's important that these foods be organic so that you can be sure they are free of pesticides, herbicides and other toxins used in nonorganic farming practices, all of which place burden on your liver.)

Wash each vegetable and then add it to your juicer or other kitchen device. Before drinking the juice, you can add a pinch of sea or Celtic salt, if you wish. Drinking a small glass of this juice on a regular basis will help stimulate your liver to flush out stored toxins.

A self-care energetic technique that you can use to help balance the liver is to massage the acupuncture point called Liver 3 clockwise for one minute twice a day. That point is found on the top of your feet. You can locate it by running your finger in the groove between your big toe and second toe, one inch below the web space, where it will sink into a small depression. This point is often used by acupuncturists to balance the liver and reduce liver stagnation.

According to acupuncture theory, regularly massaging this point can help improve a variety of conditions, including digestion, constipation, nausea, vision issues such as blurred vision or red, swollen eyes, headache, pain or tension in the upper torso, and insomnia, all of which can be caused or made worse by sluggish liver function. Additionally, massaging Liver 3 can also help ease feelings of anxiety, anger, and irritability, which Chinese medicine also associates with a stagnant, or sluggish, liver. For best results, you want to massage this point on both of your feet. In my practice, I also employ various professional care therapies to improve liver function, including acupuncture, homeopathy, and intravenous (IV) nutritional supplements.

Energy Loss Caused By Toxins

One of the primary causes of energy loss and energetic imbalances in the body, and therefore disease, is toxins. Toxin-related imbalances can result in a wide range of physical, emotional, and mental health issues. This is important to understand and address because we are constantly exposed to toxins every day.

Again, conventional medicine recognizes two classes of toxins: *exogenous* and *endogenous*. I would also add a third class: toxic emotions, which are discussed below.

Exogenous Toxins: Exogenous, or external, toxins are those that are present in the outside environment. Major exogenous toxins which affect us include:

- Tap water
- Smog
- Alcohol
- Sugar and artificial sweeteners
- Food preservatives, additives, and artificial flavorings
- Tobacco
- Pesticides
- Petrochemicals: gas, oil, fracking exposures
- Heavy metals: mercury, aluminum, lead, cadmium, etc.

- Viruses: Epstein-Barr, influenza (flu), cytomegalovirus, herpes, HIV, etc.
- Bacteria: streptococcus, staphylococcus, E. coli and salmonella (food poisoning), Lyme, etc.
- Parasites
- Prescription medications
- Over the counter medications

Endogenous Toxins: Endogenous, or internal, toxins are produced in the body as a result of compromised digestion and inefficient metabolism. They result from pancreatic digestive enzyme deficiency, poor eating habits, and wrong food combinations. Common examples of endogenous toxins are candida (*candidiasis*) and elevated blood levels of uric acid.

Toxins are discharged from the body by the liver, kidneys, lymph, colon, lungs, and skin. As more and more toxins accumulate in your system, they place severe stress on these organs of elimination. With continued accumulation, the liver, kidneys, and lymph system become less efficient in their ability to excrete these waste products, causing toxins to first accumulate in the connective tissues of the body, and then in the organs. The body tries to initially compensate by having the endocrine (hormonal) glands secrete hormones to help stimulate detoxification. Over time these glands also become inefficient and "tired." The end result is an inefficient elimination system with toxin accumulation, coupled with reduced organ function, producing an ideal environment for illness to take hold and flourish.

Illnesses caused by toxicity fall into two categories: nonspecific and specific. Again, examples of nonspecific illness include all ill-defined symptoms, such as fatigue, headaches, insomnia, bad breath, muscle stiffness, depression, allergies, etc. This group is very difficult to categorize, and can present with many possible combinations of symptoms. Many of these symptoms are also labeled as hypoglycemia, *candidiasis*, food allergies and stress.

Again, specific illnesses related to toxicity include better defined syndromes having a characteristic set of symptoms. Some examples are migraine, arthritis, psoriasis, Epstein-Barr virus, sinusitis, immune deficiencies, and tumors.

It is important to understand that other factors, in addition to toxic accumulation, contribute to illness, such as unhealthy lifestyle choices, sub-optimal nutrition, electromagnetic stress, suppressed emotions, and genetic predisposition. Such factors can amplify the harmful effects of toxic stress.

Despite how widespread toxins are in our society, most conventional doctors only focus on acute levels of toxicity caused by the intake of high levels of toxins, such as carbon monoxide levels in the blood as a result of smoke inhalation. Since the gradual accumulation of low levels of toxins cannot yet be measured by conventional diagnostic methods, many doctors ignore them or even deny their existence. Also overlooked is the fact that most conventional medical research is conducted on one specific toxin, rather than the combinations of toxins that we are commonly exposed to each day. This cocktail effect arises when different toxins in combination create a synergistic effect, which is much more detrimental than the effects of the individual toxins alone.

It is my hope that, as the use of EDS and other energy medical devices that can detect toxins early on become more commonly used, more of my medical colleagues will not only begin to pay more attention to sub-acute cases of toxicity in their patients, but will also join me in treating them before they cause serious harm.

To repeat, the liver, kidney, and lymph systems are the internal organs of elimination and detoxification. These organs are your body's primary defense against toxins. When they are overwhelmed they put in a call to the hormonal system and its associated organs, including the adrenal and thyroid glands. Hormones aid the liver, kidney and lymph systems but eventually the glands that secrete these hormones get tired and overwhelmed. At that point you've got a toxic person with tired hormonal glands, which sets the stage for toxic overload, ongoing fatigue, and disease.

As toxins accumulate in the body they compete with essential vitamins, minerals, and trace elements, preventing such nutrients from doing the jobs the body needs them to do. As a result, the body's organs, tissues, and cells are deprived of the nutrients they need and thus lose their ability to function optimally. Because of this, my first step in the treatment of my patients is frequently focused on the reduction of their toxic load. The first part of this treatment phase is called **drainage**, which you will learn more about in Chapter 6.

Once the process of drainage is accomplished it becomes easier to identify the presence of the specific toxin most responsible for reduced organ function and overall impaired health. This key toxin is frequently a heavy metal, pesticide, petrochemical, salmonella, or virus. Not only must the toxin be eliminated, but its source must be identified and removed from the patient's environment.

This is called the **detoxification phase**, which you will also learn more about in Chapter 6. After the key toxin is removed, secondary toxins are then identified and eliminated. This process is akin to peeling an onion in which toxins are removed layer by layer. Drainage and detoxification can cause energetic stress within the body, producing temporary symptoms such as headache, fatigue, depression, myalgias, sinus congestion, etc. But such issues are fleeting and can frequently be alleviated or avoided altogether by simultaneously boosting the endocrine system so that it can do its job in producing and regulating the hormones that assist the body's detoxification processes. Once the drainage and detoxification phases of treatment achieve their purpose, most of my patients rapidly go on to achieve greater states of health and well-being. In the process, they often regain a more youthful appearance, along with increased levels of energy and emotional satisfaction.

Toxic Emotions

It's well recognized that when we experience illness it can often be accompanied by emotions of sorrow, frustration, anxiety, depression, and even anger. What is less recognized is that such emotions can also affect your physical health and negatively impact your body's organs. The classic and tragic example of this is a heart attack triggered by a powerful experience of shock or anger.

The link between thoughts and emotions and both health and disease has been extensively researched since the 1970s by researchers in the field of psychoneuroimmunology (PNI), more commonly known as mind/body medicine. Numerous studies within this field have clearly documented the profound interconnection between what we think, feel and believe and our physical health. One of the experts in this field is my wife, Janet Hranicky, PhD. Here is how she explained this connection in the landmark bestseller *Alternative Medicine: The Definitive Guide,* to which she and I were both contributors:

> "In traditional psychiatry and psychology, we still have a disease model where our focus is on alleviating symptoms. In mind/body medicine, however, if we have patients focus on their problems, dissatisfactions, fears, etc, we tend to see at an energetic level that their energy goes down as they focus on what's not right in their lives. The focus in mind/body medicine, therefore, must be to strengthen the conditioning of the mind to pick a 'better' thought that feels good...This doesn't mean that there are not appropriate times to address problem resolutions. However, in mind/body medicine, energy is paramount. It takes energy for the body to heal. Excitement and passion produce high energy states, whereas hopelessness and pain create low energy levels, and fear and anxiety tend to create chaotic energy patterns."

Janet further points out that disturbances in a person's energy field occur "weeks, months, and often years before disturbances occur in cells and tissues," adding that changes in a person's consciousness via their thoughts, emotions, and beliefs can therefore alter the physical status of cells, organs, and tissues. "Spontaneous remission, for instance," she explains, "has to do with disturbances in physical matter such as tumors disappearing, often quite quickly, when healthy shifts occur in the strength, coherency, and flow in the bioenergy field."

The findings of Janet and many other scientists researching PNI are regularly proven in my own medical practice with my patients. When

OUTSTANDING HEALTH | 45

patients first consult with me, I make it a point to ask them about not only their health complaints but also about their emotional state, their fears, and whether they are passionate and excited about their lives. Invariably, as they begin to move away from fears and limited thinking and reconnect with feelings of gratitude, optimism, and their passions, their energy levels noticeably improve, so I encourage you to spend time evaluating your own life from this perspective. You'll find a list of suggestions for doing so below.

Like Energy Medicine itself, the realizations and discoveries occurring within the field of mind/body medicine are actually rediscoveries of knowledge well-known by healers from many centuries ago. The importance of healthy emotions to health has also been taught in the world's spiritual traditions. For example, in Proverbs 17:22, it is written, "A merry heart doeth good like a medicine, but a broken spirit drieth the bones."

Both traditional Chinese medicine and the medicine of ancient Greece also categorized the body's organs by the emotions that corresponded with and affected them. The Greeks, for instance, regarded the heart as the body's most important organ. They associated it with positive emotions such as love, courage, honesty, altruism and compassion, all of which they taught strengthened the heart and life force energy (*pneuma*).

Conversely, the Greeks taught that base, negative emotions like cowardice, timidity, guilt, remorse, deceit and duplicity weaken the heart and diminish vital energy, and that prolonged grief and sorrow, such as that caused by the loss of a loved one, could lead to death due to a broken heart. In addition, according to Greek medicine, the heart is very susceptible to turbulent emotions such as anger or the desire for revenge.

Everyone talks about heart attacks being related to high cholesterol and, more recently, inflammation. But when you look at it from a deeper level, the two main causes of heart attacks are not being happy and not liking our jobs. When I was an emergency room physician I frequently worked the Sunday night to the Monday morning shift. Monday morning is when more heart attacks happen than any other time of the day. Why?

I believe it's because many people really don't want to come to work. Too many people aren't very happy. We don't live with passion, we stop being grateful, and we get into this belief system that looks at aging being a downward spiral. We need to change our beliefs, just as the ancient healers advised us so long ago.

The lungs were closely associated with the heart by the Greeks and thus affected by the same positive and negative emotions and character traits. The Greeks also recognized that we need to be in a state of ease in order for the lungs to optimally function and that feelings of being denied, invalidated or emotionally smothered (what today is called a need for "breathing room") can constrict the lungs and cause respiratory problems, whereas feelings of dignity, happiness and personal satisfaction can improve lung function by causing them to expand. (You can prove this by noticing how you breathe when you are happy compared to when you feel you are being invalidated.)

In Chinese medicine, the liver is associated with anger, which causes an imbalance in its energy. If you did a liver scan you would not see any physical abnormality with the liver. Liver blood tests would be normal (normal chemical levels), but the anger might very well manifest in symptoms such as insomnia or migraine headaches. This is an example of electrical or energetic changes in the liver.

I tell my patients to think of the liver as the general of the body. When it is imbalanced, people have difficulty making decisions. The liver is also affected by weather changes. We have all heard about people whose arthritis flares up when there is a change in the weather. In Los Angeles we have the Santa Ana winds that blow hot air from the desert out to the ocean. These winds agitate the liver, and many people have sinus flare-ups, and become more aggressive and angry as a result.

In Chinese medicine, each of the twelve meridian pathways through which energy flows through the body is associated with two hours of the 24 hour clock. During this time the energy of the organ systems to which the meridian corresponds is maximized. The time for the liver is between one and three A.M. When the liver's energy is imbalanced, people either can't fall asleep or wake up between those hours.

Another area of the body where people commonly experience the link to their emotions is the intestines, which are often susceptible to emotionally-induced problems. This is particularly true of emotions such as fear, anxiety, anger, stress and emotional tension, all of which can cause gastrointestinal disturbances, such as constipation, diarrhea, and irritable bowel syndrome. This is one of the reasons why it is not a good idea to eat when you are in a distressed emotional state.

Other organs and their associated emotions according to both the ancient Chinese and Greek healers include the kidneys, which are most affected by fear, fright and shock, and are improved by feelings of security and self-assurance; the adrenal glands, which sit on top of the kidneys and are injured and drained energetically by excessive stress; and the male and female reproductive organs, which can also be affected by fears and anxiety. In men, feelings of inadequacy and "performance anxiety" can also affect the reproductive organs, while optimal health of female reproductive organs can often depend on whether or not women feel loved by, and experience emotional warmth and feelings of closeness with, their spouse or partner. Lack of trust and emotional trauma can also negatively impact female sexual health.

In my own practice, I have come to recognize the spiritual and energetic significance of many of the body's organs. What follows is a list of those organs and the positive emotions I find that most improve their energy.

- Sinuses – wisdom and proper use of power
- Teeth – courage and determination
- Tonsils – realistic assessment of life issues
- Thyroid – harmonious drive
- Heart – love of mankind
- Lungs – sense of freedom
- Breast – motherly love
- Liver – harmonious mood
- Gallbladder/bile ducts – optimism

- Stomach/duodenum – elated moods
- Kidneys – vitality
- Spleen – power to resist negative influences
- Pancreas – self-love
- Small and large intestine – perseverance
- Appendix – self-knowledge
- Ovaries/testicles – creativity
- Prostate/uterus – ability to give yourself to your sexual partner
- Bladder – self-confidence

I recommend you review the list above to notice where and how it may be applicable to you.

Finally, to conclude this section, I want to address stress. Perhaps the biggest obstacle in people's health is being in a state of emotional distress. According to researchers like Bruce Lipton, chronic stress is a primary cause of as much as 95 percent of all disease today. This fact is borne out in my practice. Nearly every patient I see tells me about how stressed they are.

Stress is not really what people think it is. It occurs when we perceive ourselves in a state of emotional discomfort. Most people view stress as something from the outside that happens to them. In reality, however, most of us are creating this state of discomfort as a result of the undesirable meaning we give to life experiences. In other words, it is not the external events themselves which cause stress, *it is how we perceive, judge, think about, and react to them.*

Learning to de-stress is a challenge. Nearly everyone today has taken on more than they can comfortably handle and consequently they are driven by what they have taken on. You can detoxify, eat right and exercise, but getting your emotional/mental state under control is what is often most important when it comes to maintaining and improving your energy and health. You've got to focus on what makes you feel good. Then use that feel good energy to help you face and solve the challenges and problems that come your way each day.

I teach my patients that they've got to make it a point to regularly express love to their spouses, partners, children, siblings, parents and friends, and to their pets if they have them. (Having and caring for a pet is a wonderful way to diminish stress, especially for people who live alone.) I also encourage them to regularly spend time engaged in activities they enjoy, whether it be hobbies, listening to great music, or rooting for their favorite sports team.

Expressing love and doing the things we love takes our minds off of our perceived problems and connects us to something greater than ourselves. Research has proven how beneficial this can be, finding that people who regularly give themselves to others in some way tend to live longer and healthier lives compared to people who are workaholics and primarily focused on themselves.

I want to also encourage you to do what children do all the time... *imagine!* Imagine being absolutely healthy every day of your life. Imagine living to 100 or longer with abundant health and energy. See yourself as an ambassador of longevity to the world.

And have fun. Some people say there is no fun in their life because there's no one to have fun with. They are alone and lonely. I tell them to make a list of all the fun things they can do by themselves, and then to set about doing them. And I encourage them to count their blessings and be grateful for what life has already given them, while concentrating on the energy of the universe moving through them. I encourage you to do the same. By taking these simple, basic steps, you can get your head and your emotions together. Then health and longevity will have a way of following.

Energy Boosting Self-Care Tips

One of the many problems affecting our nation's health care system is an over-reliance by patients on their doctors in the expectation that their doctors alone are the keys to them becoming healthier. This simply isn't so. In order to achieve and maintain good health, you need to first take responsibility for yourself and do all that you can on your own to improve your well-being.

In my practice, I take time to educate my patients in effective self-care steps they can implement on their own without my assistance. This empowers them to achieve greater control over their health and can often dramatically decrease the time it takes for them to get well. To conclude this chapter, I want to share some proven self-care steps you can take to have more energy. All of them are easy to do and can make a real difference in your health.

Take Your Shoes Off and Get Outside: All ancient healing traditions recognized the importance of spending time outside in nature. Science has long confirmed the wisdom of such advice. Time spent within natural settings has been shown to reduce stress levels, and exposure to natural sunlight supplies your body with the most useful source of vitamin D, the health benefits of which continue to be discovered.

More recently, a growing body of research has found the value of spending time barefoot on the ground. Known as "earthing" this process of walking barefoot has been shown to dramatically reduce inflammation markers in the body after as little as 20 minutes. The same health benefits have been found to accrue by resting your body against a tree trunk.

Time spent in nature will also uplift your spirit and leave you feeling more energized. So make it a point to try and spend at least 20 minutes each day outside, walking barefoot on the ground.

Breathe Deeply: Breathwork was also a component of ancient healing traditions, especially Chinese medicine and Ayurveda. According to both traditions, when we inhale, we not only take in oxygen, but also vital life force energy, improving our vitality. Modern day research has also shown that regularly making time to take relaxed deep breaths for a few minutes one or more times a day can go a long way to alleviating stress and tension in the body.

Most of us fail to breathe consciously, resulting in shallow, inefficient breathing patterns. By focusing on your breath and breathing deeply in and out through your belly (diaphragmatic breathing) a few times each day, you will find you are able to not only reenergize yourself, but also to enhance feelings of relaxation.

Another common mistake many of us make when it comes to breathing is not fully exhaling, which results in carbon dioxide and other gases and debris not being fully eliminated from our lungs. What follow are three easy-to-perform breathing exercises you can try to correct such mistakes and to boost your energy.

1. Sit comfortably with your feet on the ground in an armless chair and relax. As you inhale deeply, raise your arms straight above your head. At the completion of your inhalation, hold your breath and bend your upper body to your right so that your left arm is over your head. Then exhale deeply and completely while gently swaying your upper body. Repeat this process by bending your upper body to your left, and continue to alternate in this fashion for a total of 15 times.

2. Stand up straight and inhale deeply, rising up on your toes as you do so. Then allow your upper body to sink forward. Place your hands on your belly and exhale deeply, shaking your belly as you do so. Repeat 15 times.

3. Stand up straight and cross your arms in front of your belly. Breathe in, then exhale deeply. As you inhale, do so fully and deeply, stretching your arms sidewise as you do so and rise up on your toes. Repeat 20 times.

Take Up Yoga or Tai Chi: Both yoga and Tai chi are gentle exercise methods that involve moving vital energy through the body. Both forms of exercise have also been shown to provide a wide range of health benefits, including more energy. Most towns and cities around the country have yoga and Tai chi instructors. Courses in both activities are also available at many local community centers, and even taught at some colleges. If you are unfamiliar with either practice, the best way to get started is under the guidance of a certified instructor. Once you learn the basics, you can then continue to practice on your own. A variety of instructional DVD and online courses are also available.

Be Active: Regular physical activity can also result in increased energy levels. Unfortunately, as a nation, we are becoming increasingly sedentary. You can counteract this trend by getting into the habit of taking a walk each day. 20 to 30 minutes is all you need. Walking is an excellent form of exercise, and also good for reducing stress. Or you can engage in other activities you enjoy, such as bicycling, swimming, or sports of your liking.

Another increasingly popular form of exercise is rebounding, which consists of jumping or running in place on a mini-trampoline. Just five to ten minutes of rebounding a day can make a significant difference in your energy levels, and is an excellent form of exercise for improving lymphatic function. Whichever form of activity you choose, be sure to have fun with it and to not overdo it. (If you are not used to exercising, please consult with your doctor first.)

Make Time For Your Loved Ones: Numerous studies have demonstrated that people who have strong, loving social connections with friends and family typically also have better levels of health and overall feelings of well-being compared to people who lack such connections. Spending time with those we love and whose company we enjoy takes us "out of ourselves" and deepens our experience of our at-one-moment with Life.

Have More Fun and Make Time For Your Hobbies: All of us have something that we enjoy doing for the simple enjoyment of it. Make a list of hobbies you most enjoy and then commit to engaging in them on a regular basis throughout each week. As you do so, you will find your enjoyment levels increasing, along with your experience of fun and personal satisfaction. As this occurs, your energy levels will get a boost too.

Meditate: Meditation is another component of the world's ancient healing traditions, and many spiritual traditions, as well. Since the early 1970s, a large body of scientific research has consistently demonstrated the wide range of mental, emotional, and physical health benefits that meditating on a consistent basis can provide, including lower levels of stress, more mental clarity, enhanced creativity, and greater levels of relaxation and energy.

There are many ways to meditate, including both sitting and walking meditation methods. What all types of meditation have in common is a focusing on the breath while centering one's attention on the present moment. Initially, it is best to learn meditation from a trained instructor, although a variety of books, audios and DVDs are also available.

The simplest method of meditation is to sit in a quiet place, resting comfortably, with your spine erect (but not rigid) and your feet flat on the floor. Close your eyes and bring your attention to your breath. Allow whatever thoughts may arise to pass as you keep your focus on each inhalation and exhalation.

At first you may find this difficult to do, but with practice it will become easier and your experience of calm centeredness will deepen. Try to meditate for five to ten minutes once or twice a day at first. As you become more comfortable with the process, you can gradually increase your time to 20 to 30 minutes once or twice a day.

Harness The Power of Positive Intention: Developing positive intentions and then acting upon them will make it easier to achieve your health and other goals in life. Here are some suggestions I share with my patients about intentions that, if acted upon, can positively impact your health and energy:

- Want more for others, especially your loved ones, than you want for yourself.
- Think and act from the endpoint of your goal. Visualize yourself already having achieved the outcome you desire and act as if it has already happened.
- Be an appreciator of your life and experience and cultivate a daily state of gratitude.
- Practice ways to stay connected and in harmony with life source energy.

- Understand resistance. Effort is part of achievement.
- Practice humility.
- Keep in mind that you can never resolve a problem by condemning it.
- Throughout the day check in with yourself and ask, "Am I aligned with the field of my intention."

Working With BioScalar Energy: This cutting edge self-care technique was taught to me by my close friend, Dr. Valerie Hunt, who was also one of my patients. Valerie was a world-renowned scientist and a pioneer in every area of research she explored, which included biology, physiological psychology, science education, physical therapy, and Energy Medicine. In the 1970s, while a professor at the University of California at Los Angeles, working with NASA scientists, she developed a high frequency device which is capable of recording the electrical energy (the human aura) from the body's surface. In the process, she discovered that the energy radiating from the body's atoms emit frequencies one thousand times faster than any other known electrical activity of the body.

Valerie, who lived to be 98, spent the remainder of her life actively involved in research that uncovered the various dimensions involved in the bioenergetic transactions between humans and the environment as they relate to human behaviors, emotions, health, illness, and disease, as well as scientifically quantifying the human aura and the levels of consciousness it contains. In the process, she discovered that there exists within the human body and its energy field an energy she called *bioscalar energy.*

Valerie explained bioscalar energy in this way: "The human auric field is composed of electromagnetic frequencies which pass through the body as waves of energy. But there is also a form of electromagnetism that is organized differently. It is not a wave, but is changed to a standing energy. In physics, this is known as a scalar wave (first demonstrated to exist in 1856 by Nikola Tesla after its existence was first theorized by the physicist and mathematician James Clerk Maxwell a few year earlier), and when it exists in the body, I call it a bioscalar wave.

"If energy is introduced on a straight line from two energy sources of the same frequency at the same time, coming toward each other to meet in the middle, the frequencies get cancelled out and it becomes standing energy. This energy doesn't flow like a wave, but it does occupy space and can increase in spatial mass. When the space it occupies is sufficient, the energy expands outward in circles of energy, directly influencing the blood and the body's lymphatic system. As you know, red and white blood cells tend to clump together when there is illness or injury. According to research conducted at the Max Planck Institute in Germany, scalar energy reverses this—it 'unsticks' the cells and circulation and lymphatic flow improves, hastening healing."

The following exercise was developed by Dr. Hunt as a means of empowering others to create bioscalar energy within their bodies to promote health and healing. This is achieved, Dr. Hunt explained, "by consciously manipulating the environmental electromagnetism in the air we breathe."

> Lie down with your arms stretched straight out sideward from your body and begin focusing on your breath. Concentrating your breathing in the area of your chest, imagine that each breath is simultaneously coming from opposite sides on a straight line into your body, through your hands. Now imagine the same frequency of energy coming through each of your hands into the middle of your body. (To ensure the same energy in each hand, select a pure primary or secondary color, e.g., red, orange, yellow, green, blue, violet, or white.) As you inhale, visualize that energy entering each hand at the same time, and bring it into your body. Allow the energy to remain there as you exhale, then take in more with your next inhalation. Continue breathing in this manner.

> As you do so, you will become aware that your chest feels full, not of air, but of standing bioscalar energy. Now stop concentrating on your inhalation, and feel the bioscalar energy expanding outward in a circular motion, like that caused by a stone thrown into water. This is the automatic action of the scalar wave, and as it occurs, it separates

the compacted cells and tissues in your body, facilitating the healing phenomenon.

Soon you will notice that your creation of bioscalar energy in the center of your body has established an automatic pattern. Stop consciously creating the scalar wave and use your mind to tell the energy what you want it to do as it spreads outward, e.g., heal pain, regenerate tissue, eliminate pathogens, etc. Do not be passive about this. Use your focused intent and "command" the energy to obey your directive.

In the beginning, do this exercise for 30 minutes twice a day if you can. As you become more skillful, ten minutes several times a day should produce excellent results.

A Note About Color Frequencies: Colors have different energy frequencies and produce different effects. Dr. Hunt's research has shown that the red-orange frequency spectrum seems to have the fastest build-up, while the blue-violet spectrum tends to continue the expansion longer. The red-orange spectrum is useful for healing damaged tissue, but to calm pain, the blue-violet spectrum works best. During each session try using both at different times and see which one works best for you.

As I mentioned, all of these self-care methods are easy to implement. Choose the ones that most appeal to you and make them a part of your daily life. As you do so, you will become increasingly aware of yourself as an "energetic being," and also develop a keener sense of your personal energy flow and when you may need to spend time bringing it into balance. These techniques will help you to more easily do so. In the process, they will also help you become healthier and younger, which is the theme of Chapter 3.

Key Points To Remember

Health is first and foremost the result of the harmonious flow of energy.

Disease occurs when the flow of energy becomes disrupted or imbalanced.

All of the world's oldest and most complete systems of healing recognized the existence of vital life force energy and the primary focus of their healing methods was on restoring and then maintaining the flow of energy throughout the body and all of its cells, organs and tissues.

Conventional medicine employs a variety of Energy Medicine techniques, such as X-ray, CT scan, MRI, EEG, and EKG.

Beginning in the early 20th century, a variety of nonconventional Energy Medicine devices have been developed based upon the acupuncture system of energy (meridian) pathways. Such devices enable energetic and regulatory balances to be detected long before actual disease sets in, and often far earlier than conventional medical diagnostic techniques.

Energy loss and disruption in the body is often caused by toxins. There are two classes of toxins recognized by conventional medicine: exogenous (external) and endogenous (internal).

Addressing toxins through drainage and detoxification is often the most important first step in treating illness and restoring good health.

Your liver is your primary internal organ of detoxification and acts like your body's general due to all of the processes it is responsible for in the body.

Daily massaging the acupoint Liver 3 on the top of both of your feet can go a long way toward helping your liver optimally perform its many tasks.

A third class of toxins recognized by practitioners of Energy Medicine is toxic emotions. Our thoughts, emotions, and beliefs can affect our health in both positive and negative ways, depending on how healthy or unhealthy they are.

Each of the organs in your body is associated with corresponding emotions and spiritual values. Problems with these organs can therefore be seen as messages for issues in your mental/emotional/spiritual life that you may need to address.

There are a variety of proven self-care techniques you can incorporate into your daily life to boost your health and energy levels.

CHAPTER 3

The ABCs of Optimal Energy

As you learned in Chapter 2, your health depends upon the harmonious and balanced flow of energy throughout your body and all of its cells, tissues and organs, as well as harmony in your thoughts, emotions and beliefs. The better able you are at achieving this balance, the better your energy levels will be. As you make this positive energetic shift, not only will your health improve, but you will also start to look and feel younger and rekindle your passion for activities you may have thought you'd left behind in your past.

In this chapter you will discover additional key issues that need to be addressed along your journey to greater health, vitality and restored youthfulness. Let's start by exploring an often overlooked aspect of health—regulation.

The Importance of Regulation

While an abundant supply of energy is certainly important to your health, of itself it is not enough. Equally important is how your body is able to regulate energy as it flows through you. Both too much and too little energy flow can result in poor health and disease. This fact was recognized by ancient Chinese healers when they developed the theory of *yin* and *yang*.

In Chinese medicine balanced, good health is often represented by the Taoist symbol of harmony, which consists of a circle within which *yin*, which represents feminine, receptive energies, and *yang*, which represents masculine, active energies, peacefully coexist with each other, separated by an S-shaped curve as light and dark segments with each side containing the "seed" of the other. You can think of *yin* and *yang* as money in two different accounts in your "bank" (your body). *Yin* energy moves inward in the body and is the "money" that your body stores up in its "savings account", while *yang* energy moves outward and is the "money" you want to draw upon for energy expenditures (your "checking account").

Just as good financial health occurs when you have a healthy balance of funds in both your savings and checking accounts, so too is good physical health dependent on a balanced supply of yin and yang energies. Practitioners of acupuncture and Chinese medicine, understanding how excesses or deficiencies of yin or yang energies cause disease, focus on restoring the balance between yin and yang rather than merely attempting to relieve disease symptoms. As a practitioner of both acupuncture and Energy Medicine, I do the same thing, and help my patients to do so for themselves, as well.

Our bodies are designed to maintain this optimal flow of energy through a variety of regulatory processes. These processes, combined together, are known as *homeostasis*. Regulation, which is a cardinal feature of optimal health, is the ability of an organ or tissue to respond appropriately to a stimulus.

One of the easiest examples of regulation to grasp has to do with your body's core temperature. It needs to be maintained within a specific, narrow range in order for all of your metabolic processes to function properly. Therefore, your body is constantly regulating its temperature in response to the external temperature to which you are exposed. In warm weather, your body will cool itself, primarily through the skin via perspiration. But in cold weather, your body seeks to warm itself and maintain its core temperature, drawing upon your liver and muscles in order to do so, under the direction of hormones transmitted by your pituitary and thyroid glands. This process of internal temperature regulation is also aided by receptor sites in your spleen and gut, which act as constant internal sensors so that your body adjusts its regulatory responses according to what is required to maintain its health.

Another example of this process occurs when you are exposed to harmful pathogens (germs) such as bacteria or viruses. When such pathogens enter the body, the body's regulatory processes immediately go into action to eliminate them. One of the primary ways that the body does this is by raising its core temperature. We called this response a fever. Fever, in turn, stimulates white blood cells, which comprise your immune system's first line of defense, helping them be more effective in eliminating the infectious agents.

The systems of your body that have the most profound effect on regulation are the autonomic nervous system and the endocrine system. The autonomic nervous system functions rapidly, making adjustments within seconds. The endocrine system acts more slowly, with its effects taking from minutes to hours to develop. Each system has an effect on the other.

The main link between the nervous system and the endocrine system is the hypothalamus, a small gland in the brain that acts as the hormone control center. Messages from the brain are sent to the hypothalamus, which in turn releases hormonal messages to the pituitary gland, located just below the hypothalamus. The pituitary gland then produces hormones that stimulate target glands (such as the adrenals, thyroid, ovaries, and testes) to secrete their hormones.

Both the small and large intestines, as well as the healthy intestinal flora they contain, and the lymphatic system, are also involved in the process of regulation. Together, they work to ensure that your body is able to optimally assimilate the nutrients you obtain from your food, and to aid in the elimination of internal and external toxins. They also play essential roles in helping to maintain and regulate your immune system. As mentioned, though, it is the autonomic nervous system and the endocrine system that are of most importance when it comes to regulation, so let's take a closer look at both of them.

The Autonomic Nervous System: The autonomic nervous system (ANS) is also known as the automatic or subconscious nervous system. It controls the activity of the heart by lowering or raising the pulse rate. It also controls blood pressure and breathing, as well as the activity of the intestines, and temperature regulation to name just a few of the many other functions it oversees and regulates. Additionally, it is in direct contact with both the central nervous system (brain and spinal cord), and the peripheral nervous system (motor and sensory nerves). The ANS is of great importance in Energy Medicine, because it controls all other mechanisms of regulation and thus your body's ability to react and adapt to stressors and changing circumstances.

The ANS has two integrated parts—the sympathetic nervous system and the parasympathetic nervous system. Think of the ANS as an information transport system. If you think of the brain as the central switchboard, the ANS is like the telephone lines leading to all the branches. The sympathetic nervous system is responsible for energy production and your body's stress coping mechanisms, as well as the "fight or flight responses" and immune stimulation triggered by emergency situations. It is more active during the day. The parasympathetic system, by contrast, is engaged in energy recovery, repair, regeneration, and relaxation, and is more active at night.

Think of the sympathetic and parasympathetic systems like this: sympathetic equals performance and parasympathetic equals recovery. In sports we are only concerned with performance, for example, how fast can an athlete run the 100 yard dash, not with how long it takes him to catch his breath. Yet often it is the second issue that best determines overall athletic achievement. Similarly, from the perspective of Energy Medicine, the stronger the parasympathetic nervous system, the healthier the patient is, as well, because he or she is able to perform well without an excessive expenditure of energy.

Since the sympathetic nervous system controls the level of tension in muscles, and since it is frequently over active in many people, when it is imbalanced in comparison to the parasympathetic system, it commonly leads to health complaints such as muscle tension, muscle fatigue, and muscle spasm. Magnesium will lower sympathetic activity (as opposed to calcium which will increase sympathetic activity), and can be quite helpful therapeutically. Conventional medicine understands this well, which is why conventional doctors often prescribe calcium channel blockers for patients with high blood pressure.

Since the parasympathetic system is usually the one that is in most need of attention, I make it a point to educate my patients about simple self-care measures they can take to stimulate and restore it to optimal functioning. Such measures include:

- Eating potassium-rich foods (avocado, bananas, dark leafy greens, legumes, wild caught salmon) and using potassium supplements
- Consuming warm drinks and avoiding cold drinks and drinks that have been sweetened
- Drinking peppermint, lavender, and linden (tilia) teas
- Taking time throughout the day to perform deep breathing exercises
- Gargling
- Singing loudly
- Stimulating your gag reflex
- Practicing yoga
- Meditating

Here is another exercise you can do that is also effective. Take a deep breath in and hold it. As you do so say out loud the vowels A, E, I, O, U. This may seem like an odd thing to do, yet I encourage you to try it because it really works.

The overall functioning of the autonomic nervous system can be assessed very easily with an in-office test called Heart Rate Variability (HRV). For this test a sensor is attached to the chest area to record the heart beat for two minutes while the patient is lying down, and for another two minutes when the patient stands. The results are then plotted, or graphed, to reveal the activity of the sympathetic and parasympathetic nervous systems, with values ranging between +4 to -4 for both systems.

Heart rate variability refers to the difference in length of each heart beat. For example, you would conclude that if a person had a pulse rate of 60 beats per minute, then each beat would last for one second. If each of the 60 beats lasted for one second, however, this would be a case of no heart rate variability, and the patient would have definite symptoms of chronic disease.

If one beat lasted for 1.0 seconds, followed by the next beat at .98 seconds, followed by the next beat at 1.02 seconds, followed by the next beat at .97 seconds, however, this would indicate excellent heart rate variability, and this patient would be considered quite healthy (with a positive reading on the parasympathetic nervous system). A decrease in, or lack of, heart rate variability is a common risk factor for virtually all chronic diseases, regardless of a person's ages. (You will learn more about heart rate variability, and HRV testing and its importance as an effective diagnostic tool in Chapter 9.)

The Endocrine System: Your endocrine system is made up of the adrenal, pineal, pituitary, thyroid, parathyroid, and sex glands, as well as the hypothalamus and the pancreas. All of these glands and organs release hormones into your body's bloodstream under the direction of the brain and nervous system in order to maintain your body's harmony and balance.

Hormones act as electrochemical messengers in your body and are involved in a variety of functions, including helping to regulating your body's biochemistry and maintaining homeostasis. Energetic disruptions in the body due to toxins, stress, nutritional deficiencies and other factors interfere with proper hormone production, and can even cause endocrine glands to shrink in size.

For most people, these negative impacts on the endocrine system are also a consequence of aging. When they occur, a wide range of health problems soon follow, from poor sleep, loss of muscle mass, mood swings, unhealthy weight gain, and decreased immunity. In women, hormone imbalances often show up when they near, and then enter, menopause, and can also increase their risk of developing fibroids and breast cancer. In men, the most common hormone tested is testosterone, lower levels of which can result in an increase in abdominal (belly) fat, lack of energy, low libido, impotence, and an increased risk of prostate cancer.

Restoring hormone balance and improving hormone levels is an important element in my overall approach to medicine. As I address my patients' hormone levels, the improvements in their overall health soon become apparent, not only to themselves, but to others. Their bodies typically becoming leaner, with better muscle tone, their skin improves, they have more energy, and they report a rejuvenation of their sex lives, enjoying sexual satisfaction as they did when they were in their 20s and 30s.

As with all other health processes of the body, the mechanisms of regulations are first and foremost mechanisms of proper energy flow. Ignoring this fact is where conventional medical approaches to treating regulatory problems arise. That's because conventional, drug-based approaches rely on chemical drugs to attempt to correct such issues.

Meet Your Mitochondria—Energized Cells for a More Energized Life

Having read this far, I'm confident you understand that everything your body does, including the simple act of reading this page, requires energy. But have you ever wondered where this energy comes from? As I explained in Chapter 2, our lives are made possible because of the existence of a vital life force energy that surrounds and flows through our bodies. Yet this life force energy is not the sole source of energy you need to live and function each day. You also need its physical energy counterpart. And where does this physical energy come from? For the most part, the answer lies in your cells.

It is estimated that the adult human body contains approximately 100 trillion cells. Within most of these cells (red blood cells being a notable exception) there exist tiny "energy factories" known as *mitochondria* that work every minute of your life to produce approximately 95 percent of all the energy your body uses on a daily basis. These microscopic pow-erhouses accomplish this by taking in the nutrients delivered to the cells from the bloodstream. They then break the nutrients down (metabolize them) and combine them with oxygen to produce *adenosine triphosphate* (ATP), the main chemical fuel supply for your body's energy needs. This process is known as *cellular respiration*. Mitochondria are the only com-ponents of the cell where food molecules and oxygen can be combined.

Not only are mitochondria essential for supplying your body with adequate energy, they also play important roles in protecting against disease and helping you to live longer. In addition, they are involved in a range of other processes, such as cell signaling and cellular differentia-tion, as well as the control of the cell cycle and cell growth and division, and normal cell death (apoptosis). They also regulate cell metabolism. Depending on the type of cell, along with other factors such as your body's nutritional status, the number of mitochondria inside a cell can range in number from 2 to 2,500. Overall, the adult human body con-tains an estimated 500 trillion mitochondria.

A remarkable characteristic of mitochondria that is unique among all other cellular components is that they possess their own DNA, which is distinct from the DNA found in the nucleus of the cells. This means that mitochondria have the ability to increase their number inside each cell. This fact has important implications, as scientists now believe that overall health and longevity in humans depends in large part on the amount of mitochondria within human cells, and on how well the mito-chondria function. More high-functioning mitochondria in your body mean better health and a greater chance that you will live a long life.

Unfortunately, their very function—metabolizing nutrients with oxygen to generate ATP for energy—make mitochondria highly suscep-tible to impaired functioning and premature death due to accelerated degradation and destruction of their DNA. The reason for this is simple: Because of the large amount of oxidative activity that mitochondria re-quire to produce ATP, they are constantly exposed to large amounts of free radicals, one of the primary causes of aging and disease. Cellu-lar DNA is defended from free radicals by the cells' double-membrane structure that shields it from the rest of the cell, along with a plentiful supply of protective proteins. The DNA of mitochondria lacks such protections and therefore has few defenses against free radical damage. As a result, and not surprisingly, as we age mitochondrial function tends to decline, as does the overall number of mitochondria in our cells.

Over the last four decades, a growing body of research has found that the decline of mitochondria in the body and impaired mitochondrial functioning are primary causes of many disease conditions today, ranging from cancer, diabetes, heart disease and stroke, and kidney and liver conditions to neurodegenerative conditions such as Alzheimer's and Parkinson's disease. Because of how essential mitochondria are for good health, abundant energy, and long life, doing all you can to protect them is vitally important. Fortunately, doing so is not very difficult, although it does require a commitment to following a healthy lifestyle. Here are some proven ways you can begin.

Diet: When it comes to keeping your mitochondria functioning properly, there are two dietary rules you need to obey: *Eat well* and *eat less*.

As mentioned, the foods you eat are processed by mitochondria into energy. In a very real sense, this means mitochondria act as engines for energy production. As with any engine, the more work mitochondria have to do, the faster they are likely to wear out. Therefore, be sure to eat foods that are nutrient-rich and not nutrient-deficient. Nutrient-rich foods, which include fresh fruits and vegetables (preferably organic), nuts, seeds, lean meats and poultry (free-range, if possible) and wild-caught fish, provide mitochondria with a plentiful supply of raw material from which they can produce energy. Nutrient-deficient foods, on the other hand, such as junk and processed foods and simple (white) carbohydrates, cause mitochondria to work just as hard, yet supply little that can be used to produce energy. In addition, drink plenty of pure, filtered water throughout the day, along with green tea, and fresh-squeezed vegetable juices if possible, while limiting your intake of unhealthy beverages such as soda, commercial juices and teas, and alcohol.

Along with eating well you should also do all you can not to over-eat. That's because research has shown that caloric restriction not only protects mitochondria (again, the more calories you take in, the harder mitochondria have to work), but can actually stimulate the production of new mitochondria. One simple way you can accomplish caloric restriction without feeling hungry is to chew your food thoroughly (at least 20 times per biteful) before swallowing. Doing so not only makes it easier for your body, and thus your mitochondria, to digest the food you eat, but can also help you feel full without the need for larger meals.

Other ways to help prevent overeating include having your last meal of the day at least three-four hours before bedtime, and skipping meals on occasion. More recently, a growing body of scientific research has pointed to the benefits of intermittent fasting. This means eating all of your meals within an eight hour period each day. This provides your body with more time to digest the foods you eat and can result in increased levels of energy.

Exercise: Regular exercise is also important for keeping your mitochondria healthy. This is particularly true of short-burst aerobic exercises, also known as high-intensity interval training (HIIT). HIIT is easier to achieve than you may think. One of the easiest methods of effective HIIT exercise is to alternate the pace of a daily walk. Start out by walking at your normal pace for two-three minutes and then walk as fast as you can for 30-45 seconds. Then return to your normal walking pace for another two minutes, then accelerate for another 30-45 seconds, and continue walking in this manner for a total of ten minutes or so. (**Note:** If you aren't used to physical activity or have a pre-existing health condition, consult with your doctor before beginning any type of exercise program.)

Nutritional Supplementation: Just as your car engine needs to be properly fueled and lubricated in order for it to perform and prevent unnecessary wear and tear, your mitochondria also requires the correct fuel and lubrication. Two nutrients taken together have been shown to provide such benefits for mitochondria. The first nutrient is Acetyl-L-Carnitine (ACL), an amino acid that has been shown to boost energy production in the cells, thereby reducing mitochondria's workload. However, ACL taken alone can increase the risk of free radical damage within mitochondria. Researchers have found that another nutrient, alpha lipoic acid, when taken along with ACL, prevents this from happening. That's because alpha lipoic acid is one of the most potent antioxidant nutrients ever discovered. It's so powerful, in fact, that it is often referred to as the "universal antioxidant" because of its ability to protect all parts of the body from free radical damage. Continuing our analogy of an engine, ACL helps rev the mitochondrial engine, while alpha lipoic acid acts as the "oil" that keeps that engine lubricated. You can find both of these nutrients at your local health food store.

Another very useful nutrient for helping to maintain mitochondrial health is coenzyme Q10 (CoQ10). And recent research suggests that the benefits of CoQ10 can be significantly boosted by another nutrient known as *pyrroloquinoline quinine,* or PQQ. What is most exciting about PQQ is the fact that it has now been shown to create new mitochondria in the cells. (HIIT exercises and caloric restriction can have also been shown to create new mitochondria.) Clinical studies have demonstrated that taking PQQ in combination with CoQ10 protects mitochondrial DNA from damage, and can therefore help the conditions associated with mitochondrial decline and impairment. PQQ is found in certain foods, such as egg yolks, meat, green peppers, papaya, and citrus fruit, as well as in organic green tea. In my opinion, however, the best way for most people to get PQQ is in a supplement. A typical dosage range is 10 mg of PQQ taken with 50-100 mg of CoQ10 once a day with meals.

But perhaps the most important nutrient for your mitochondria, and therefore your body's production of energy, is magnesium, a mineral nutrient that nearly everyone in the US is deficient in. Without enough magnesium, your body simply cannot meet all of its energy needs. As I mentioned above, mitochondria are responsible for producing ATP, your body's primary source of chemical energy. This fact is well known. What is not so well known is that before ATP can be used by the cells it must first be activated by magnesium, its primary cofactor. This task is accomplished when magnesium ions bind to ATP molecules. When this occurs, the shape and electrical charge of ATP changes, forming a new compound called Mg-ATP (Mg denotes magnesium). Simply put, by activating it, magnesium brings ATP to life. Without magnesium, your cells, and therefore your body, would lack the energy needed to keep you alive and healthy.

Unfortunately, the supply of magnesium can be rapidly depleted due to a variety of factors, especially stress and poor diet. In addition, commercial farming methods have seriously depleted our cropland's supply of magnesium and other minerals, meaning that the amount of magnesium found in even magnesium containing foods is not enough for most people to obtain their daily needs. That's why I recommend magnesium supplements to my patients.

Magnesium supplements come in various forms. Those I most recommend are magnesium citrate, magnesium malate, magnesium glycinate, and magnesium taurate, all of which are better absorbed by the body compared to other types of magnesium. You can also obtain magnesium by soaking in a hot, soothing bath with Epsom salts, or by using magnesium lotion, which delivers magnesium directly to your cells through the skin.

Now that you understand how vital mitochondria are to your health, and what you can do to help maintain their proper functioning, let's take a look at three vital organ systems that are keys for becoming healthier and younger.

Thick Versus Thin Blood

Another often overlooked key to good health has to do with the thickness, and stickiness, of your blood, a measurement known as blood viscosity. Blood thickness and stickiness, just like blood pressure, is not the same at all times. It fluctuates with every beat of your heart, becoming greater and lesser and back again as blood leaves and enters the heart chambers. Overall, however, in order to be healthy, you need thin blood with less stickiness.

People with cancer, people with heart disease, and people with strokes all have thick blood. People with chronic infections have thick blood. Blood should flow like wine not like ketchup. When blood is thick, the oxygen and nutrients it carries can't get to the cells. Without a sufficient supply of oxygen and nutrients, cells start to age and die prematurely, setting the stage for a wide range of disease conditions. Conversely, when your blood is healthy and thin, your cells are able to obtain more oxygen and nutrients, resulting in better health and more energy.

To better understand the importance of thin versus thick blood, consider your home's water pipe system. When water is clean (thin), it flows freely through the pipes and out through your faucet whenever you need it. Moreover, because of how easily it flows, it does not cause damage to the pipes themselves. But when water is contaminated and thick like sludge, the flow of water through the pipes is much slower, requiring more energy and force to get it to move. This can result in clogged, damaged, and even burst water pipes.

The above analogy is akin to what happens within your entire cardio-vascular system and its miles of arteries, veins and capillaries. Healthy, thin blood flows freely, requiring a reduced output of energy from the heart. But as it thickens and becomes stickier, more energy is needed to move (pump) it, and the more likely it is that cellular debris and other waste matter will begin to stick to the blood. This, in turn, will increase blood pressure levels, and can damage the arterial walls and/or lead to the buildup of debris along the walls, while simultaneously diminishing the cells' ability to obtain the oxygen and nutrients they need, and to eliminate wastes building up inside them. As this happens, inflammation levels in the body will begin to rise, and, in order to repair damage to its arterial walls, your body will start to secrete plaque around the damaged sites, resulting in a narrowing of the arteries, a further increase in blood pressure levels, and a continued loss of cellular energy.

For all of the above reasons, I make it a point to measure my patients' blood viscosity levels, and I encourage you to have your doctor do the same. An effective indirect way of estimating blood thickness is to have your doctor order a cardiac CRP (C-reactive protein) blood test, which gives an indication of inflammation in the body. If it is very high (over 4), this would indicate that the blood is too thick.

In order to improve blood viscosity levels, I also recommend the use of various nutritional supplements, including fish oil, garlic, gingko biloba, vitamin E, and a supplement called nattokinase, an enzyme extract derived from fermented soybeans (natto), which has long been used in Japan and other Asian countries to good effect. These supplements are especially important if you live a sedentary lifestyle, especially if you are in your 40s or older. Since lack of exercise can also increase blood viscosity, as can a poor diet, I also recommend that you get regular exercise and follow the dietary recommendations I share in Chapter 7. Doing so can go a long way toward keeping your blood thin and healthy.

Drug Therapies Versus the Energy Medicine Approach

From the conventional medical perspective, the body and its health are considered to primarily be an interplay of biochemical reactions that can be manipulated by medications. What this approach fails to recognize is that such medications create not just chemical reactions in the body, but also energetic reactions. From the perspective of Energy Medicine, it is essential that the interplay of energies (that of the drugs and that of the body's own energetic makeup) occurs harmoniously if health is to be achieved. Unfortunately, this rarely happens with pharmaceutical drugs, which explains why conventional medications are so fraught with the risk of serious, side effects.

Simply put, the energetic reactions these drugs can cause in the body are very often contradictory to what the body really needs to restore itself. As a result, although new classes of drugs continue to enter the marketplace, the incidence of disease in the US and elsewhere continues to climb, as does the incidence of drug-induced side effects. In the US alone over 100,000 people die every year as a result of using medications that their physicians properly prescribed while taking them according to their doctors' instructions, and more than two million more people are hospitalized. Such grave consequences do not occur with the use of Energy Medicine.

Another significant advantage of Energy Medicine is that it allows doctors like me to detect imbalances in the body's regulatory processes much sooner than the use of conventional diagnostic methods does. This, in turn, means that I am able to determine when, where and how such imbalances are occurring long before they result in actual disease.

While drug-based medicine certainly has its place, the over-reliance on drugs in our society is one of the leading factors contributing to how and why annual health-care costs in the US is now close to $3 trillion. Today it is quite common for many Americans, especially as they get older, to be taking at least one and often as many as five or more prescription medications every day. Even with health insurance, the cost of such medications is not cheap. More importantly, in addition to the high risk of side effects associated with such drugs, with very few exceptions, such medications do not address the *cause* of illness, they only manage *symptoms*.

Additionally, all drugs, including aspirin, when used regularly, place a burden on your liver, the importance of which we discussed in Chapter 2. That's because all drugs contain inorganic ingredients that are, of themselves, toxic—a significant percentage of pharmaceutical drugs, for example, are known as *petrochemicals*, meaning that they contain petroleum (oil); other medications are derived from coal tar, and still others contain fluoride derivatives—leaving your liver to have to deal with them on top of all of the other toxic burdens it must cope with every day.

There is a saying among integrative, holistic physicians that I sometimes share with my patients: *No illness in the history of the world has ever been caused by a pharmaceutical drug deficiency.* I point this out because, in order to truly address disease, physicians must determine actual deficiencies, whether they are dietary, nutritional, or hormonal, and then seek to correct them. Detecting such deficiencies is another area in which Energy Medicine can be both advantageous and effective, compared to conventional diagnostic tests.

Here are some of the other significant advantages Energy Medicine has over drug-based medicine:

- Energy Medicine looks for and treats the causes of illness.
- Energy Medicine is safe and free of harmful side effects.
- Energy Medicine is more economical (less expensive).
- Energy Medicine evaluates a person's health status from a whole-person, energy based perspective; drug-based medicine focuses on specialized, segmented care that ignores the entire body.
- Pharmaceutical drugs interrupt cellular communication; Energy Medicine creates coherence within and around the cells, enhancing cellular communication.
- Drugs, because they mask symptoms, cause energetic and other disturbances in the body; Energy Medicine restores and balances such disturbances.
- Regular use of pharmaceutical drugs causes tissue acidity; Energy Medicine does not.

Based on the above facts, in my practice I typically will only prescribe pharmaceutical drug treatment for cases of acute illness for which symptom care is essential, and for serious bacterial or viral infections, in which case properly prescribed antibiotic or antiviral drugs may be necessary. Once the acute phase of illness has passed, I then will often apply the drainage and detoxification methods you read about in Chapter 2, while also seeking to improve their overall energy levels. This is where your cells' mitochondria come in to play.

Key Points to Remember

In order to be healthy, your body's regulatory system needs to function optimally.

The two key systems that oversee regulation in the body are the autonomic nervous system and the endocrine (hormone) system.

The autonomic nervous system is divided into two parts—the sympathetic and parasympathetic systems. Of the two, imbalances in the parasympathetic system are far more common and therefore most often in need of attention.

Key glands within the endocrine system are the pituitary gland, adrenal glands, the pancreas and its islets of Langerhans, and the thyroid gland.

Energy Medicine offers many advantages over conventional drug-based therapies when it comes to evaluating and treating these glands.

Your cellular "energy factories", the mitochondria, are another key component to good health. Without healthy mitochondria your cells cannot produce all of the energy your body needs to perform its many.

Another important key to good health is keeping blood thin as opposed to thick. Doing so improves blood flow, reduces wear and tear along the entire cardiovascular system, and keeps cells healthy by providing them with an abundant supply of oxygen and nutrients, thereby producing more energy and protecting against disease.

PART TWO

Knowing
The 6 Essential Keys To
Outstanding Health

CHAPTER 4

The Breakthrough Action Plan

Now that you have read the chapters in Part One and have a deeper understanding of your body's energy system and the key factors that influence your health, it's time to take the next step on your journey to a younger, healthier you. In the remaining chapters of this book you will find detailed instructions for how you can begin that journey by addressing each of the six key essentials that require your attention in order to create a lasting foundation for your optimal well-being. Here are some important guidelines that will help you maximize your results.

Upgrading Your Health and Energy

My goal in writing this book is to provide you with the tools and information you need to experience a dramatic improvement in your health and energy levels in as little as eight weeks. Does this mean that two months from now you will be completely free of whatever health issues you may be experiencing today? Not necessarily. Yet it does mean that you will be much closer to achieving and maintaining optimal health than you are now, *so long as you faithfully apply the information that I am sharing with you.* If you do, I can promise you that you *will* soon begin to feel better than you do right now. And isn't that the hope you had when you picked up this book?

My patients and I are living proof that these tools work, but I don't want you to take my word for it. I want you to prove it for yourself, and for your loved ones, by heeding my advice. If you do, I can promise you that it will make a significant difference in your health.

The program that you will be following is designed to be both comprehensive yet easy to follow. During the weeks ahead you will be addressing the key elements upon which lasting health rests in a way that works with your entire self—body, mind and spirit. As your journey unfolds, you will soon discover the pace that best suits you. That is the pace you need to follow. Don't overdo things. Stay focused on the journey itself instead of being impatient to reach the destination, because the destination itself will continue to change as your health changes too. As with life itself, when it comes to your health there is and will always be one more step to take. Don't forget that all climbers must rest. So I encourage you to view the journey you are undertaking as an adventure. Have fun with it!

At the same time do all that you can to stay motivated. Like all adventures, there will come times when you may find yourself feeling frustrated, wanting to give up, or tempted by the unhealthy yet comfortable lifestyle choices you are used to from your past that have taken a toll on your health. To succeed, you need to make a commitment to yourself, taking each step one at a time so that you get to where you want to be. Consistency is what matters most, for you will find, as you continue to make progress, that you will soon be generating your own momentum, making it easier and easier to keep going. And once the positive changes in your health and energy begin to take hold you will know how valuable and worthwhile your new, energetic lifestyle really is.

Evaluating Your Current State of Health: The Tests You Will Need

As with all journeys, when it comes to improving your health you need to know where you are starting from in order to both keep track of your health gains and to fully appreciate your progress. In order to do so, I highly recommend that you do all that you can to evaluate your current state of health, and to discover which areas of your health and of your lifestyle are most in need of improvement.

You began this process when you answered the questions of the questionnaire in Chapter 1. (If you have not yet answered them, then go back to Chapter 1 and do so now.) Your scores for each section of the questionnaire are indications of which aspects of your health are strong and which aspects are not. As you begin your eight-week make-over, place particular emphasis on the weaker aspects that are in need of strengthening.

Ideally, I recommend that you also work with your doctor to check your current health status. In particular, I recommend the following blood panel test: CBC, Platelet Count, Electrolytes, BUN, Creatinine, Glucose, HgbA1C, Calcium, Phosphorous, Fibrinogen, Homocysteine, ALT, AST, GGPT, Albumin, Globulin, Total Protein, Bilirubin, Alkaline Phosphatase, Uric Acid, LDH. Leptin, Sed Rate, Cardiac CRP, ANA, Rheumatoid Factor, 25 OH Vit D, Ferritin, Magnesium RBC, RPR, Blood Mercury, Blood Lead, PSA and Free PSA (men), Advanced Lipid Panel, Blood Type. Your doctor can order this test for you and then go over the results so that you understand what they mean.

In addition, I also recommend that you have a comprehensive urinalysis, as both urine and blood markers can provide you with a comprehensive picture of your current health status. Both tests can also identify correctable risk factors you may have for diseases such as diabetes, heart disease and cancer. Given the amount of information these tests provide, I regard them as vital components of a complete health care program, and recommend that they be given at least once a year.

Because blood tests can be expensive for people without insurance and for those with insurance plans with a high deductible, another option for testing that can save you money is the Life Extension Foundation (LEF) in Fort Lauderdale, Florida. LEF is one of the oldest and most reputable organizations devoted to uncovering the latest research related to health and longevity. It offers membership to the lay public, as well as a variety of services and product offerings, including a monthly magazine, a wide array of nutritional supplements, and a variety of blood tests that are priced much lower than what you can expect to pay at most medical labs that physicians commonly use. These tests are available in every state except Maryland to both members and nonmembers of LEF. (Nonmembers pay a bit more.)

Ordering LEF blood tests is easy. Simply contact LEF to order the tests you want. Once your order is placed, you will be directed to a medical lab near you to have your blood drawn, after which your blood will be sent directly to LEF for analysis. You will then receive your results and have the option of discussing them with an LEF health adviser at no extra charge. For a full list of the blood tests offered by LEF, visit www.lef. org/Vitamins-Supplements/Blood-Tests/index.htm. You can also contact LEF by calling (800)-208-3444. LEF is located at 5990 North Federal Highway, Fort Lauderdale, Florida 33308.

In addition to the tests above, I also strongly recommend that you obtain the following hormone tests: TSH, Free T3, Free T4, Thyroid Peroxidase Antibodies, Thyroglobulin Antibodies, FSH, LH, Estradiol, Progesterone, Testosterone, Free Testosterone, DHEA-S, Cortisol, Prolactin, Insulin, SHBG.

There are two ways to have your hormone levels tested: blood tests or a saliva hormone panel, or assay. LEF also offers blood hormone testing, and your doctor can order these tests as well. I use the saliva hormone assay to accurately assess adrenal gland status, because the saliva hormone assay provides a more accurate indication of cortisol and DHEA-S levels throughout an 24 hour period, showing when they are most elevated and when they are at their lowest levels.

Unlike blood hormone tests, which occur with a single blood draw, the adrenal saliva hormone assay is performed by taking saliva samples at specific times throughout a 24-hour cycle. This provides a more complete overview of your adrenal hormone status, since hormones fluctuate throughout the day. By knowing your adrenal hormone status during each of the specific times of the day for which saliva samples are collected, especially during nighttime, you will have a clearer picture of whether or not your adrenal hormones are most active when they need to be, or if they are out of balance. For example, cortisol levels should be at their highest level in the morning when you wake up, yet all too often they are out of balance and peak during sleep hours, making restful sleep difficult and resulting in fatigue throughout the day. Saliva testing can detect such imbalances more accurately than blood testing can.

There are other advantages to saliva hormone testing too. In addition to being painless and noninvasive, the saliva test can be performed in the comfort of your home. Because blood testing for hormones requires a blood draw that needs to occur at a doctor's office or at a lab, patients often cannot have this procedure conducted in the morning due to their or their doctors' or medical labs' schedules.

More importantly, saliva hormone samples provide a measure of the biologically active, or "free", hormones that influence cells. The saliva test is also usually less expensive than blood hormone tests, and can be more easily performed more frequently, if necessary, to monitor hormone changes that result once health treatments begin. For this reason, I recommend that you first obtain a baseline measure of saliva hormone prior to beginning your health program, and then retest within two months to monitor how well you are progressing.

Saliva hormone tests can be ordered by your doctor, or by yourself. If you wish to order them by yourself, I recommend you contact one of the following labs:

Sabre Sciences (888) 490-7300 www.sabresciences.com
Diagnos-Techs (800) 878-3787 www.diagnostechs.com
ZRT Labs (866) 600-1636 www.zrtlab.com

Before You Get Started: A Few Questions to Ask Yourself

When patients come to see me for the first time, I ask them to answer a series of questions. I find that their doing so helps them to become more conscious of their current health status and of the factors, including their lifestyle choices and the types of stress they are habitually exposed to, that may be influencing their health and overall well-being. I recommend that you answer the same questions for the same reason. The questions are:

1. What percentage of your body's healing power do you feel you are using now?
2. How long do you think it will take for you to regain your health?
3. What lifestyle/dietary changes do you think you need to make to feel better?
4. What emotional or stress-related factors are of concern to you currently?
5. What do you do to reduce stress in your life?
6. How will your life be different when you regain your health?
7. What do you need to do to reach a state of outstanding health?
8. Do you consider yourself to be healthy?
9. If not, what would you need to see happen in order to consider yourself to be healthy?
10. How would you like to see your health improve?
11. Do you take supplements?
12. Do you exercise? If so, what type of exercise?
13. What excites you; what are you passionate about?
14. What are you grateful for?
15. Are you living your dream?
16. What is your main health or life complaint, and why, and how does it trouble you?
17. Do you have pain? If so, rate it on a scale of 1-10.
18. What do you expect this type of medicine, and particularly the diet changes, to do for you?

19. Were you breast fed as an infant? If so, for how long?
20. As a child, were you susceptible to infections?
21. Have your tonsils or adenoids been removed? Or have you had an appendectomy?
22. As a child, did you have eczema, any other skin problems, or allergies?
23. Do you have mercury fillings or root canals?
24. Have you had a lot of antibiotics?
25. What vaccinations have you received?
26. Are you following any particular diet?
27. Do you often feel very tired after a meal?
28. Do you often get attacks of intense hunger, so that you simply have to eat something?
29. Do you have regular bowel movements?
30. Are there any foods that you do not tolerate, or are especially fond of?
31. How much, and what, do you drink every day?
32. Do you sleep well? Do you snore?
33. What are you most afraid of?
34. What do you consider to be the cause of your health problem(s)?
35. Imagine that a wizard came along and could grant you one wish, but you can't request a wish for healing or to receive magical powers to change everything. What would you wish for?

What to Tell Your Doctor: Integration with Conventional Medicine

Before beginning any type of new health program, including this one, I strongly advise you to inform your primary physician that you are doing so. Although the vast majority of physicians who only practice conventional medicine today are unfamiliar with much of the information and health care approaches you are learning about in this book—indeed, most conventional MDs don't even have a basic knowledge of diet and nutrition—your doctor still needs to be kept abreast of what you are doing. If you think it may be helpful to get them to better understand your decision, you can show them this book and let them know that everything that I am recommending is both completely legitimate and verifiable.

Don't be surprised, however, if your doctor expresses doubt or resistance to what you want to do, at least initially. People, especially experts, often have a difficult time grasping or accepting new concepts that don't fit into what they've been taught. That's okay, and is simply an aspect of human nature. At the same time, recognize that the most beneficial relationship with your doctor is as teammates, with both of you collaborating and working together to achieve better health for you. From that perspective, it's useful to realize that the word *doctor* is derived from the Latin word *docere*, which means *"to teach"*. This means that one of the most important roles doctors ought to play is that of being a teacher for their patients. This is something I am very mindful of with my own patients, and is the role I consciously took on when I wrote this book.

The best teachers in life are usually the ones who are most willing to learn from their patients. They are open to new ideas and willing to explore them. Hopefully, you have access to a physician like that. Either way, I encourage you to remember that your doctor is someone who works for you, not the other way round. So, keep him or her informed of what you are doing and ask them to monitor your progress by using the tests above, as well as the additional testing methods that I will be sharing with you in the chapters ahead.

At the same time, recognize that, when it comes to your health, there is only one person who should be in charge of it, and that person is you. Take responsibility for that fact and act accordingly. And should you find your doctor is unwilling to work with you on this new health journey you are embarking upon, seek to work with a more receptive physician instead, ideally one who has a background in both conventional and integrative medicine. (You will find a list of organizations made up of such physicians, including how to locate ones in your area, in the Resources section of this book.)

Introducing the Six Essentials Keys To Outstanding Health

The healing journey you are about to begin consists of six interrelated essential keys: Creating emotional mastery cleansing your body, addressing the health of your gut through healthier eating and drinking, creating a more energized lifestyle, boosting your body's energy levels with Energy Medicine, and strengthening your endocrine glands and balancing your hormones. What follows is an overview of each of the six essentials.

Creating Emotional Mastery: When it comes to healing, your mind and emotions are your most powerful allies. This part of the program will enable you to become more conscious of your habitual thoughts, beliefs, and emotions and empower you to transform them so that they align with your health goals. You will learn how to program your mind to help keep you healthy, and also how to master your fears. In addition, you will discover how to create a more meaningful life for yourself, one that is truly aligned with your life purpose and spiritual values.

Cleansing Your Body: This part of the program focuses on the various types of toxins you are exposed to and teaches you how to eliminate them from your body. We will also be examining tissue acidity and the steps you can take to reduce it. This is where you will learn how to employ the drainage and detoxification measures that I discussed in Chapter 2.

Addressing the Health of Your Gut: Your overall health and vitality depend in large part on the health of your gut (your body's gastrointestinal tract). The third essential explains the significance of your GI tract to health, outlines the causes of an unhealthy gut, and then provides you with the tools you can use to improve gut health and address issues such as bacterial imbalances, leaky gut, and irritable bowel syndrome. It will also teach you what to eat, when to eat, and how much to eat, along with the best nutrients and other supplements you can use to create lasting gut health.

Creating A More Energized Lifestyle: This part of the program is all about how you can revitalize yourself and create a more energetic lifestyle using exercise, meditation, and breathwork. It also examines the link between the health of your brain and your energy levels, and shows you how to tailor your diet and nutrition to keep your brain healthy at every age. In addition, you will also learn self-care tips for improving your sleep and banishing stress.

Boosting Your Body's Energy Levels with Energy Medicine: Here is where you will learn how to boost your energy in as little as 15 minutes a day, and also learn about the energetically based professional therapies that you can also use to keep yourself healthy, including acupuncture, homeopathy and applied kinesiology.

Strengthening Your Hormone Glands and Balancing Your Hormones: This last essential element of the program is one of the most important. Here you will learn how to prevent and reverse adrenal fatigue and exhaustion, optimize your thyroid health, and discover which nutrients and herbs can increase and balance your body's hormone production. In addition, I will provide you with the guidelines you need to properly utilize bioidentical hormone therapy and to safely and effectively supplement with human growth hormone.

By incorporating each of these six essential aspects of my rejuvenation program you will be sure to address all aspects of your health in a truly holistic, whole person manner. In doing so, most likely you will soon discover new levels of health and energy that once might not even have seemed possible to you.

What To Expect

Expect your health and energy to change dramatically for the better. Make a decision to feel well. Thoughts that make you happy, make you well. If you believe it, you will see it. This will allow you to live and enjoy the present moment. By passionately believing in what doesn't exist, you create it.

Forgive yourself for your prior lifestyle and nutrition choices that have contributed to you not feeling well. Remember that life is *FOR GIVING*.

My greatest value to you is in providing a further measure of believing in your own well-being. You are reading this book with an enthusiastic desire to be well. Because we both believe in your wellness, you will get well. And always remember that life is not always measured by the number of breaths we take, but by the moments that take our breath away.

Key Points To Remember

By faithfully following all of the essential elements of my rejuvenation program you can create significant improvements in your health and energy levels in as little as eight weeks. The key to doing so is to take action.

Before beginning my program, it is important that you first know your current health status. You can find out by ordering a complete blood panel along with a hormone panel or assay. To most effectively determine and monitor your adrenal hormone levels, a 24-hour saliva hormone assay is recommended.

It is vitally important that you inform your doctor about the steps you are taking to improve your health, working with him or her as a partner and collaborator. Should your doctor prove resistant to this program, you always have the option of working with a different physician, ideally one who is trained in both integrative and conventional medicine.

There are six essential elements to my makeover program. They are interrelated and are intended to address all of the major aspects of your health from a holistic "body, mind, and spirit" approach. By making use of all six of them, you can expect your health to improve in ways you may not have previously imagined for yourself.

As you progress through your healing journey, you can expect various outcomes to occur at different times. These are all part of the healing process. As they arise, recognize them for what they are, and, if appropriate, inform your physician of them. And don't give up. There is no final destination when it comes to your health, just greater and greater degrees of well-being, all of which can be yours so long as you are willing to continue along your healing journey.

CHAPTER 5

Essential #1: Cleanse and Fortify the Mind

"If someone wishes for good health, one must first ask oneself if he is ready to do away with the reasons for his illness. Only then is it possible to help him."

~ Hippocrates

The first essential for achieving and maintaining ageless vitality involves taking conscious control over your thoughts, emotions, and beliefs. I call this step cleansing and fortifying the mind. The statement by Hippocrates that opens this chapter is instructive in that regard. However, it may seem confusing to you. If you are sick or lacking energy you most likely believe that, of course, you are ready to do away with whatever is causing your health problems. But are you really?

Before you answer that question, take a moment to honestly assess whether or not you truly are willing to do all that it takes to get well.

I raise this point because, during my many years of practicing medicine, I find that many patients initially, yet usually unconsciously, derive benefit from their health issues. For them, being sick becomes the major theme of their "story", the tale that they tell themselves and others.

You likely know or have met at least one chronically, yet not seriously, ill person who makes their health issue the centerpiece of every conversation you have with them. Usually this occurs in the form of complaints, yet underneath the complaint there is often a cry for attention, sympathy, or love that their illness or pain provides for them in ways that they did not receive when they were healthier. By the same token, often a health complaint provides a convenient and self-justifiable excuse to avoid taking action in other areas of one's life, including following one's passion, which, in my experience, is a hallmark of many people who are in good health.

Excuses are often part and parcel of how people handle their health issues. For example, though we all know the importance of regular exercise, how often have you avoided exercising by telling yourself you were too tired or don't have the time for it? In my Los Angeles medical office I offer several stress reducing treatments that last from 10 to 30 minutes. What amazes me is that many patients will tell me that they don't have enough time to experience these wonderful treatments, and instead rush out of the office to their next destination. I constantly hear, "I don't have enough time right now." Maybe the reason why so many people experience so much stress in their lives, have trouble sleeping, and are in poor health is because of their preoccupation with the idea that time is running out.

But if you connect with the purpose of your life and allow it to guide you, you soon discover that there *is* enough time to do everything you truly want and need to do. That's because the simple yet powerful act of committing to your life purpose automatically starts to enable you to prioritize making time for what is most important to you. As you do so, there is less stress, you can sleep more easily, your mood improves, and you start to notice you are experiencing better health and more energy. When we continue to focus on purpose, passion, and all that we have to be grateful for, we feel whole and happy, and life flows smoothly.

So what gets in the way of that?

In most cases, the answer lies in our thoughts, which in turn influence our beliefs, emotions, and ultimately the health of our bodies. So, to return to what Hippocrates taught, are you ready to do away with the reasons for your lack of vitality and optimal health? The rest of this chapter is designed to empower you to be able to answer this question with a resounding, unqualified Yes!

Let's begin by examining the role that your mind plays in your health.

The Power of Your Mind

Take a moment to perform this exercise. Close your eyes and imagine your favorite food set on a plate before you. Give yourself free rein to imagine it as completely as you can. Sense its aroma and its taste as you imagine yourself biting into it.

As you performed this simple visualization, you likely soon found your salivary glands were activated, with an increase of saliva in your mouth. For many people, this happens just from reading the words above, even before they perform the exercise. Even though the food did not exist before you, your body still reacted as if it did. This shows you the power your mind and your thoughts have to influence your body.

Unnoticed by you as you performed the above exercise were the many biochemical and enzymatic reactions that occurred that led to your mouth watering. Similar reactions occur in your body in response to all of your thoughts and emotions. Which is why, as I mentioned earlier in this book, I tell my patients, "Thoughts that make you happy, make you well." This isn't just a pie-in-the-sky, New Age platitude. It's a fact that has repeatedly been proven by scientific research.

In mind/body medicine, the emotional status of an individual is viewed as importantly as their physical status. How someone is feeling emotionally has everything to do with their physical prognosis, their energy for healing, their pain level, and so forth. From the perspective of both mind/body and energy medicine, emotions are viewed as revealing the state of consciousness of a person. Changes in consciousness can shift the body's bioenergy field which, in turn, can influence health.

One of the leading pioneers in this field was the late Candace Pert, PhD, author of the book *The Molecules of Emotion*. Dr. Pert spent most of her professional life researching cell receptors. These receptors are single molecules situated within cell membranes. A single nerve cell, or neuron, can have upward of a million or more receptors.

Based on her research, Dr. Pert likened cell receptors to the cells' "brains", and discovered that they act as the interface between our emotions and their effects on the body. The "messages" that receptors transmit are influenced by compounds known as *peptides*. A *peptide* acts as a biochemical key that fits within the receptor in a process called binding. Dr. Pert described this process as "sex on a molecular level."

Examples of peptides are insulin and other hormones, and neurotransmitters such as serotonin, which are primarily produced in the brain to carry information across the gap (synapse) between neurons. Dr. Pert coined the phrase "molecules of emotion" in response to her finding that 85 to 95 percent of the neuropeptide receptors are found in the emotion centers of the brain.

Building on research dating back to the 1920s, which found that strong emotions could be generated by electrically stimulating certain parts of the brain, Dr. Pert and the team of scientists she oversaw also discovered that high concentrations of neuropeptides exist in most locations of the body where information from the five senses is transmitted to the nervous system. Additionally, she and her team found that for almost every peptide that exists in the brain, receptors also exist for them within the immune and endocrine systems, and that these peptides are released during different emotional states. What this means is that, while previously emotions were thought to be solely psychological in nature, science has now proven they are directly linked to specific chemical processes that take place throughout the body, not just within the brain, and that the neuropeptides that correspond to emotions affect the functioning of all body systems, including the immune and endocrine system.

Based on Dr. Pert's research, we now know that neuropeptides play a significant role in how we retrieve or repress memories, as well as how we deal with them. We also know that memories are literally stored throughout the cells of the body, not just in our brains, and that our emotions and moods are triggered by various peptides. What we experience as an emotion is also a mechanism in both the brain and body to generate a particular behavior. Research has conclusively established that our behavior, as well as all memory processes, are emotion-driven, and that peptides, in Dr. Pert's words, "are the sheet music containing the notes, phrases, and rhythms that allow the orchestra—your body—to play as an integrated entity."

So, what does all of this mean in terms of your health?

Simply (yet profoundly) put, it means that you have the power to influence your health and overall well-being by consciously using the power of your mind by way of the thoughts and emotions you choose to have. This, too, was proven by Dr. Pert and her team of scientists. They found receptors on immune cells for almost every peptide or drug-like chemical found in the brain. Immune cells make and secrete the same neuropeptides that the brain produces to control mood. Dr. Pert's findings proved that the brain, glands, and immune system are linked together within a mind/body "intelligent information network," and that emotion-affecting peptides actually control the routing and migration of immune cells that are essential for good health. For example, viruses use the same receptors as neuropeptides to enter a cell. Depending on how much of these peptides there are for that cell's receptors, the easier or more difficult it will be for a virus to get into the cell. More neuropeptides makes it much harder for viruses to take hold, while less peptides increases your risk of infection. This means that your emotional state, along with the quality of your thoughts, can determine whether or not you will get sick.

Based on the above, you can understand why the biggest obstacle for most people's health is being in emotional distress. Almost every patient I see tells me about how stressed they are. Yet stress is not really what people think it is. Stress occurs when we perceive ourselves in a state of emotional discomfort. Most people view stress as something from the outside that happens to them. In reality, most of us are creating this state of discomfort as a result of the undesirable meanings we give to life experiences.

There are three main causes of chronic stress. First we have long term unhealthy beliefs that cause us to perceive life events as "dangers", and thus trigger an alarm, or fight or flight, response. Second, we have persistent deprivation of our emotional need for "bonding" or closeness. Lastly, we do not get enough of our psychological needs met in our daily environments, that are unique to our specific personality type. Some of us need to have fun and excitement; others need acknowledgement of their values; others need acknowledgement of their ability to think clearly and logically; other people need solitude; and some of us need our senses to be richly stimulated.

Learning to de-stress is a challenge. This is especially true as we get older. Just as our physical bodies decline with age if we neglect them, so too does our ability to cope with our daily exposures to stress if we neglect learning how to effectively manage and reduce stress. When that is the case, situations that we might have shrugged off without a thought when we were in our teens or 20s can trigger a cascade of harmful stress hormones in us by the time we reach our 30s and beyond. That's why it is so important for you to regain the resiliency of your youth in the face of stress.

Most people today have taken on more than they comfortably can take on and consequently they are driven by that. So you can detoxify and exercise, but getting your emotional/mental state under control is most important. You've got to focus on what makes you feel good. Then you need to use that feel good energy to solve your problems. This can be done in many ways, often without even having to deal with the problem directly, at least not initially.

As an example, have you ever experienced a solution to an issue you were faced with after expressing love or gratitude to someone you care about? Or after you turned away from the problem at hand in order to spend time doing something fun and enjoyable? Usually, after doing such things you will notice that you feel better, as well. And, indeed, you are, because emotions of love and gratitude, as well as participating in activities you enjoy, not only reduce stress but also flood your body with health-enhancing peptides, hormones, and other biochemical compounds. Research has shown that even a short, ten-minute walk acts to increase feelings of happiness by boosting these compounds.

So I encourage you to tap into those feelings of love and gratitude every day, and to regularly make time for activities you enjoy. Doing so will help foster ongoing positive emotions and thoughts. As that happens, I've found, both for myself and for my patients, that better health and longevity have a way of following.

In concluding this section, I want to emphasize that, no matter what your current state of health may be, there is never a lost cause. There is always a way to improve your health, and it starts with using the power of your mind.

As a doctor, the worst thing I can do is give a patient a diagnosis of a disease without also giving them hope. Otherwise they will likely start to panic, which leads to feelings of helplessness, depression, and other negative emotions that ultimately weaken their immune system. The wise doctor must never destroy the hope of the patient. All patients have resources within them that they can draw upon by using their thoughts and emotions. My job is to help them conquer their fears and unleash those resources.

A lot of people ask me what's more important, the patient's belief in the doctor or the doctor's belief in the patient. I know it's the doctor's belief in the patient. In fact, one of the most overlooked aspects in medicine is the role of physicians in their patient's progress. Their beliefs about the patient and about the recommended treatment will dramatically influence the outcome of the therapy, whether it be conventional treatment or holistic therapy. Research has shown that physicians' strong beliefs in their therapy and in their patients will cause the patients to also believe more in the therapy, as well as to believe in themselves, thereby improving patient outcomes.

A physician can do much to help guide the patient toward adopting a more loving and positive attitude, and into a state of receptivity, which will permit the body's regenerative forces to work more effectively. That's because, when the doctor believes in the patient, the patient gets it immediately. Once the patient gets it, all things are possible.

I want you to know that I believe in you just as much as I believe in my patients. And my hope is that you will believe in yourself, as well. Doing so can make all the difference in your health.

Fear is the Killer, Not Disease

In 1954 Roger Banister was the first person to run a four-minute mile. Until then, nobody believed it was possible. Then, in the next five years, 30 or 40 other people ran a four minute mile. This illustrates how, once a belief system starts changing on a large level, all sorts of new, previously unheard of possibilities start to occur. I keep this thought in mind with patients, by doing all that I can to help them change their limiting belief systems and help them get rid of fear.

In my opinion, fear is what most holds us back from our dreams, including optimal health. We are afraid of poverty, criticism, ill health, and old age. We fear death and we fear cancer. Every day I have patients come to me and every ache, pain, or digestive complaint that they have convinces them they have cancer. The cancer fear is huge. Our bodies can be in either one of two modes: survival or growth. If you are totally in survival mode there's no way you can get yourself into a growth mode or anti-aging mode. Eliminating fears, especially the fear of diseases like cancer and other serious illnesses, is crucial for all people to move into growth mode.

This is an important point to consider, because in many cases it is the fears people have about their disease conditions, not the diseases themselves, that is most detrimental. Their fears keep them in survival mode and therefore prevent them from effectively mobilizing their internal resources to get better. Very often, too, these fears arise from the belief that their condition is hopeless, leading them to no longer follow their doctors' recommendations, Sadly, such a belief usually becomes a self-fulfilling prophecy. In fact, in most cases it is a limited or erroneous belief that creates fear in the first place, not anything that is objectively real.

My experience as a physician has taught me that I can bring almost anyone back to an excellent state of health if they are willing to work with me and do what it takes to change their beliefs and move away from fear and hopelessness. I have an underlying faith that people are more resilient than they might believe, and that with proper guidance, education, and tools that I am sharing in this book, we have everything that is necessary to create lasting good health and vitality. The key is getting people to fortify their minds and then do whatever else is appropriate.

The results in my practice bear this out. I've worked in the arena of anti-aging and Energy Medicine for 28 years and the results that my patients and I have achieved together make a mockery of the standard health statistics. For example, statistically in the U.S. one of every 8 women will develop breast cancer. Yet in my practice it's closer to one out of 1,000 women. Why is that? Is it because of what I know? Is it because my practice attracts a health-conscious patient? Is it because of the synergy between myself and my patients?

I believe it is all of these factors. My patients really do want to get better and they are willing to do away with their reasons for being ill. Moreover, as I guide them in managing their beliefs, thoughts and emotions, they develop a consistently positive, health-affirming mindset. Consequently, the levels of disease in my practice are much less than that of the general population.

When it comes to helping my patients manage their beliefs and overcome their fears and feelings of hopelessness, I often make use of the discoveries of, and techniques developed by, my wife, Dr. Janet Hranicky, a well-known psychologist specializing in the relationship of emotional attitudes to the occurrence and treatment of cancer. One of Janet's key contributions to this field has to do with her exploration of what she has termed "the pleasure-freeze response." While we are all familiar with the fight or flight response in relation to stress, the pleasure-freeze response is equally important, yet often overlooked.

"Not only can one fight or flee in response to stress," Janet explains, "one can also detach as a way of neutralizing danger. We naturally move towards pleasure, or comfort, emotionally and physically, unless we have learned to 'hold back' because of previous pain. Detachment is a defense response to neutralize physical pain, anger, and fear so as not to feel discomfort. When we use detachment on a regular basis, we get good at numbing our normal feedback mechanisms that would ordinarily signal us to make some changes behaviorally. Long-term 'freezing' of, or holding back from, emotions prevents them from being fluid. When any of our emotions become frozen the energy they contain is not discharged from the body, which can lead to serious health consequences. For example, the endocrine system weakens when there is a dominance of repressed, frozen, and denied emotions such as pain, anger, and fear." Dr. Hranicky has developed a unique program called *The Key To Me In Getting Well: Personalized Stress Management* to help guide people to heal their repressed or frozen emotions.

Dr. Hranicky and other researchers have found that denial of our fears and feelings of hopelessness is the emotional state that most often precedes the development of cancer. "We experience hopelessness when we do not get our emotional and psychological needs met over long periods of time," Janet adds. "Because deprivation is a painful experience, we learn to protect ourselves by repressing and denying the pain, anger, and fear that are the real emotions associated with deprivation. We begin to give up unconsciously about ever getting what we really want. Eventually, we may completely lose awareness of our deep-rooted sense of hopelessness."

When you experience emotional pleasure or comfort the parasympathetic nervous system is engaged, and your body experiences chemical changes which create a state of physical ease mixed with normal levels of excitement (unfolding growth potential). Optimal physical health occurs in this state. Conversely, when your sources of pleasure are blocked or are perceived as blocked, the natural movement towards growth is inhibited. The natural pursuit of emotional pleasure will not occur, and you will instead "freeze" that desire rather than discharging it. This "pleasure-freeze" sets up a physical and emotional state of tension that can adversely affect your health.

An emotionally healthy person will move away from emotional pain, but this is impossible if emotional pain is being produced by a mechanism such as the "pleasure-freeze," which is, itself, also a mechanism protecting against another source of pain. Here the alternatives in action are one type of pain or another type of pain, and the only possible relief lies in "freezing"—choosing neither—thus creating a potential cycle of ongoing pain and other detriments to your health that are easily ignored or unnoticed because of the pleasure-freeze response.

A proper understanding of the relationship between fear and its other attendant emotions and disease reveals that both fear itself *and its denial via the pleasure-freeze response*, are equally detrimental to your health. This is why honestly admitting to and addressing fear head on can make such a powerful difference in improving your health, as well as your ability to experience more pleasure and comfort in your life. Since fear is primarily the result of our thoughts and beliefs, the key to managing and eliminating fear lies in consciously creating better quality thoughts and beliefs. You will learn how to do so later on in this chapter. For now, let me leave you with this tip from Pope John XXII: "Consult not your fears, but your hopes and your dreams. Think not about your frustrations, but about your unfulfilled potential. Concern yourself not with what you tried and failed in, but with what is still possible for you to do."

There is a lot of wisdom in this quote, and I encourage you to start applying it in your daily life.

The Beliefs and Emotions of Outstanding Health

The general state of your health is directly related to your consciousness. A change in your health, for either better or worse, always involves a corresponding change in your consciousness. The following quote from the Dalai Lama helps illustrate this fact: "There is something about the dynamics of self-absorption, or worrying about ourselves too much, which tends to magnify our suffering." When we focus on worrying about our problems, including those related to our health, it *does* usually increase our feelings of being ill at ease, fearful, and so forth. Fortunately, when we choose to focus instead on the positive aspects of our lives and what we are grateful for, we tend to feel healthier, happier and more energetic.

Your body is constantly renewing itself, repeatedly forming completely new versions of your cells, tissues, internal organs, and even your skeletal system over the course of your life. Science has proven that your consciousness, which consists of your thoughts, emotions, and beliefs, can and does affect this process of regeneration, either positively or negatively.

An example of this fact recently crossed my desk. It involved a study published in the medical journal *Stroke* of more than 6,700 healthy adults between the ages of 45 to 84, all of whom completed a questionnaire to indicate their stress levels and the degree to which they experienced feelings of anger, depression, and hostility. Such emotions are a measure of one's cynical views about life and other people. Researchers then followed the participants for between eight to 11 years, examining the relationship between these psychological factors and study group's risk for stroke.

At the conclusion of the study, the participants who demonstrated the highest levels of cynicism were found to have a more than 50 percent greater likelihood of having a stroke compared to those who were less cynical. The study also found that chronic stress increased the risk of stroke by 59 percent. Most shocking of all, those in the study group who most often experienced feelings of depression had their risk of stroke increased by 86 percent. The results of the study were consistent even after researchers accounted for other known risk factors of stroke, such as the participants' age, race, sex, lifestyle choices and behaviors (smoking and drinking habits, and their level of physical activity), and blood pressure levels.

Alarming as this study's results are (and there are literally hundreds of previous studies that show a similar correlation between habitual negative attitudes and emotions and a significantly greater risk for disease, including heart disease and cancer), it also contains a very positive silver lining, in that is shows us how we can all drastically reduce our risk of stroke by adopting a more optimistic attitude about life and others, and regularly cultivating positive emotions.

In my experience, there are seven primary positive emotions, along with seven emotions that can be considered to be negative. The seven positive emotions are desire, enthusiasm, faith, hope, love, romantic feelings, and sexual attraction. Whenever we experience such emotions, we are in growth mode and typically experience greater levels of energy and overall well-being.

The seven negative emotions are anger, greed, fear, hatred, jealousy, superstition, and revenge. The Buddha perfectly summed up the detrimental effects of these emotions when he said, "Holding onto anger is like grasping a hot coal with the intent of throwing it at someone else; you are the one who gets burned," and "You will not be punished *for* your anger. You will be punished *by* your anger."

You can substitute any of the other negative emotions for anger and the end result will still be the same: Such emotions hurt and punish you far more than they do anyone else. Thus, if you truly wish to be and stay healthy, you must do all that you can to let go of such emotions for, as science has now proved, they can indeed cause you to become ill.

This does not mean that you are expected to live a perfect life, never experiencing negative emotions ever again. Such an expectation is unrealistic. All of us will continue to experience such emotions from time to time. The key is to train yourself to become more conscious of them when you do experience them, and then make the choice to release them. Doing so is actually easier than you may believe once you commit to being more observant and conscientious about your thoughts and behavior.

Thoughts and emotions "just happen;" in truth they always arise from our choices. For the most part, those choices occur unconsciously, leaving us *reacting* to our life experiences rather than *consciously creating them*. As you practice being more observant about your thoughts and behaviors, you will soon discover that you can consciously change them at any time, simply by deciding to do so. This will not happen overnight, yet the more you focus on being more conscious, the easier you will find it is to shift away from negative thoughts and emotions to those that are more positive and which truly serve you and your health.

For, as the Buddha also said, "Every human being is the author of his own health or disease," which is why he taught that the key to creating and maintaining good health lies in learning how to discipline, or program, the mind.

Programming Your Mind to Be Healthy

The famous yogi saint, Paramahansa Yogananda, who was largely responsible for popularizing both yoga and meditation in the U.S., once wrote, "When you can convince your mind of its accomplishing power, you can do anything." That is certainly true when it comes to your health.

And it is also true when it comes to ill health. For example, my wife, Dr. Hranicky, has spent decades researching and working with cancer patients and has found that they are more apt to have a long-standing belief system that keeps them in a state of emotional pain. They distance themselves from people close to them, and from nature. They are not interested in play and having fun. They tend to harbor resentment and self-pity, and have more difficulty creating meaningful long-term relationships.

However, when they learn to change and let go of their limiting beliefs and emotions, open themselves up to loved ones, and reconnect with activities they enjoy, they often get better. In some cases they even experience what is known in the medical literature as a "spontaneous remission", or complete healing of their cancer that cannot be accounted for by their treatment.

Research about spontaneous remission has found common elements among all patients who experience it. Among those elements are the patients' acceptance that there is a Divine Intelligence that has given them life, and that it is in charge of their bodies and capable at all times of healing them independent of their own will; their understanding and acceptance of the fact that their thoughts, emotions, and beliefs contributed to their illness, and their willingness to change their way of thinking; and their commitment to "reinvent" themselves in order to reconnect with and commit to the people and activities that are most meaningful to them, leaving behind anyone and anything that did not fulfill them. In some cases this meant ending relationships or leaving their jobs because neither situation was in alignment with their true values and passions.

Creative Visualization: Another common factor among cancer and other patients who spontaneously heal is active and creative visualization. The power of creative visualization is one of the major healing tools in your possession. When it is used to bring about pure love in one's heart, as well as forgiveness and contentment, the elements are in place to create mental and emotional peace and true healing. But when it is used to focus on worries, fears, or past negative experiences, the opposite occurs.

Many people with serious health concerns have a highly developed ability to recall in detail past memories and vividly visualize them. Dr. Hranicky's research has shown that there is a tendency for patients to hold more pain-related memories and to relive them over and over. This is an example of using creative visualization to unhealthy effect. However, it can just as easily be used to create significant, even remarkable, healthy outcomes.

Also referred to as guided imagery, creative visualization has produced many well-documented healings among cancer and other patients. One of the pioneers in this regard was the late O. Carl Simonton, MD, a radiation oncologist with whom my wife worked very closely for many years. Dr. Simonton taught his patients to use imagery to enhance their treatments, often suggesting that his patients imagine cancer cells as "anything soft that can be broken down," and their bodies' immune cells as "aggressive and eager for battle."

Dr. Simonton's first use of imagery occurred in 1971 with a throat cancer patient whose condition was regarded as hopeless. The man was 61 years old, extremely weak, had trouble breathing, and was dangerously underweight. Though he was scheduled to receive radiation treatment, his doctors worried that the treatment would only make his condition worse given his already poor health.

Dr. Simonton developed a program of relaxation and creative visualization for this man and had him devote between five to 15 minutes to it three times a day, imagining his radiation treatment as "bullets of energy" that killed off his cancer cells while simultaneously strengthening his healthy cells. The man was also instructed to visualize his cancer going away as his health returned to normal. As a result of this process, not only was the man able to tolerate the radiation with little discomfort, his appetite returned and he regained his lost weight and strength. Two months later, he was completely cancer-free.

Many others cancer patients of Dr. Simonton also achieved remarkable recoveries from cancer using the visualization methods he taught them. And even when patients were not cured, they reported that the visualization exercises they performed provided them with other benefits, including loss of anxiety, pain relief, increased feelings of self-esteem and well-being, and an increased sense of having control over their bodies. They also were able to tolerate chemotherapy or radiation treatments, and, in addition to coming to grips with their illness, they often were able to resolve personal issues and heal conflicts with their loved ones.

Today we know that creative visualization can be applied to all aspects of one's life for greater well-being, including virtually all other disease conditions.

Though critics dismiss the health improvements and cures achieved by patients who have used creative visualization as little more than the placebo effect, even if they are correct, does it matter? In my opinion, such a dismissal is simply a way for such critics and skeptics to explain away something that does not fit into their limited belief systems. Moreover, the placebo effect has long been accepted as real by conventional, as well as holistic, medicine. In fact, within a research setting, a medicine or treatment is considered effective only if it has a significantly greater benefit than otherwise obtained by the placebo effect.

A positive placebo effect is created when a person believes in and trusts the treatment's benefits. This belief can enhance the effect of the intended treatment, even if that therapy was previously proven to be ineffective. For years, the conventional scientific community regarded all successful results of healing by holistic practitioners as placebo effects. This was partly true, since holistic practitioners, including me, all encourage their patients to heal by believing in their recovery. The positive placebo effect can be enhanced considerably by creative visualization.

So, every time you take a remedy, visualize the action of the remedy helping you get better. And make it a habit to spend at least five minutes at least twice a day actively visualizing greater health for yourself. Doing so will not only enhance your body's ability to heal and stay well, it will also generate more regular connections to positive emotions and thoughts. All told, creative visualization is one of the most powerful, yet easy-to-perform, methods for programming your body and mind for better health.

Examining and Reprogramming Your Beliefs: Another important key to programming your mind to be healthy is to consciously examine your current habitual beliefs and then to diligently work to replace those that don't serve you with healthier, more positive, life-affirming beliefs. What follow are guidelines for doing so developed by Dr. Hranicky based on her many years of experience helping others improve the quality of their thoughts, beliefs and emotions.

To evaluate some of your beliefs, use the following criteria to see if they fall into the category of superior beliefs that engender greater health and personal satisfaction. Superior beliefs:

Empower you.

Support your health, well-being, and longevity.

Protect your survival.

Test well in reality (are based on fact, not perception).

Give you energy.

Engender more self-love and love for others.

Lead to greater pleasure and less pain, anger, and fear.

Add value to others and to our planet.

How do your beliefs test out? If you are uncertain start with analyzing your most routine, or habitual, emotional responses, the ones that characterize you. For example, if you routinely feel sad, ask yourself what causes you to be sad? Inevitably the answer is your beliefs about something or someone in your life. An example of a belief that could create sadness might be, "I don't believe that I am loved just for being me."

The next step in this process is to evaluate this belief using the eight criteria for superior beliefs mentioned above. If your belief doesn't meet those criteria, then it is limiting and you would do well to change or replace it.

To change your limiting beliefs or habitual thought patterns:

1. Identify the belief itself. For example, "I can't get well."
2. Identify the disempowering emotion associated with it, for example, fear or anxiety.
3. Determine the experiences or past references that support the unwanted or disempowering belief. For example, "My doctor told me that I will have to live with my condition for the rest of my life."
4. Use questions, statements, stories, or metaphors of counter-examples to create doubt about the remaining experiences, and thus about the belief. For example, who are some people you could meet who have a similar diagnosis and are doing well?
5. Demonstrate to yourself how the belief violates your efforts to reach your short-and long-term goal or goals (thus violating your sense of personal power).
6. Make a commitment to change the belief.
7. Create new experiences that challenge that belief.
8. Practice the new belief with consistency.
9. Anchor your new belief by reinforcing it with new experiences.

One other important concept to understand when it comes to your health is this: The quality of your life has nothing to do with what is going on around you; *it has everything to do with how you evaluate your life experiences.* The people who are most successful in staying well usually have the ability to evaluate things more effectively.

You can increase your ability to evaluate your experiences more accurately and effectively by practicing asking yourself better questions throughout each day. Your brain is like a computer; it will give you information on whatever you ask of it. Notice the questions that you asked yourself in the past that may have caused you to be in an unhealthy or unhappy state. What would be some questions that you could ask yourself about your current life challenges, including those related to your health, that would make you feel better no matter what else is going on?

Remember, what you focus on determines the quality of your life and health. Asking better questions daily forces your brain to make better evaluations. How you evaluate things is going to determine how you feel and what you do. This requires you to hold specific images of what you want—*not of what you don't want*. Reality follows image. Many people spend much more time during the day thinking about the things they are afraid of that might happen, rather than focusing specifically on what they want.

As you experienced when I asked you to imagine your favorite food, your body does not know the difference between what is real and what is imagined. When your mind holds pictures or images of perceived anxiety- or stress-producing outcomes, your body gears up for a survival response, preventing you from being in growth mode. When we continually hold images in our minds that create pain, anger, or fear, our bodies remain in an overly activated defense response which eventually drains us of our energy, impairs our health, and can actually get in the way of our survival.

Here are some other tips for preventing such outcomes by improving the quality of your thoughts and beliefs:

1. Recognize that your beliefs are optional, not set in stone.
2. Transform your vocabulary. Pay attention to what you say. If you eliminate some of the negative words in your vocabulary, you will begin to eliminate some of the unhealthy beliefs often associated with negative and painful emotional experiences.
3. Change the way you view your personal history. By giving better meanings to your past, you will give different and more optimis-

tic meanings to your future, helping to create a more empowered belief system of increased hope and faith.

4. Practice paying attention to what you focus on and what you ignore. The process of framing can help you learn how to change the meanings of situations in your life. You can do this in two ways—pre-framing and re-framing. Pre-framing involves telling yourself something to pay attention to that is desirable in advance, and visualizing how you want to feel as a result. Re-framing involves changing something that you view as a problem to something with a better meaning. By creating better meaning for your experiences you will have more references to support your empowered beliefs.

5. Open up to experiencing more pleasure in your life, in place of emotional pain.

6. Express any lingering emotional pain, anger, fear that is getting in the way of "my feeling love and pleasure."

Affirming Better Health: You can further reprogram your mind by the use of affirmations. Affirmations are positive thoughts that you repeat to yourself (either verbally, in thought, or in writing) throughout the day in order to produce the outcomes you desire. The more you associate strong emotions to your affirmations, the more powerful they become. Over time, affirmations work with the unconscious mind to reprogram it with the thought and belief patterns you consciously select to influence your behavior. Here are some excellent affirmation statements selected by Dr. Hranicky:

I am entitled to pleasure without pain. I am lovable.

I am good enough, without having to be perfect.

I have needs. My needs are real and important and deserve to be fulfilled.

I have feelings. It is safe and appropriate to express them.

I have all the time I need to make the changes I want to make in my life.

I have everything I need to get well.

As I enrich my life, my health improves, my body's immune system is enhanced, and my ability to live a long and energetic life is increasingly maximized.

You can also create your own affirmations that are specifically tailored to your needs. When working with affirmations, always state them in the present tense and keep them positive. For example, use "I am getting healthier each and every day," as opposed to "I am no longer sick." Also keep your affirmations short and simple and no longer than two sentences. To enhance the positive benefits of affirmation, make the process as vivid and real as possible by also visualizing what you are affirming *as if it is already accomplished*, allowing yourself to feel all of the positive emotions associated with it.

What's Your Purpose? Creating Meaning For Your Life

"Your purpose in life is to find *your* purpose and give your whole heart and soul to it." This statement is as true today as it was when the Buddha first taught it approximately 2,500 years ago. Creating a meaningful, purposeful life that supports you and empowers you is the foundation upon which health and personal fulfillment is built and maintained.

In my experience, people with a strong sense of purpose tend to have greater levels of health and energy, and are more resilient in the face of whatever challenges life may present to them. Their sense of purpose gives them a greater degree of confidence and determination about their life goals and their ability to achieve them. A purposeful life, which literally means "living on purpose," also typically results in greater feelings of contentment and a deeper connection with others and life in general. It also engenders a desire to want to keep on living as long and energetic as possible, so that you can continue to make meaningful contributions to the world, another trait of people who embody the characteristics of outstanding health.

If you are already clear about what your purpose in life is, congratulations. If, however, you have not yet determined what your purpose is, most likely it is because you have simply not taken the time to consider what it might be. Socrates, the great Greek philosopher, taught that "The unexamined life is not worth living." Too often, however, that is precisely how many people go about their lives—unaware of, or even uninterested in, the reasons why they are alive and doing what they are doing. Yet, should they decide to explore those reasons, very often they come to realize the true nature of the gifts they were born with and how they can best use them to create more meaning and fulfillment in their lives. As they do so, their lives tend to change for the better, and their health typically improves, as well.

There are two main clues to what your life purpose may be—the gifts you were born with (your talents and aptitudes) and the activities you most enjoy or have the inclination to investigate. For example, from the time I was young, I had a strong interest in helping others and in exploring the workings of the body and what is necessary to keep it functioning efficiently. I also possessed the skills, or gifts, necessary to further my exploration, including a talent for learning and a desire to share what I learned with others for our mutual benefit (helping others has always been of benefit for me, too, because of the personal fulfillment I derive from it). As I look back at my life, it seems inevitable that I would become the physician I am today, dedicated to helping as many people as I can stay young and healthy for as long as possible.

Knowing your purpose in life is something that only you can determine for yourself. Certainly friends and family members you trust can be helpful because of the feedback they can provide based on how they know you, yet ultimately the answers about your purpose lie within you. To that end, I often advise patients who are looking for more meaning in their lives to first create two lists. I call them the What My Gifts Are and the What I Most Enjoy lists.

Creating both lists is simple. Start by writing down all of the talents and gifts you have. Then write down all of the things, activities, etc. that you most enjoy and are most passionate about and grateful for.

Many people find that it is easier to create the second list than it is to describe their talents. Usually, that is because they may not recognize their gifts and talents. If you fall into this category, you may find it helpful to create the list of what you most enjoy first. Initially, don't worry about the order; just list as many of the things you most enjoy (at least ten).

Once you have your enjoyment list completed, take some time to consider what talents or gifts are brought out in you as you engage in such activities. As they occur to you, write them down to create your talents list. You can also ask those who know you well about what talents they recognize in you. Their responses may surprise you, yet usually you will find them to be true, so write them down, as well. When you create both lists, be sure not to censor yourself.

Once you have completed both lists set them aside for a day. Then go back to them and rearrange your listings in order of their importance to you. In other words, list your best talents and gifts first, and then do the same for the things that you most enjoy.

After you complete this step, examine both lists side by side and consider how and where your talents overlap with the activities you most enjoy. As you link your gifts and talents up with your most enjoyable activities, ask yourself how many various ways you might possibly be able to live on purpose by combining your gifts with what you most enjoy doing.

Creating a meaningful livelihood is obviously an essential component of living on purpose, yet it is not the only one. Your career or work is an area where you can define yourself and you can find satisfaction, and it is certainly wonderful to be able to do something you are really good at doing. Yet, for many people today, work, even when it fulfills them, has become something they overly focus on at the expense of other equally important aspects of their lives, especially their relationships and their health. Over-working is not honoring your body. The goal in life is balance.

Famed peak performance and personal development expert Tony Robbins has identified six basic human needs that must be met to create a truly purposeful and fulfilling life:

1. Certainty (a sense of comfort, security, and stability in our lives),
2. Variety (without change, surprise, and new experiences, we stagnate, and stagnation leads to poor health and premature aging),

3. Significance (a sense of personal achievement),
4. Growth (an ongoing process of expanding our horizons, and cultivating and developing new skills and interests),
5. Contribution (life is for giving of ourselves in a win-win manner), and, most importantly,
6. Love, which includes being intimate, passionate, vulnerable, and knowing your connection to the unified Wholeness of life.

One of the first things I advise my patients whose needs aren't being met is to slow down. This is something that all of us can benefit more from. I counsel my patients to breathe deeply, to try meditation, to do yoga or take walks, to take vacations, and to laugh and enjoy themselves more. All of these activities act as potent de-stressors, and I find that they also help people reconnect to who and what is most important to them.

What follows are some of the other questions I ask my patients as we go deeper and work together to reconnect them to their purpose. I encourage you to ask them of yourself, as well.

Do you make time each day to meditate, pray, or simply sit still to contemplate your life and all you have to be grateful for? Are you in a relationship? If so, how is your relationship with your significant other? Do you like your work? Why do you think you are on planet earth? Do you feel connected to God or a higher power? What is your support system like with your family and friends? Are you having enough fun in your life? What turns you on and excites you? What are you grateful for? Ask yourself what you can do, beginning now, to improve your experience in each of the above areas of your life.

When someone tells me they are not happy or satisfied with their life, I find that asking questions such as the ones above usually helps them get clearer about what they need to do to make their lives more meaningful. From my perspective, the three major areas of a purpose-filled life are to be happy, to be of service, and to experience who you really are through the use of your gifts and talents. Certain people may have a different order of what is most important, but the big question is, Where does one find joy? I think most people don't really realize that the main purpose in their life is to be happy, and to use their gifts to create a livelihood for themselves that also contributes back to the world in some way.

Finally, as I also counsel my patients, *always remember that life is not measured by the number of breaths we take, but by the moments that take our breath away.* You will find that you will experience more of such moments the more that you connect with and live the purposeful life.

The Purpose of Illness: For most people, illness also serves a purpose. Consider the following real-life example of what happened to a cancer patient once she consciously worked to understand the underlying purpose of her illness.

Like many other cancer patients, this woman was emotionally "blocked" and had a lot of unresolved frustration in her life. When she was asked directly if she truly wanted to be cured of her cancer, she became very thoughtful. Finally, she answered, "No." She realized that if she were cured, she would lose all the gains her illness had brought her. Her husband had quit working overtime to be available to help her. Her three daughters, who previously rarely visited, were now visiting daily. When it was explained to her that it might be possible to receive similar attention in another way, by doing volunteer work and by visiting her daughters regularly, she suddenly realized that she no longer needed to have cancer in order to get the love and attention she craved. She recovered completely within several months.

It is important to understand that illness is a warning sign, and that there is a lesson to be learned from it. Something is wrong physically, emotionally, or both. If we only heed the warning signal and not the underlying cause, the body will find another way to warn us by evoking another warning signal (another disease). Because of this fact, I often ask my patients to pause and reflect upon their lives to see if they can determine the "message" that their illness or health challenge carries with it.

Ask yourself: Are you headed in the direction that is right for you? What are you neglecting, or what price are you paying, as you go about your current life routine. For many people, the price can be exorbitant and include loneliness, because they are too busy to socialize or have time for a relationship; lack of sleep, because they have too much to do or think about; lack of relaxation time, such as listening to music, reading a good book, going on vacation, or just doing nothing; and lack of appropriately rewarding themselves with a massage, jacuzzi, sauna, or other healthy relaxing activities. Illness is often a way for a person's unconscious to point out just how much a person is neglecting or straying from their true life purpose. Once that message is received, understood and appropriately acted upon, very often illness disappears—often of its own accord in ways that baffle physicians—because it is no longer necessary.

But it would be foolish to wait until you get sick to get such a message. Regardless of your current state of health, it pays to regularly assess your life by asking yourself:

Do you freely and appropriately express yourself, or do you keep most of your worries and frustrations inside?

Are you creating too much pressure upon yourself because you've over-extended yourself, have too many deadlines, or believe that "there's not enough time?"

Do you take a few minutes every morning to reflect on and plan your day?

Do you set goals? Are they realistic, both short- and long-term, and do you have what you need in place to keep you on target for achieving them?

Do you make time each day to exercise, eat right, manage stress, and nurture your relationships?

Do you take time before sleep to evaluate how your day went and reflect upon what you could have done to be more positive, loving, and constructive?

Do you wake up grateful to be alive for another day, and are you in the habit of daily recognizing and expressing thanks for all you have to be grateful for?

Are you content with what you have, or are you always striving for more in order to feel secure?

If you do not get what you want, what is the price you pay in your health as a result of anger, depression, lost hope, and feelings of insecurity?

Do you see the positive side of events, even when they appear not in your favor?

Are you able to perceive life challenges, obstacles and "accidents" as new opportunities to grow and to learn?

Do you empower others by telling them what you appreciate about them?

Do you take time to reflect upon and relive the beautiful moments in your life, the moments of success and joy?

Do you operate from a win-win mindset where both you and others can be happy and satisfied with your achievements, or do you prefer to win regardless of whether or not it is at another's expense?

What would you like to change in your life, if you could? Do you really believe it is possible?

Now is the time for you to make a plan and set goals for changing the things in your life that you want to change. Once you understand the role your thoughts, emotions, beliefs, life choices and actions play in the creation of disease, and how illness is often a message about what you have been ignoring, you will be much closer to achieving a deeper understanding about health, have a deeper commitment to doing what is necessary to achieve and maintain it, and be more aligned with your purpose so that you meet each day with renewed enthusiasm and gratitude.

Spiritual Aspects of an Energized Life

Ultimately, our lives, including our health, is a spiritual adventure and journey. As the saying goes, you and I are "spiritual beings having a physical experience." Recognizing and connecting with your spiritual nature can make a profound and lasting positive difference in your health and in your energy.

In the deepest sense, all *dis-ease* can be seen as a disconnection between ourselves and our true, spiritual nature. From that perspective, outstanding health encompasses not only greater energy and an absence of physical and emotional ailments, but also an intimate connection to ourselves, our families and friends, and our communities, as well as an abiding awareness of God, Spirit, or however you wish to define the divine energy that created the Universe. It really doesn't matter how you define it. What matters is that you come to know and attune yourself to its guidance (your intuition) in all areas of your life.

I find when this deeper connection takes place people automatically experience a release of their fears, self-defeating behaviors, and emotional problems, and develop a greater capacity for self-love and self-acceptance, coupled with a renewed enthusiasm and sense of purpose for their lives, along with a greater capacity to interact with others without judgment. They also develop a deeper and more conscious awareness of and commitment to their community and environment.

There are a variety of ways to deepen your awareness of your spiritual nature. Two of the oldest and most common approaches are prayer and meditation. Research has established that regular performance of prayer and/or meditation results in a greater sense of well-being, improved stress reduction, and the triggering of what is known as the "relaxation response," a term coined by the famed Harvard researcher and mind/body expert Herbert Benson, MD, after he discovered how both prayer and meditation deactivates the body's stress mechanisms to engender greater levels of relaxation and contentment.

A wide body of research has demonstrated that both prayer and meditation can improve the likelihood of recovery from disease. Meditation, in particular, has also been shown to provide numerous other health benefits, including improved cardiovascular and immune function, and pain relief.

There are two other important, yet often overlooked, methods for cultivating and expanding your awareness of yourself as a spiritual, socially connected human being—spending time in nature and the daily practice of gratitude.

The Healing Power of Nature: Nowhere is the beauty and creative power of Spirit more evident than in nature. When we spend time in nature, whether it be in a park, a walk in the woods, a hike in the mountains, or a day at the seashore, we are able to most directly experience the four elemental forms of energy—earth, water, fire, and air. Earth is energy in its most condensed form, water represents receptiveness, fire is the energy of transformation, and air is the blend of these other elements into subtle life force energy, which is why conscious breathing exercises have always been an integral aspect of healing methods such as yoga, tai chi and qigong, resulting in a greater experience of *qi* or *prana*.

These four elements also manifest in your body as organic matter (earth), blood and other body fluids (water), metabolism and energy production (fire), and oxygen, carbon dioxide, and nitrogen (air). Time spent in a nature setting helps to balance and enhance these elements. In fact, in recent years, an entire new field of health therapy known as *earthing* has arisen after researchers found that as little as 15 to 20 minutes spent walking or standing barefoot on grass, soil, or sand at the beach can dramatically reduce inflammation levels in the body, and do so to a greater degree than anti-inflammatory nutrients such as fish oil and other vitamins and minerals. The significance of this discovery cannot be overstated, given that chronic inflammation is a primary cause of a wide range of serious disease conditions, including arthritis, cancer, diabetes, and heart disease.

Research has also shown that spending time in nature can lower blood pressure, ease symptoms of depression, anxiety, and anger, and even increase the body's production of various natural killer (NK) cells and anticancer proteins and their activity. Because of these and other findings, I encourage my patients to go barefoot in the grass for 15 minutes or more at sunset or right before sleep to discharge the excess positive charge that builds up in the body as a result of stress. If they can, I also tell them to walk the beach to inhale the energizing negative ions there. I encourage you to do the same. Get out into nature as often as possible.

Practicing Gratitude: Robert A. Anderson, a co-founder and past president of the American Holistic Medical Association, once described gratitude as "the Great Attitude". As he explained, "Gratitude produces feelings of joy and self-acceptance, and is an attitude that anyone can choose to have, just as we can choose to see the glass half full or half empty. Being grateful for what you have, instead of worrying about what you lack, enables you to let go of negative thoughts and attitudes more easily...If you make the effort to release these painful emotions and choose to be grateful instead, positive benefits can be achieved."

I wholeheartedly agree with Dr. Anderson, and see these positive benefits all of the time, both in my patients and in my own life, when we take time to focus on all that we have to be grateful for. To that end, I make it a practice of noticing and giving thanks for all the experiences and people I am grateful for each day. I highly advise that you get in the habit of doing the same. You can do so simply by ending your day by mentally reviewing and inventorying all of the things happened that day for which you feel grateful. Or you might consider keeping a "gratitude journal" in which you write about what you are grateful for each day before you go to bed. Whatever approach works best for you, by regularly cultivating gratitude you will soon find yourself experiencing more joy and contentment in your life.

As you continue to cultivate the spiritual aspects of your life here are some other benefits you can expect to begin experiencing more often:

New insights about life issues.

A clearer understanding and eventual healing of past emotional trauma.

Heightened creativity.

Greater levels of inspiration.

Greater compassion for others.

A deeper connection to your own intuitive abilities and your own inner guidance.

When I contemplate my spiritual nature I am often reminded of the nursery song Row, Row, Row Your Boat. I'm sure you are familiar with the lyrics:

Row, row, row your boat
gently down the stream,
merrily, merrily, merrily—
life is but a dream.

I find the lyrics to be both instructive and helpful in keeping me attuned to Spirit. From my perspective, the boat is my body and my physical life, and they are also, whether I am consciously aware of it or not, being "rowed", or guided, by my Soul, or Higher Self. Additionally, I am encouraged by the lyrics to pay attention to my dreams—both in terms of my life goals and aspirations, and also to the dreams I have when my body sleeps for the messages and guidance they provide.

I also find that simply mentally saying the lyrics to myself during life's challenging moments very often is enough to prevent the triggering of a stress response, and even to provide me with a new, more insightful and empowering perspective. Try singing the song to yourself the next time you are facing a challenge and see what happens. The results may pleasantly surprise you.

Giving Back: Hand in hand with the practice of gratitude is giving back and being of service to others. In all of the world's religious and spiritual traditions, this is commonly known as practicing charity. It is also referred to as being altruistic.

As the saying goes, "charity begins at home." Being there for your family members and loved ones is a perfect way to begin practicing being charitable. There are many ways and opportunities that being with your family and other loved ones can afford you to be of service to them. It can be something as simple as greeting family members with a smile or a hug, helping them with their daily chores, or lending a kind and attentive ear to them when they are going through struggles. Such charitable acts deepen the bonds of love and strengthen family relationships and friendships. They can also be quite healing.

You can also extend your practice of charity to others you meet during the course of your day. Even something as simple as smiling and saying hello to a passersby can often make a difference in others' lives.

You can also donate your time or food items to your local food bank, or participate in community activities that improve your neighborhood. As with your family and friends, the opportunities to be of service to others are many once you start to look for them.

Another way of giving back is by donating money to worthwhile causes. In religious traditions, this is known as tithing, a practice that is of particular importance during this time of economic hardship for so many people. My co-author and I are both firm believers in tithing, which is why we have chosen to donate a portion of this book's sales to the charity Feeding America, an organization that was brought to our attention by Tony Robbins. (For more information about the wonderful work this charity does helping to feed America's hungry, visit www. feedingamerica.org.) There are many other worthwhile charities that you can donate to, as well. Find one or more whose causes you support and give what you can when you can.

As I mentioned, regularly finding ways to give back to others can be a very healing experience. This fact has been proven by scientific research. A number of studies have found that altruistic people have better overall health outcomes, including greater longevity and improved mental and emotional health, compared to people who are focused only on themselves. So I encourage you to find ways to give back within your relationships and in your community. Not only will you being doing good to others, you will be doing good for yourself, as well.

Other Helpful Methods for Healing and Fortifying Your Mind

What follow are various proven and effective treatment methods for healing troubling emotions and past traumas, positively reshaping beliefs, and enhancing your ability to use your mind to create greater levels of well-being in body, mind, and spirit.

Counseling and Therapy: People who are not happy are usually also not clear about their life purpose, and can be greatly burdened by past issues and traumas in their lives that they are unable to resolve on their own, or with the support of their families and friends. Counseling and therapy can often be effective in helping to turn such people's lives around. Professional counselors and therapists can often help people find their way to a better understanding of their behaviors and limiting thoughts and beliefs, and then help empower them to move beyond them.

Such professional care providers can also objectively help people look at how they are interacting with the other people in their lives. Most of us spend time with our significant other or with the people at work. If either of these relationships are not working, it's going to be pretty hard for a person who isn't that conscious to find the satisfaction they are looking for in their lives.

There are a range of counseling and therapy options to choose from, running the gamut from psychotherapy, to family and marriage counseling, to cognitive therapy, to working with spiritual counselors (priest, ministers, rabbis, etc.). Unfortunately, the field of psychiatry today has increasingly become a symptom-care, drug-based profession that fails to address actual mental or emotional issues, beyond medicating, or numbing, such problems away with drugs. While such medications can be helpful in serious cases of mental illness, overall I do not agree with this approach, both because emotional and mental health issues are not due to a deficiency of drugs, and, more importantly, because all such psychiatric drugs carry the risk of very serious, even life-threatening side effects. Equally important, by focusing on drug treatments for psychological issues, many psychiatrists deprive their patients of the opportunity to truly heal.

Should counseling or therapy appeal to you, I recommend that you choose an approach that is holistic in nature. Hallmarks of such approaches are that they not only address psychological problems, but also help clients discover and commit to their life purpose, their unique talents, and their interests and desires in life. Such a therapeutic approach helps to both uncover solutions to current life issues and to empower clients to mobilize their gifts and inner resources to achieve a greater sense of control over their lives, and to be able to reframe past painful experiences as opportunities for learning, growth and personal transformation.

Flower Essences: Flowers have always been regarded and used as symbols of beauty and the development of our highest human faculties. Human development over the course of our history owes much to the energies we draw from the plant kingdom. Flower essences make use of plants' healing energetic properties to resolve and heal various emotional issues.

Flower essence therapy originated in the early 1930s. It was developed by the renowned British physician, researcher, and homeopath, Dr. Edward Bach, after he recognized that many of his patients' ills were related to their various negative states of mind. He noted that fear, anger, lack of confidence, jealousy, hopelessness, resentment, guilt, and uncertainty so depleted a person's vitality that the body lost its natural resistance to infection and other illness.

Dr. Bach felt that illness was a reflection of disharmony between a person's personality and his or her Higher Self, or Soul. He taught that we come into this world with a certain soul purpose. We then develop a personality that is a reflection of how we interact within this world. Frequently our personality is in conflict with our soul purpose. Dr Bach felt that the subtle vibrational energies of flower essences could assist in realigning our personality with our soul, or life, purpose and thus create greater harmony within us. By correcting these emotional factors, he reasoned, patients would increase their physical and mental vitality and be aided in resolving any physical illness.

Dr. Bach discovered the effects of various flowers through observation of how they affected him. Living in the English countryside, he took long walks in search of the emotional healers within nature. His sensitivity to subtle energies was so great that by touching the morning dew from a flower to his lips, he could experience all of the physical symptoms and emotional states to which the flower's essence was an antidote.

Dr. Bach discovered 38 flower remedies, along with an all-purpose remedy he called Rescue Remedy. He prepared each remedy by placing a specific flower upon the surface of a bowl of spring water for several hours in sunlight. The subtle effects of sunlight were critical in charging the water with an energetic imprint of the flower's vibration. The 38 Bach remedies related to seven emotional states—fear, uncertainty, insufficient interest in the present, loneliness, over-sensitivity to outside influences and ideas, despondency, and being overly concerned with the welfare of others.

The flowers used by Dr. Bach to create his remedies each embody a certain soul quality, meaning, in energetic terms, they have a particular energy wavelength. Each of these plant-based, soul qualities is in tune with a certain soul quality in a person, i.e., with a certain frequency in the human energy field. Following his discoveries, Dr. Bach used his flower remedies as his principal form of treatment with his patients, finding that, as they effectively resolved their underlying emotional issues, their physical illnesses and ailments would automatically begin to resolve themselves. Since Dr. Bach's time, a number of other researchers have added to his understanding of the healing properties of flower essences, and have also developed additional flower essence formulas. Such essences are now used by a growing number of holistic healers and counselors all around the world.

A firsthand experience I had while working as an emergency room physician in 1988 showed me the value of Bach Flower remedies. The paramedics had just brought in a lady in a state of acute pulmonary edema (water in the lungs secondary to congestive heart failure). I used all the standard ER procedures to try and help her, which included oxygen, morphine, diuretics, and breathing treatments. Nothing worked, and she was going downhill. I then gave her five drops under the tongue of the Bach Flower Rescue Remedy. Within 30 seconds, her anxiety dissipated, her breathing slowed, and she was soon fine. In that moment I became a firm believer in Bach Flower remedies as an effective form of Energy Medicine (and so did the paramedics and ER nurses).

Energy Psychology: The field of energy psychology is an exciting addition to the overall field of mind/body medicine. It was originally developed by the late Roger Callahan, PhD, a clinical psychotherapist who also had an understanding of the energetic meridian pathway systems of acupuncture and traditional Chinese medicine (see Chapter 2). One day, while working with a female patient who suffered from a deep-seated, longstanding water phobia that he had been unable to help her resolve despite working with her for more than year, the woman revealed that, as they addressed her phobia, she was starting to experience stomach symptoms. Knowing that the meridian that passes through the stomach originates at an acupuncture point just below the eye, on a hunch, Dr. Callahan began lightly tapping that acupoint with his fingertip. To both his and his patient's surprise doing so not only resolved the woman's stomach problems, it also caused her water phobia to completely disappear, never to return.

Intrigued by this, Dr. Callahan began to further investigate the relationship between acupuncture points, the meridian system, and mental and emotional issues, and eventually developed a system of mental/emotional healing called Callahan Thought Field Therapy, or TFT. One of his former students, Fred P. Gallo, PhD, dubbed this approach to healing, *energy psychology*. Since TFT's inception, a number of other forms of energy psychology methods have been developed. Among the most popular methods today are emotional freedom technique (EFT), Tapas Acupressure Technique (TAT), and Eye Movement Desensitization and Reprogramming (EMDR).

A full explanation of how and why energy psychology methods work and how to use them is beyond the scope of this book. Suffice it to say, however, that a growing body of research continues to demonstrate that these methods can be highly effective for healing deep-seated emotional issues, ranging from anxiety and depression, to fears and phobias, to post-traumatic stress disorder (PTSD). Moreover, researchers have also found that, as people's mental and emotional issues are healed and resolved by the use of energy psychology techniques, their physical health issues also tend to resolve and lessen.

Many types of energy psychology techniques are easy to learn and incorporate into your daily life as effective self-care tools. You will find a list of contact organizations offering training in these methods in the Resources section of this book.

To end this section, let me offer a few other suggestions for a creating happier, healthier and more mentally fortified life:

Commit yourself to doing more of what you love; as you do so, health and healing will follow.

Surround yourself with people that make you feel good.

Heal your relationship with your parents, family members, spouse or partner.

Make fun and relaxation a daily priority.

Learn to love and accept yourself. Once you learn to forgive yourself, it's easy to forgive others. Remember that life is for-giving.

Recognize that your home is your sanctuary. Fill it with things that support and nurture you.

Enjoy sex as a loving and sacred communion.

Make decisions that give you the greatest peace of mind.

Do the best that you can, and let go of judgment of others.

Connect with your spiritual nature as often as you can. Tap into it as often as possible for it is your primary source of knowledge, inspiration, and guidance.

Treat the earth well and spend time in nature as often as possible.

And get in the habit of regularly asking yourself, Am I letting in:

Source Energy

Well-being

God Force

Clarity

Abundance

Enthusiasm

Vitality

Balance

Release of financial struggle

Friends

Loved ones

Relationships

My spouse or partner?

I will close this chapter with the following story. When asked what surprised him most about humanity, the Dalai Lama answered, "Man. Because he sacrifices his health in order to make money. Then he sacrifices money to recuperate his health. And then he is so anxious about the future that he does not enjoy the present; the result being that he does not live in the present or the future; he lives as if he is never going to die, and then dies having never fully lived."

Although this depiction by the Dalai Lama is true for so many people in the world, it need not be true for you. Make a commitment to yourself to apply the information you learned in this chapter. As you do so, expect your thought, beliefs, and emotions to change for the better, and your health and energy to change dramatically for the better, too. Make a decision to feel well. If you believe it, you *will* see it. This will allow you to live and enjoy the present moment, and further support you in your ongoing journey and adventure of outstanding health.

Key Points To Remember

Your thoughts, emotions, and beliefs have a profound influence on your health, both positively and negatively.

Many people unconsciously become attached to the "stories" about their illness or health ailment. By doing so, they derive benefits from their stories.

Recognizing and learning to let go of such stories and all else that holds back healing is an essential part of the overall healing process.

Numerous studies have not only proven that thoughts, emotions, and beliefs influence our health, but also that there are cell receptors in the body that correspond with our thoughts and emotions, acting as their physical counterparts. Pioneering mind/body researcher Candace Pert showed that these receptors act as the interface between our emotions and their effects on the body.

Fear is far more dangerous to your health and well-being than actual disease. Your fears about illness can greatly suppress your body's ability to heal. Positive thoughts and emotions, on the other hand, can dramatically improve your body's ability to heal, and even result in "spontaneous remissions".

In addition to the "fight or flight response" in the face of actual or perceived stressful life events, you also need to be aware of the "pleasure freeze-response". This response can cause you to detach, or numb, yourself to stress and other uncomfortable life situations, resulting in an inability to move forward to experiencing pleasure, comfort, and joy, as well as a fluid movement of your life energy toward what you truly want in life.

There are seven positive primary positive and seven primary negative emotions. By learning how to consciously choose to experience the seven primary positive emotions, you can significantly improve your health.

Creative visualization, examining and reprogramming your beliefs, and the use of positive affirmations are all effective self-care approaches you can use to fortify your mind and improve your health.

Reconnecting with and living from your true life purpose is another very important necessity when it comes to healing and personal fulfillment. When you are ill, this includes understanding the purpose of your illness and heeding and acting upon the messages that your illness may carry for you.

Healing also requires a deepening of your connection to your underlying spiritual nature. Effective means for doing so include prayer, meditation, spending time in nature and the regular practice of gratitude.

Various other methods for mentally and emotionally healing and fortifying your mind include counseling and therapy, flower essences, and energy psychology techniques such as EFT.

CHAPTER 6

Essential #2: Cleanse and Renew Your Body

We live in a world that is filled with toxins. Virtually everyone alive today, including newborn babies, carry within their bodies a toxic cocktail of industrial chemicals, pesticides, food additives and preservatives, and a wide array of health-sapping heavy metals, along with residues of pharmaceutical drugs and synthetic hormones, which are found in our food and water supplies. Because of this alarming fact, the essential first step in creating better health, more energy, and a more youthful dynamic for yourself is to reduce your body's toxic burden so that its organs, starting with your liver, can once again return to full, optimal functioning.

In this chapter, you will learn more about how and why toxins are so detrimental to your health, and then be guided in the proper use of the most effective methods for eliminating them using proven drainage and detoxification techniques, many of which you can do by yourself in the comfort of your own home.

The Ultimate Agers: Toxins and Tissue Acidity

To fully understand why toxins are so dangerous, you first need to understand an aspect of health that is all too often overlooked by doctors—tissue acidity. Tissue acidity is a condition in which tissues, and thus the organs they make up, have a low, or acidic, pH. pH refers to the concentration, or level, of hydrogen ions in body fluids (blood, urine, or saliva). In terms of health, pH is used as a measurement of the ratio of acidic, alkaline, and neutral components of the body's fluids and tissues. For good health to be maintained this ratio must be balanced. When it is out of balance—either too low (overly acidic) or too high (overly alkaline), the body's internal environment is negatively affected, setting the stage for disease.

pH is measured on a scale of 0 to 14, with a pH of 7 being neutral. Any measurement below 7 indicates acidity, while measurements above 7 indicate alkalinity. In a state of optimal, thriving health, the pH of your blood needs to be in a slightly alkaline state, with a pH between 7.35 and 7.45. (By contrast, normal saliva pH levels can fluctuate between 6.0 and 7.4, while urine pH levels can range from 4.5 to 8.0.) Should pH blood levels move below or above this very narrow range, illness, can soon follow. For this reason, your body, via the mechanism of homeostasis, does all that it can to maintain blood pH within this narrow range.

There are various protective mechanisms that your body must call upon in order to cope with acid buildup. In the face of chronic over-acidity—a condition that affects most people today—these mechanisms must work overtime, diverting alkalinizing minerals, such as calcium, magnesium and potassium, from bones in an attempt to buffer, or neutralize the acid. This, in turn, means that these minerals are less available to meet the literally hundreds of other tasks they help regulate in the body. Eventually, the body's various regulatory systems start to become compromised, setting the stage for disease and premature aging.

One important example of this is what occurs with your body's enzyme systems. Every biochemical activity in your body is initiated by specific enzymes, and all enzymes are active within a very narrow pH range. When this range changes for any length of time, which is what happens with over-acidity, neither the enzymes nor the processes they activate can function properly. This is one of many reasons why it is so important to maintain a healthy pH balance in the body so that is not strained with the burdens of chronic acidity.

The three main organs involved in maintaining proper acid-alkaline balance in the body are the kidneys and the lungs, along with, to a lesser extent, the skin. The kidneys help to maintain blood pH by eliminating acids such as sulfuric and uric acids. In the presence of elevated acidity, the kidneys are forced to excrete more hydrogen ions, resulting in a low urine pH (5.0). In order to eliminate such acids the kidneys rely upon alkalinizing minerals that are primarily stored in and around your bones.

Ideally, the supply of such minerals is added to daily by a diet high in mineral-rich foods. All too often, however, dietary sources of these minerals are lacking due to poor eating habits. When that is the case, the kidneys must deplete the body's store of these minerals.

The lungs help keep body pH levels normal by eliminating carbon dioxide (CO_2). The lungs' involvement in maintaining acid-alkaline balance can provide a clue as to whether or not your body is too acidic. If it is, typically your respiration, or breathing rate, will be elevated (greater than 20/minute). People whose bodies are not overly acidic tend to have lower respiration rates.

Your body also eliminates acids through its sweat glands when you perspire. Compared to the amount of acids eliminated by the kidneys and lungs, however, the amount of acid eliminated by the skin is rather modest, since sweat is unable to eliminate acids at the same levels of concentration as the kidneys and lungs can. But the skin, too, can provide clues to whether or not your body is burdened with excess acidity. Typical symptoms of over-acidity include excess body odor, and a flare up of skin conditions, including acne, eczema and psoriasis.

No matter how hard the kidneys, lungs, and skin work to accomplish their buffering and elimination of acids, there is only a certain amount of acidity that they can cope with in every 24-hour cycle. Whatever amount of acids is left over, especially in the case of the kidneys, has to be dealt with by the body's mineral stores. If these stores are low, they are soon depleted, resulting in acid build up in the body, a condition known as *cellular acidosis*.

Chronic acidosis sets the stage for a wide range of health problems, starting with the disruption of healthy cell function. All cells need to be in a state of acid-alkaline balance in order to properly carry out their many tasks. When this balance is lost due to acidosis the cells' ability to perform their numerous functions is impaired. This is especially true with regard to the cells' mitochondria, the "energy factories" that you learned about in Chapter 3. Acidosis results in a loss of energy production by the mitochondria, resulting in cellular fatigue and premature cell death. This chain of events then spirals outward to the body's tissues and organs, eventually impairing their functioning, as well.

Here are some of the most commonly occurring health issues caused by over-acidity in the body:

- Loss of calcium in the urine, the dissolution of bone, and the development of osteoporosis.
- Reduced bone formation.
- Increased levels of blood parathyroid hormone, a hormone that, in excess, can cause bones to become brittle and prone to fracture.
- Depletion of potassium and magnesium stores from the body.
- Depressed protein metabolism, resulting in the inability to fully repair cells, tissues, and organs.
- Irritation of the urinary tract and bladder.
- Suppression of growth hormone, insulin-like growth factor, and other pituitary hormones, causing suboptimal tissue renewal and hormone dysfunction
- Increased production of *free radicals*—unstable molecules that cause cellular damage—resulting in inflammation, lowered immunity, and the increased risk of degenerative disease and premature aging.
- Weakening of connective tissue due to increased free radicals generated by chronic inflammation, leading to muscle weakness and pain.
- Increased risk of kidney stone formation.
- Disrupted balance of intestinal bacteria, and related gastrointestinal problems.

- Loss of oxygen in the blood, cells and tissues, creating a fertile breeding ground for bacteria, fungi, and viruses, all of which thrive in an anaerobic (low oxygen), acidic environment.
- Impaired brain and cognitive function due to loss of the brain's energy reserves.
- Decreased ability to perform exercise at a high level of intensity.
- Increased acidity of the mouth, leading to imbalanced oral bacteria, dental decay and periodontal (gum) disease.
- Low thyroid function .

Test Yourself for Acidosis: Here is a simple test you can perform at home to determine whether or not your body is in a state of chronic over-acidity. To perform this test you will need to buy pH strips, also known as Hydrion paper, which is available at most drugstores. pH strips change color when coming in contact with various substances, according to their level of acidity or alkalinity. The color the strip turns is then compared to a color chart that comes with the pH paper that corresponds to different pH levels ranging from 5.5 to 8.0.

Before you eat, collect a bit of your first morning urine, and then briefly wet the pH strip with it. Be careful not to over-saturate the strip. A quick dip into the urine is all that is necessary. Then wait a few seconds as it changes color. Once it does, compare the color to the corresponding pH chart. This will give you a fairly accurate measurement of your body's pH. I recommend that you perform this test every morning for a period of one to two weeks, so that you can determine your average baseline pH reading. Any reading below 6.0 is an indication of over-acidity in your body. If your reading is consistently between 6.5 to 7.5, you most likely have a healthy pH.

Don't be surprised if your baseline measurement indicates over-acidity, as today that is the rule for most people, rather than the exception. If you are overly acidic, you can do a lot on your own to move to a more balanced pH level simply through your diet, by following the dietary guidelines you will learn about in Chapter 7. As you do so, you can use this home pH test to monitor your progress. Most people will note an improvement in their morning urine pH levels within a few weeks of following such a diet. However, if there is no improvement within one to two months' time, this may be a sign of an underlying condition that requires medical attention.

The most important point to remember from this section is this: An acidic environment is the foundation for all illness to develop. The more acidic and the more toxic you are, the weaker your liver is, and the weaker your hormonal system is, and ultimately your cells wind up not being able to create sufficient energy, and could result in cells that can only ferment sugar. Ultimately, if this process is left unchecked, they can become cancer cells. Therefore the first step to a healthy, cleansed body is to become less acidic. In addition to changing your diet to one that consists primarily of alkalinizing foods (again, see Chapter 8), this means addressing and reducing your body's toxic load, especially with regard to one of the most common types of environmental toxins, heavy metals.

Mercury and Other Heavy Metals

Heavy metals are a huge problem in our society. You and I are exposed to heavy metals and other environmental toxins in concentrations that are far greater than previous generations faced. This fact was brought home by a 2005 paper published by the Environmental Working Group. Entitled *Body Burden: The Pollution in Newborns*, the report stated, "Not long ago scientists thought that the placenta shielded cord blood—and the developing baby—from most chemicals and pollutants in the environment. But now we know that at this critical time when organs, vessels, membranes and systems are knit together from single cells to finished form in a span of weeks, the umbilical cord carries not only the building blocks of life, but also a steady stream of industrial chemicals, pollutants and pesticides that cross the placenta as readily as residues from cigarettes and alcohol."

The paper was the result of a study conducted by researchers at two major laboratories. The paper reported that the researchers "found an average of 200 industrial chemicals and pollutants in umbilical cord blood from 10 babies born in August and September of 2004 in U.S. hospitals. Tests revealed a total of 287 chemicals in the group. The umbilical cord blood of these 10 children, collected by Red Cross after the cord was cut, harbored pesticides, consumer product ingredients, and wastes from burning coal, gasoline, and garbage." Of the 287 detected chemicals the researchers wrote, "We know that 180 cause cancer in humans or animals, 217 are toxic to the brain and nervous system, and 208 cause birth defects or abnormal development in animal tests."

To me, the most disturbing aspect about this study's findings is that in every case, mercury was found in the babies' cord blood. The presence of mercury was attributed to pollution from coal-fired power plants, mercury-containing products, and certain industrial processes. Mercury also accumulates in seafood, and is the most common element in dental amalgam fillings, which consist of 50 percent mercury, along with the heavy metals silver, tin, and copper.

Mercury is far more prevalent in our environment and food and water supply than most people realize. In part, this is due to the high levels of mercury that are being spread by the massive industrial development now occurring in China and India, which now account for about 30 percent of mercury pollution in the U.S. Mercury and other heavy metals and pollutants from these countries' coal-fired power plants soar high into the atmosphere to circle the globe via transcontinental air currents, adding to the already substantial amount of mercury pollution created by our nation's own factories, power plants, and mines.

Another little known source of mercury toxicity is cement kilns, which are largely unregulated in the United States. It is estimated that cement kilns in the U.S. emit more than 20,000 pounds of mercury compounds into the air each and every year, the largest amount after that produced by coal-fired power plants. Waste incineration further adds to this problem.

Once in the atmosphere, mercury enters the food chain when it is deposited on our nation's soil and waterways to be consumed by fish and mammals. According to the Environmental Protection Agency (EPA), approximately one-third of our nation's lakes and 25 percent of its rivers are so polluted with mercury that the EPA now advises that people, especially children and pregnant women, either significantly limit their intake of fish caught within them or avoid them altogether. Health safety warnings about mercury have also been issued by regulatory agencies in 45 states.

Overall, fish consumption has become another common source of mercury exposure. While certain types of fish provide a variety of important health benefits, eating fish selectively makes good sense these days, as does focusing on fish that have the least amount of mercury content. An online calculator created by the National Resources Defense Council can help you monitor your mercury intake from a variety of fish. For more information, go to www.nrdc.org/health/effects/mercury/calculator/calc.asp.

Another source of mercury toxicity is various vaccines, which contain mercury, in the form of thimerosal, as a preservative. Many vaccines also contain a variety of other toxic substances, and although both the pharmaceutical industry and the United States government continue to insist that vaccines are safe, there is no question that a correlation can be made between the dramatic rise in autism and other developmental disorders in children and the corresponding increase in the number of vaccines that are prescribed for children from the time they are newly born until they are two to three years old. Moreover, although it is now a law that vaccine manufacturers cannot be sued for damages caused by vaccines, the U.S. government has quietly awarded tens of millions of dollars to the families of children injured as a direct result of vaccination through its Vaccine Injury Compensation Program. In most of these cases a major culprit behind such injuries, which range from autism to seizures, has been thimerosal.

Mercury In Dental Amalgam Fillings: So-called silver dental amalgam fillings are another common source of mercury toxicity. As mentioned above, such fillings contain 50 percent mercury, which has been recognized as a poison since the 1500s. Yet, even though the EPA declared scrap dental amalgam a hazardous waste in 1988, such fillings continue to be widely used by American dentists, despite being banned in other countries, including Germany, Denmark, Norway, Sweden, and Russia. Both the European Union and U.S. State Department have also called for a complete phase out of the use of mercury in amalgam fillings, although no set time table for this has yet been agreed upon. So it remains a continuing controversy in medicine that a very toxic substance such as mercury can be considered totally harmless once it is placed in the teeth. This debate has been going on since dentistry began using mercury many decades ago.

Energy Medicine has demonstrated that a high percentage of persons with chronic disease have mercury as their Key Toxin. In most cases, the mercury was leaking from their fillings. The reason dental amalgams containing mercury and other heavy metals pose such a health threat is because of how these toxins get released as vapors through such activities as chewing food or gum, brushing teeth, flossing, drinking carbonated drinks and warm beverages, and teeth grinding. Additionally, over time, mercury and other metals in dental fillings can corrode. . As all of this occurs, the released mercury migrates into the root of teeth, into the jaw, the thyroid gland, and the nerves, as well as entering into the bloodstream by the act of swallowing, to be deposited into the tissues of various organs and glands, where it acts as a chronic disruptor of many biological and enzymatic processes.

Many patients also have problems caused by a secondary phenomenon called oral galvanism, in which an electrical current is created in the mouth when two or more metals are used for fillings. This electrical current has a stronger intensity than the natural electrical currents generated in the brain, and thus can contribute to emotional issues and insomnia. These currents can also get amplified by cell phones and computer screens, resulting in a wide array of symptoms caused by electromagnetic field disturbances (EMF's)

Years of research in Energy Medicine has shown that:

1. Mercury is toxic in any form.
2. Mercury fillings can induce serious side-effects in individuals overly sensitive to mercury.

3. Long-term exposure to mercury in most people will cause chronic stress in the body.

4. For those people in whom mercury is the Key Toxin, metabolic processes are blocked, along with the immune system.

5. Patients without mercury fillings are more responsive to treatment than those with mercury fillings.

Based on these observations, it is safe to say that mercury should not be used in dental fillings. If you have amalgam fillings, I strongly encourage you to do further reading on this subject, and decide for yourself whether to replace your mercury fillings with more appropriate materials such as porcelain, gold, or other nontoxic composites when the opportunity arises.

With allergic patients, persons who have autoimmune illness (rheumatoid arthritis, lupus, multiple sclerosis, etc.), and patients with immune system weakness, extra precautions should be taken before removing the fillings. These patients should be seen by "Biological Dentists", who use rubber dams, high vacuum suction, negative ion generators, and inhaled oxygen during removal of the fillings. Patients should also take chlorella 1,000 mg daily for several days before mercury removal.

Chlorella, is a single-celled micro-algae that is available at most health food stores. Chlorella has an interesting molecular structure that enables it to bind to certain heavy metals, including mercury, along with various other toxic compounds, while leaving health-enhancing minerals in the body untouched. Other health benefits of regular supplementation of chlorella include enhanced oxygenation to cells and tissues, blood purification, elimination of molds and fungi (both of which have a tendency to cling to, and flourish in the presence of heavy metals), and overall cleansing of the body's elimination systems, including the bowels and liver. Chlorella also promotes the healthy growth and repair of tissues. You can also take chlorella prior to eating fish, so as to protect yourself from mercury and toxins in the fish.

Patients should take Selenium 200 micrograms daily as long as they have mercury fillings in their teeth. Selenium is an anti-oxidant, and can help block the adverse effects of mercury.

The fillings should be removed one quadrant at a time per visit. Patients should take 4,000 mg of Vitamin C orally at the end of the dental visit. There should be a 4 week interval between visits, so as to allow the body to fully recover from the procedure. Many patients will feel better after all the mercury fillings have been replaced. The next step involves the removal of the mercury from the tissues of the body, as the mercury has leaked out of the fillings over time. This can be accomplished with products such as cilantro, chlorella, homeopathic chelation, and in selected cases intra-venous and oral chelation products that contain sulfur, the safest of which is glutathione. Intravenous Vitamin C is also very helpful. With these therapies combined with homeopathic drainage (especially the kidneys) and detoxification (see Chapter 10), these reserves will be eliminated. It often will take up to six months to remove all traces of mercury, but the rewards are great.

It may be difficult to find a dentist who is aware of these serious problems. The American Dental Association (ADA) has positioned itself in favor of amalgam fillings, and discourages their members from removing fillings for reasons of toxicity. If your dentist refuses to remove your fillings, you can contact an organization called the International Academy of Oral Metal Toxicology (iaomt.org) to find a biological dentist in your area. It often takes time for medicine to acknowledge that a mistake has taken place. With the mercury issue, lack of cooperation between the medical and dental professions has made things even more difficult. Mercury may cause symptoms months or years after amalgam fillings are implanted in the oral cavity. Patients then seek out physicians who make no connection between their symptoms and their earlier dental work. Once a treatment is considered safe, it often takes much suffering before a change is effected, especially when the side-effects are difficult to notice. Yet the evidence exists: Many patients have greatly improved their general health after removing their mercury amalgam fillings.

Because of how widespread mercury is in our environment, it is not surprising that it is the number one source of heavy metal toxicity in most people, as documented by the EPA. The health issues and diseases mercury can cause is quite extensive. In addition to causing symptoms of every known neurological disease, including amyotrophic lateral sclerosis (Lou Gehrig's disease), Alzheimer's disease, multiple sclerosis, and Parkinson's disease, mercury toxicity can be associated with cancer, especially breast and prostate cancer, because of how it acts as a xenoestrogen. Mercury toxicity has also been linked to impaired brain function (especially in newborns and young children) and mental retardation, behavioral disorders such as ADD/ADHD, kidney problems, high blood pressure, and thyroid problems.

As the thyroid isn't very far from the lower jaw, I often come across a condition called Hashimoto's thyroiditis in my patients with mercury amalgams. This is an autoimmune disease in which the body attacks the thyroid gland with antibodies. Other autoimmune diseases can also be triggered or exacerbated by mercury toxicity.

Research has also established that mercury can cause high blood pressure and elevated cholesterol levels, and can double the risk of death caused by heart attack and other cardiovascular diseases. Studies have also shown that mercury damages and inhibits the repair of DNA, negatively affects the activity of enzymes needed for all biochemical reactions in the body, impairs immune function, interferes with proper endocrine function and hormone production, impairs healthy digestion by killing off "friendly" bacteria in the gut, and displaces and deactivates vital mineral nutrients, including calcium, magnesium, and zinc. Mercury can even cause harmful bacteria to become resistant to antibiotics, and has been shown to be involved in cases of psychological/emotional upset because of its harmful effects on the brain.

The prevalence of mercury in our environment is bad enough on its own. Unfortunately, this problem is greatly compounded by other heavy metals that we are also commonly exposed to on a regular basis. Arsenic, cadmium and lead toxicity are also very common in much of the population today, as is toxicity caused by exposure to aluminum.

We've all been exposed to lead in the gasoline that used to be in the pump, and from the paint in our homes and old lead pipes and radiators, and so forth. Lead is also often found in children's toys and jewelry, especially those manufactured and imported abroad. It is also found in dust and soil, including many outdoor playgrounds across the nation, as well as in tap water, various cosmetic products, leaded crystal, and car batteries, to name just a few other sources. As a result, studies show our bones have 1000 times more lead than the bones of those who lived 100 years ago.

Cadmium exposures range from cigarette smoke (including second-hand smoke), automobile exhaust, metal plating, and plastics, where it is used as a stabilizer. Cadmium is also released into the environment through mining and smelting, as well as through various other industrial processes, and can enter the food chain from uptake by plants grown in contaminated soil. Nonorganic rice, cereal grains, and potatoes are particularly susceptible to cadmium uptake. Cadmium is also found in phosphate fertilizers and sewage sludge.

According to the EPA, arsenic ranks second to only mercury as the most common heavy metal in the U.S. One reason for this is because of how prevalent arsenic is in much of our nation's water supply, especially in the groundwater of states in the south- and northwest, as well as Alaska. Nonorganic wine often contains arsenic, as do nonorganic poultry and certain types of seafood, especially cold water fish and bottom-feeding finfish. Arsenic is also found in commercial insecticides, pesticides, and wood preservatives, and is emitted into the atmosphere during industrial processes such as smelting and glass production. Like cadmium, it is also contained in cigarette smoke.

Another common heavy metal is aluminum, which is found in aluminum foil, canned foods and beverages (both beer and soda, for example), as well as in many types of pots and pans and cooking utensils. Various types of aluminum are also used in food packaging, antiperspirants, antacids, and cosmetic products, and aluminum is also found in various vaccines, and as a coloring agent in certain pharmaceutical drugs. It can also be found in tap water and in buffered aspirin products. In recent years, aluminum has been implicated in the rising incidence of Alzheimer's disease and dementia, after researchers found aluminum in the neurofibrillary tangles in the brains of patients with Alzheimer's disease. Tangles are nerve cells that become bunched together and knotted in the presence of aluminum.

Other Heavy Metals and Their Harmful Effects: According to the Centers for Disease Control and Prevention (CDC), other common heavy metals to which we are commonly exposed include antimony, barium, beryllium, cesium, cobalt, molybdenum, platinum, tungsten, thallium, and uranium. Like mercury, all of these heavy metals can wreak havoc inside the body, leading to a wide range of health conditions, including:

- Neurotoxic damage to brain structures; lower IQ; lowered dopamine levels
- Kidney damage
- Impaired immune function
- Cardiovascular problems: hypertension; elevated cholesterol, heart attack
- Anemia and chronic fatigue
- Bone and tissue deposits
- Yeast and fungi overgrowth
- Hormonal disruption - thyroid, adrenals, sex hormones
- Cognitive problems - ADHD, Alzheimer's, dementia
- Mood disorders: anxiety, depression, obsessive compulsive disorder (OCD)
- Impaired metabolism: energy decline, weight gain
- Type II diabetes
- Raynaud's disease.

Although some people can be exposed to mercury and other heavy metals and be able to excrete them without much consequence to their health, the vast majority of people are non-excreters, meaning that their bodies cannot get rid of these toxins without assistance, which is why ongoing drainage and detoxification measures are so important. The bottom line is that in today's world, we really can't avoid ongoing exposure to heavy metals and other toxins, but we certainly can take steps to constantly clean our bodies. What follows are some of the most effective methods to remove toxins from our bodies.

Drainage: The First Step To Purifying Your Body

All chronically ill persons have a very high accumulation of toxins in their bodies. Many healthy persons also have a high level of toxicity. High levels of toxicity cause stress on the tissues, slowing down the metabolic processes and interfering with the function of the immune system. The stronger the body's constitution and the more balanced one's mental condition, the longer it is possible to maintain relative health with a high toxic load. Ultimately, however, we all pay the price.

The first essential key to health is to clear toxins from the body, while minimizing stress, and adopting a healthy lifestyle. As you learned in Chapter 2, the initial step in getting toxins out of the body is called drainage. This is the process of stimulating the organs of elimination, such as the liver, kidneys, lymphatics, colon, and skin.

The following metaphor bests explains the concept of drainage. Before repainting a house, the first thing to do is to remove all signs of dirt and dust which have accumulated since it was previously cleaned. The walls are first washed and the floors swept . This needs to be done before applying fresh coats of paint. If you do repaint a dirty and dusty house, you will have done yourself a disservice.

Drainage is the process of stimulating the organs that excrete toxins. I have created herbal and homeopathic formulas that are used daily in my practice to accomplish drainage. Mild discomfort can occur during drainage due to the release of toxins into the circulatory system. These can include headaches, irritability, sinus congestion, depression, insomnia, fatigue, "brain fog", and acne. These reactions are temporary and can be avoided or minimized.

Drinking eight glasses per day of purified water helps the kidneys and bladder to flush out freed toxins. Exercise can also be of considerable help. A diet avoiding red meats, additives, refined sugars, alcohol, and coffee should also be followed. Most reactions occur for one or two days, and are minimal. If they do not go away in a few days, consult your physician.

I recommend that patients begin their day by drinking a 12-16-ounce glass of pure, filtered water to which the juice of a fresh-squeezed, organic lemon has been added, not only during the drainage and detoxification process, but as an ongoing part of their daily health regimen. I advise you to do the same, in order to help reduce acidity in your body, boost your metabolism, and to help your liver expel toxins. Then wait at least ten minutes before having breakfast.

During the drainage and detoxification process, I also recommend that you help your liver by using the nutritional supplements and herbal remedies mentioned in Chapter 2: vitamin C, alpha lipoic acid, and N-acety-cysteine (NAC), dandelion root, milk thistle, peppermint, and turmeric. Daily use of chlorella is also recommended.

Besides the liver, the primary areas of focus during the drainage phase are the kidneys and the lymphatic system. Since most people are well-familiar with the liver and kidneys let's deal with them. Here are my drainage recommendations for each of these organs.

Kidney Drainage: Drink healthy, non-distilled pure filtered water every day. The standard recommendation is to drink eight -8-ounce glasses of water each day. For some people, more than that may be necessary.

One of the world's leading authorities on water and its relationship to health was the late Dr. Fereydoon Batmanghelidj, author of the book *Your Body's Many Cries For Water*. Dr. Batman, as he liked to be called, devoted the last three decades of his life solely researching the numerous ways in which adequate water intake each day could improve health. Based on his findings, he recommended that a person divide their body weight in half, and then drink that amount of water in ounces each and every day. As an example, a man weighing 200 pounds would drink 100 ounces of water per day, while a woman weighing 120 pounds would need to drink 60 ounces. To increase hydration from water, Dr. Batman also advised adding a pinch of sea salt to each glass of water. Doing so helps carry water more efficiently into the cells, thus improving the cells' ability to flush out toxins, and also providing you with a wide spectrum of important trace minerals.

To strengthen your kidneys and help them drain, you've got to be drinking healthy water. This means avoiding both tap water, unless it is first filtered through a good quality water filter or filtration system, and distilled water, which is dead water, because it has no minerals. (It is also very important to have filters for your shower heads so that you do not absorb toxins in your skin when you shower and bathe.) I have found that Volvic water, which comes from France, can be helpful because it is slightly alkaline and contains both healthy electrons and the right amount of minerals. It's active vibrant water. You can find Volvic water at most health food stores. Fiji water is also very good. Alkaline water has also become increasingly popular.

To further support kidney drainage, be sure to eat a plentiful supply of organic fresh fruits and vegetables. Such foods act as natural cleansers because they are high in fiber and help in the digestion process. They also are rich in vitamins, minerals and other nutrients. Kidney-friendly foods include asparagus, blueberries, cranberries, cucumber, grapes, kale, spinach, string beans, and watermelon. Eat them raw or lightly steamed. You can also make fresh-squeezed juices from many of these foods. Herbs such as dandelion, ginger, nettles, and parsley are also recommended. Horsetail tea also promotes kidney drainage.

Liver Drainage: In addition to drinking fresh-squeezed lemon water upon arising, you need to incorporate a variety of foods each day that assist liver function. Such foods include apples, artichokes, beets, broccoli, cabbage, carrots, dandelion greens, grapefruit, lemons, limes, squash, watercress, and zucchini. Cruciferous and dark green, leafy vegetables are also important.

Cruciferous vegetables, which include broccoli, Brussels sprouts, cabbage, and cauliflower, contain compounds called *glucosinolates*, which aid in enzyme production in the liver. These liver enzymes help flush out carcinogens, and other toxins out of our body, and have been shown to lower the risk for cancer. Dark, leafy greens are rich in chlorophylls, and help eliminate environmental toxins from the bloodstream. They also contain compounds that help to neutralize heavy metals, chemicals and pesticides, thus providing an important protective mechanism for the liver. Bitter greens, such as arugula, chicory, and dandelion and mustard greens, also help increase the production and flow of bile, which further helps remove toxic residues from the body's blood and organs.

Other liver-protecting foods include avocados, which are a rich source of essential fatty acids and other nutrients, and which helps the liver to produce glutathione, a compound that is necessary for the liver to be able to eliminate toxins, and healthy grains such as quinoa and millet, which are excellent alternatives to grains that contain gluten. Cold-pressed organic oils, such as coconut, flaxseed, hemp, and olive oil can also help because of the healthy fats (lipids) they contain, which also aid liver function. The liberal use of garlic and turmeric is also recommended, as both of these herbs provide a variety of healthy benefits for the liver, as does organic green tea.

Lymphatic Drainage: Since most people are unfamiliar with the lymphatic system, providing you with an overview of this important system is in order. Simply put, without your lymphatic system you could not live. The fluid circulating in the lymphatic system is called lymph and is derived from blood plasma but it is clearer and more watery. The body has twice as much lymph as blood, and twice as many lymph vessels as blood vessels. Besides lymph vessels, the lymphatic system includes lymph nodes, the appendix, tonsils, and the spleen.

Closely related to the cardiovascular system, the lymphatic system has several major functions, including aiding in immune function by filtering out disease-causing organisms, manufacturing white blood cells, and generating antibodies. The lymphatic system is also important in the distribution of fluid and nutrients all over the body, because it drains off excessive fluids and protein (left behind by the capillary circulation), so that the tissues do not swell.

All of the soft tissue of the body is bathed in lymph fluid. This second circulatory system is important in cleansing other body fluids; lymph nodes filter out bacteria and, along with the spleen, produce disease-fighting lymphocytes. The lymphatic system also plays an important role in the digestion of fats, as well as in the transport of nutrients and wastes. This is the system that preserves the fluid balance throughout your body.

Unlike blood that is pumped by the heart, lymph has no pump. Continuous pressure to move is exerted as new tissue fluid drains into the spaces between the cells, pushing out the fluid that is already there. The contraction and the expansion of nearby arteries and muscles also exert a forward pressure on lymph. The process of breathing creates a partial vacuum in the chest. This partial vacuum causes both blood in the veins and lymph to flow upward, and return to the blood stream from which it came.

In its basic operations, blood finds a powerful ally in the lymphatic system. Lymph fluid serves as a bridge across which oxygen, nutrients, and wastes pass between the capillaries and the body cells. As the bloodstream unloads its cargoes through the capillaries, 50 percent of them in the course of a day, also escape under the force of blood pressure. Once they have broken out, they cannot get back directly into the blood stream. The lymph facilitates this, directing them through a special circulatory system of its own, composed of lymphatic capillaries and ducts, into veins near the shoulders, which pass them into the heart. Lymph also carries along a number of chemical products, including droplets of fat and cholesterol which are absorbed during the process of digestion.

Lymph nodes can become enlarged and tender in response to draining sites of infection, as in enlarged" neck glands" of sore throats and ear infections. The swelling indicates that the nodes are working overtime. Based on all of the above, you can understand why keeping your lymphatic system healthy and properly functioning is so important.

The easiest way to facilitate drainage of your lymphatic system is to take deep breaths. Try to make it a point to engage in deep breathing exercises for five to ten minutes at a time at least three times a day.

Breathe in an out through your abdomen, completely expelling the air in your lungs during each exhalation.

Daily exercise is also important. All forms of exercise can help lymphatic drainage because of how muscular contraction moves lymph. But a particularly enjoyable type of exercise involves jumping on a mini-trampoline, or rebounder, for five to ten minutes twice day. As you bounce, the lymph nodes expand as you rise into the air, and then compress when you hit the trampoline. This creates the pumping activity that improves lymph flow. Once you are done rebounding, lie on the floor for five minutes with your legs raised. Or you can rest on a slant board if you have one. Jumping rope or jumping jacks are also excellent forms of exercise for the lymphatic system.

During the drainage process continue to drink an adequate amount of water each day to help the lymph move and flush out toxins, since the lymphatic system eliminates toxins through urine. Also continue to eat a plentiful supply of raw fruits and raw or lightly steamed fresh vegetables, and avoid all dairy products during the drainage and detoxification phase.

Another excellent measure for improving lymphatic function is skin brushing. Skin brushing not only helps keep lymph flowing properly, it also helps rid the outer layer of skin of accumulated dead skin cells and other debris, while enhancing overall circulation and helping your skin to "breathe" easier. For this reason, I recommend daily skin brushing before you shower or bathe.

Skin brushing is easy to do. You will need a dry skin brush. Starting with your arms and hands, brush towards your heart in long, firm strokes. Then do the same with your feet and legs, starting from your legs and brushing upward. Then brush all along your chest and abdomen, again moving the strokes towards your heart. As you brush, be sure to take full, deep, relaxed breaths. Once you finish brushing, take a bath or, more ideally, a shower. (Be sure to use a shower filter to remove toxins that may be in your water supply.) (For more on skin brushing, see Chapter 13.)

Other Drainage Self-Care Tips: To get the most benefit from your drainage self-care program, here are some other suggestions I recommend you follow:

- Get at least seven to eight hours of sleep each night, and try to go to bed no later than 11 PM, and ideally before that.
- Take measures to ensure that you get appropriate rest each day, and avoid stressful situations as much as possible.
- One day each week, consider doing a fresh vegetable juice fast. Vegetables are preferable to fruits when it comes to juicing fasts because they do not contain the same amount of natural sugars that fruits contain. By combing a variety of vegetables, you will also be obtaining a wider array of nutrients. For an added zing to the juicing combinations you make, juice a piece of raw ginger.
- As an alternative to fasting, you can eat only raw or lightly steamed vegetables one day a week, along with one or more bowls of miso soup. Fruit is permissible as a snack. Also continue to drink plenty of pure, filtered, vitalized water.

As you move through the drainage process note any reactions you may be experiencing, as well as any improvements to your health and energy levels. Most people will do well to continue with the drainage phase for one or two weeks or more, depending on the results they experience and how they feel. From there, it is time to move on to the deeper phase of detoxification.

Going Deeper: The Detoxification Phase

Once you have completed the drainage phase of the cleansing process, the next step is the detoxification phase. Detoxification refers to removing toxins from their binding sites in the tissues. From there the toxins enter the lymphatic system and then the bloodstream, before being eliminated in the stool and the urine. If you attempt to detoxify before doing drainage, people will get very sick, because the organs of elimination (liver, kidneys and lymph) cannot handle the extra toxic load. The analogy would be having a bowel movement on a toilet that won't flush. This is why many people get sick when they start to fast.

During the detoxification phase you are going to go deeper to accelerate the cleansing process, eliminating even more toxins so that your body and its organs can be rejuvenated and made stronger. Ideally, during this phase, you want to be under the supervision of a doctor or other health care specialist with experience in detoxification. However, most people can safely undergo the following self-care detoxification steps on their own, although informing your doctor that you are doing so is advised. As always, though, if problems arise, seek medical attention.

The first component of the detoxification phase is to adhere to a detoxification diet. What follows are a list of food and beverage groups you can and cannot include on such a diet, as well as a sample meal plan for the day.

Foods and Beverages to Include:

Milks: Sesame, rice and almond milk, fresh or store bought, unsweetened.

Fruits (organic only): Apples, berries (blueberries, blackberries, strawberries, raspberries), lemon, lime, watermelon.

Vegetables (organic only): Organic, non-starchy vegetables should comprise the bulk of your food intake, each day. Eat a wide variety of such vegetables to ensure that you are obtaining a broad spectrum of vital nutrients.

Juices: Wheatgrass and other green juices, fresh or store bought. You can add some carrot juice or beet juice for taste. Keep your juices as green and full of chlorophyll as possible. Green powders are also excellent, and can be used throughout the day.

Alkaline Proteins: Almonds and almond butter, chestnuts, tempeh (fermented soy), tofu.

Alkaline Sweetener: Stevia. (Organic honey, although lightly acidifying, can also be used.)

Alkalizing Spices/Seasonings: Chili, cinnamon, curry, ginger, miso, mustard, sea salt, tamari.

Beans: Black beans, chick peas, kidney beans, lentils, pinto beans, red beans, white beans.

Animal Protein: Lean poultry, lamb, wild-caught fish. (Avoid fish high in mercury such as tuna and swordfish, and make sure all animal protein is as organic as possible. Also limit your total protein intake to no more than 50-60 grams per day.)

Nuts: Cashews, almonds and almond butter, pecans, walnuts.

Grains: Quinoa, brown rice, millet, organic, non-GMO corn.

The "No, Don't Even Think About It" List:

Sugar, artificial sweeteners

Maple syrup

Wheat and wheat products

Simple carbohydrates

White flour

Vinegar (except apple cider vinegar; be sure it contains "the Mother")

Dairy

Processed or preserved foods

Coffee/alcohol/soda.

Meal Plans

(Begin your day with a 12-16-ounce glass of pure, filtered water with the juice of one fresh-squeezed, organic lemon.)

Breakfast Choices: Protein Shake with Protein Powder (Pea Protein or Whey if not allergic), Almond Milk, Berries. 20 minutes later:

Eggs, Spinach, Mushrooms and Tomatoes

Spinach and Tofu

Tempeh with Tamari

Or:

Hot Grain Cereal with Rice Milk (if no gluten sensitivity)

Oatmeal with Rice Milk (if no gluten sensitivity)

Spelt Toast with Butter.

Lunch Choices:

Salad with avocado and fish

Grilled veggies

Salad and salmon

Chicken Soup

Beef Barley Soup

Seaweed Salad

Hot Vegetable soup with oat bran muffins (if no gluten sensitivity)

Spelt pasta and spicy tomatillo sauce

Baked sweet potato and salad

Mid-Afternoon Snack: Fresh green juice, or protein shake with green chlorophyll powder.

Dinner Choices:

Rice and sauteed vegetables

Broiled chicken and salad

Sweet potato and steamed greens

Quinoa, corn and salad

Spelt spaghetti with fresh tomato basil sauce

Evening Snack: Nuts (eat sparingly)

Also be sure to drink plenty of pure filtered water throughout the day, along with organic green tea and/or fresh-squeezed vegetable juice. For best results, also take digestive enzymes before each meal, along with a high-potency probiotic supplement once a day away from food.

The Liver/Gallbladder Cleanse

During the course of your detoxification phase, you may wish to go one step further in detoxifying your liver by doing a liver/gallbladder cleanse. The benefits of such a cleanse can be significant, due to how it can improve the numerous complex functions of the liver. Many malfunctions of the body are, at least partly, caused by impaired liver function.

The liver/gallbladder cleanse is designed to improve liver function and to eliminate gallstones. It is widely believed that gallstones are found only in the gallbladder. This is a common misunderstanding. In fact, most gallstones are actually found within the liver, where they can form from thickened gall to a gelatin-like, rubbery or even hard consistency. Relatively few stones actually appear in the gallbladder.

Many people today, particularly those who suffer from chronic diseases such as heart disease, arthritis, multiple sclerosis, diabetes, and even cancer, also have gallstones which clog or even block the bile ducts of their liver. The presence of gallstones in the liver and gallbladder substantially disturbs various processes in the body, such as digestion of food, elimination of waste products, and decontamination of harmful substances in the bloodstream. Gallstones can also lead to inflammation in the gallbladder, and to cramp-like contractions of the gallbladder.

A common yet erroneous belief among conventional physicians is that gallstones can only be removed by surgery. But according to experts such as Dr. Thomas Rau, medical director of the famed Paracelsus Clinic in Switzerland, where the liver/gallbladder cleanse has been performed for many years, very frequently even large stones (up to three centimeters in diameter) can be completely expelled without pain when the cleanse is properly performed. As the cleanse unblocks the liver bile ducts the body's cells are able to "breathe" better again and better receive and process the nutrients they need, while at the same time becoming better able to expel waste products and to maintain optimal communication with the body's nervous and hormonal systems.

The liver/gallbladder cleanse is performed as follows. For six days, drink one to two quarts (32-64 ounces) of organic apple juice per day. Apple juice softens gall stones and enlarges the gallbladder ducts, thus facilitating their expulsion from the gallbladder. Due to its strong effect, however, it can also lead, in the first few days, to a bloated feeling and and/or to thin stool. If too many unpleasant reactions arise, you can dilute the juice with water. Drink the juice slowly throughout the day, between meals. (Avoid drinking the apple juice directly before or after the meals, or in the late evening.) In addition to the juice, continue to also drink pure filtered water each day.

During the six days avoid all animal protein, milk and all dairy products, coffee, non-herbal teas, table salt, soda, sugar, wheat, and simple (white) carbohydrates. Follow this dietary guideline exactly.

Begin each day with a glass of lemon water or organic apple juice. Wait 20 minutes, then, for breakfast, select between: fresh fruit (avoid citrus fruits, except 1/2 grapefruit); avocado with fresh lemon juice and cold-pressed, organic olive oil; porridge prepared with filtered water, not milk, with fresh fruits or berries.

For lunch select between: raw or steamed vegetables (zucchini, artichokes, carrots, broccoli, red beets, lettuce, celery, etc.), with lemon juice, cold-pressed, organic olive oil, sea salt and/or herbal spices; potatoes or yam (in small quantities); sprouts (alfalfa, lentils, mungbeans, etc.); a bowl of brown rice, or quinoa with vegetables.

At dinner, you should generally eat as little as possible. Dinner selections include: vegetable juices, green vegetables, carrots, steamed spinach and/or other steamed vegetables; finely cut salads with lemon juice and organic, cold-pressed olive oil or flaxseed oil; or vegetable soups. At every meal, be sure to chew all foods thoroughly.

At some point during these six days, or before, you will also need to buy a bag of Epsom salts (available at most drug stores).

On the morning of the seventh day begin the cleanse by slowly drinking one or two glasses of pure, filtered water slowly. Fifteen minutes later, take two tablespoons of organic, cold-pressed olive oil, mixed with the same quantity of freshly squeezed lemon juice. Then wait at least 30 minutes before having a light breakfast. At noon, have a light lunch.

From 2 PM on do not eat or drink anything (except pure, filtered water). Around this time, in a glass pitcher or jar, prepare a mixture of four tablespoons of Epsom salt and three cups of water. This makes four ¾ cup servings. Set the mixture in the refrigerator.

At 6 PM, drink one serving of this mixture. You can drink some lemon juice after the first few sips, in order to take the bitter taste away.

At 8 PM, drink the second serving. At 9:45 PM, prepare the following mixture: Squeeze one or more grapefruits or lemons to make 3/4 of a cup of juice, straining out the pulp. Mix the juice with ½ cup of organic, cold-pressed olive oil. Shake the mixture well, until it is watery. At 10 PM, drink this mixture while standing up, and finish drinking within five minutes. Afterwards, lie down in bed with the upper body elevated, with an extra pillow or cushion.

Remain absolutely calm for the next 20 minutes. Should you feel nauseous, try lying on your right side, again with your upper body elevated and your knees pulled in. Mentally support yourself by imagining the gallstones leaving your body. Breathe in and out from your diaphragm (belly breathing). Then go to sleep for the night.

Do not be concerned about cramps or pain as the Epsom salts act as a muscle relaxant for the bile ducts and the gall bladder, opening them up and allowing for the easy passage of the stones. You may have a bowel movement at night, but it probably will not occur until the next morning.

Upon awaking, take your third dose of the Epsom salt mixture, but not before 6 AM. If you have indigestion or nausea wait until it is gone before drinking it. After you drink the mixture, you may go back to bed if you wish. Two hours later drink the fourth and last serving of the mixture.

At some point during the morning you should have your first bowel movement. You will possibly get some soft stool, or diarrhea, as the gallstones are expelled. Look for gallstones in the toilet. They will tend to float on the surface of your toilet, are recognizable from their color (green, brown or black), and can range in size from a tiny pea or smaller to up to three centimeters in diameter. In many cases, large quantities of stones can be expelled at one time. In other cases, stones can continue to be released with subsequent bowl movements.

Two hours after your first bowl movement, have a glass of lemon water or organic, fresh squeezed vegetable juice. Half an hour later eat some fruit. One hour later you may eat regular food but keep it light (salads, steamed vegetables, etc.). By supper you should feel fully recovered and can resume eating normally.

Juicing for Detoxification

Whether or not you choose to do the liver/gallbladder cleanse is up to you. However, during your detoxification phase (and for the drainage phase, as well, should you wish), I strongly encourage you to drink at least 16 to 32 ounces of fresh-squeezed, organic vegetable juices each day due to the many detoxification benefits such juices can provide. The following are some of the best vegetables you can include in your juice drinks, along with some of the benefits they provide:

- **Broccoli** – aids the liver in eliminating toxins
- **Asparagus** – aids the kidneys and acts as a natural anti-inflammatory agent
- **Beets** – aids the liver and gallbladder to eliminate bile and other toxins
- **Cabbage** – aids the liver and lowers LDL ("bad) and total cholesterol
- **Cucumber** – acts as diuretic and boosts collagen
- **Dandelion greens** – strengthens the liver
- **Kale** – helps flush toxins and debris from the kidneys
- **Wheatgrass** – immune system booster and effective at lowering blood sugar.

The Master Cleanse Fast

Another helpful detoxification measure is known as the Master Cleanse fast, which was developed by Stanley Burroughs, a naturopath, in the mid-20th century. In recent years, this cleanse has gained in popularity after being endorsed by celebrities such as Beyonce, who used it to get in better shape for her appearance at the Academy Awards.

Also known as "the lemonade diet," the Master Cleanse is a fast that can be safely undertaken from anywhere from three to ten days or more. The main ingredients of the drink are grade B maple syrup, fresh lemon juice (be sure the lemons are organic), cayenne pepper and pure, filtered water. The basic proportions are: two tablespoons each of grade B maple syrup and fresh squeezed organic lemon in eight ounces of healthy water, with a pinch or more of cayenne pepper, according to your taste. You need to drink between 64 to 96 fluid ounces of this mixture each day, and can drink more if you continue to feel hungry.

Because the act of digesting food consumes about 35 percent of our energy on an ongoing basis, it follows that the elimination of solid food for short periods of time will make the energy normally used for digestion available for the process of detoxification. Thus the first step is to stop eating food so that the lemonade drink can commence its work.

Because the lemonade drink is easily assimilated, it places little or no demand on the digestive system. Fresh squeezed lemon juice is a powerful cleanser for the body, and is also high in vitamins. The maple syrup provides energy from unprocessed sugar, which still contains many of its original nutrients, and the cayenne pepper breaks up mucous and acts as a cleanser for the digestive, respiratory, and circulatory systems. Initially, I recommend that you undertake the Master Cleanse for no more than three days, and then, if you wish, build up to longer durations as you gain more experience with it.

To obtain the most benefit from the Master Cleanse, you will need to help support your colon in eliminating the toxins that the cleanse will break down and dump into your gastrointestinal tract. There are two ways to do this, either by enema or by what is known as a saltwater flush.

Enemas have a long history of use in traditional healing systems around the world because of their ability to eliminate stored waste matter in the colon, or lower large intestine. To perform an enema you will need to purchase an enema kit, which you can find at your local drug store. The kit consists of a two-quart enema bag, an attached hose, a plastic hanger, and a rectal speculum.

To get started, fill the enema bag with warm (not hot) water that is close to body temperature. Then add one tablespoon each of baking soda and salt to the water (to prevent the water from being absorbed by the intestine), letting it dissolve. Next, hang the enema bag to a towel rack in your bathroom so that it hangs three to four feet above the floor. Lubricate the speculum and attach it to the hose, then kneel comfortable on the floor, raising your buttocks in the air and placing you head on the ground, inserting the speculum into your rectum. Once this is done, release the clamp on the hose and allow the water mixture to flow into you, taking in as much as is comfortable.

Once you have taken in the water mixture, rest comfortably, gently massaging your lower abdomen over the colon area. Five to fifteen minutes later—or sooner, if necessary—sit on the toilet and void the solution. To help elimination, continue to massage your lower abdomen. You may find that you need to return to the bathroom more than once after the enema is performed. This is normal and nothing to be alarmed about. However, for this reason the most appropriate time to administer an enema is in the evening after you have taken care of your daily activities and responsibilities.

On the last day of the Master Cleanse, substitute acidophilus for the salt and baking soda. Doing so will help recolonize any healthy intestinal flora that may have been depleted by the enemas. Simply add an eight of a teaspoon of powdered acidophilus or the contents of four to five acidophilus capsules to the water and let it dissolve.

A safe and effective alternative to an enema is a daily saltwater flush. The saltwater flush has a number of advantages compared to enemas. For one, it is easier to do and does not require the purchase of an enema kit. It can also be performed at any time, both during fasts and while eating solid food. In addition, unlike enemas, which primarily cleanse only the colon or lower intestine, the saltwater flush helps to move toxins and waste matter out of the entire gastrointestinal tract. Because of its convenience and effectiveness, many health conscious individuals perform the saltwater flush on a weekly or monthly basis as a method of detoxification.

To perform a saltwater flush combine two teaspoons of sea salt to 32 ounces (one quart) of warm to mildly hot water. Drink the entire solution within 15 to 20 minutes, then sit or walk comfortably until you feel the urge to go to the bathroom (usually within 10 minutes to half an hour—if you do not need to go to the bathroom within this time frame, drink more warm, salt-free water to trigger the elimination process).

Once you go to the bathroom you will expel water along with fecal matter. Continue to drink regular, filtered water until the liquid you are expelling is nearly clear. On day two and beyond of the Master Cleanse, it is only necessary to drink 16 ounces of the salt and water solution to start elimination.

The final key to successfully performing the Master Cleanse lies in how you break your liquid fast. The most common mistake first-time fasters make is to quickly resume normal meals. Doing so is a big mistake and can significantly interfere with the benefits achieved by fasting. Therefore, it is vitally important that you reintroduce foods gradually, starting with foods that are easily digested and then, over the course of a few days, slowly resuming eating of more complex foods.

What follows are guidelines for properly breaking your fast. Be sure to abide by them. Otherwise, you will most likely experience uncomfortable abdominal bloating and cramping, as well as other potential gastrointestinal problems, such as constipation.

The first foods to begin eating after you break your fast are those foods that require little effort by your body to digest. As your body begins to adjust to the process of eating again, you can then slowly start to introduce more complex foods. Initially, begin with fruits and non-starchy vegetables for at least a day. (The vegetables can be eaten raw or lightly steamed.) Then proceed to adding starchy vegetables, such as squash, yams, whole grains, and seeds, before moving on to legumes and fatty foods. Eventually, you can reintroduce protein foods, such as fish, poultry, meats, and nuts (wait at least three days before adding these types of foods).

Other Detoxification Aids

The following aids can further enhance your detoxification experience.

Bentonite Clay: Bentonite clay, which you can find at many health food stores, as well as online, is composed of aged volcanic ash, and is an effective detoxification aid. The internal use of bentonite clay is not new. It has been used for centuries as a healing agent by indigenous peoples all around the globe.

When added to water, the clay swells up and is stretched open like a highly porous sponge, to produce a negative electrical charge that enables it to attract, absorb and bind heavy metals and other toxins, including pesticides, herbicides, and harmful viruses. Once bound, the toxins, along with the clay, pass safely out of the body through bowel movements. The clay also helps get more oxygen into the cells because of its ability to pull excess hydrogen out of cells, allowing them to re-place it with oxygen. Among the toxins bentonite clay has been shown to bind and eliminate are arsenic, aluminum, cadmium, copper, lead, and mercury, as well as formaldehyde, which is used as a preservative in many vaccines.

The best way to use bentonite clay is to add it to a small glass of water or juice and take it on an empty stomach at least one hour before or after meals. Bentonite is available as a gel, or in capsule and powder form. Start with one tablespoon (or its equivalent) of bentonite clay each day. After one week gradually increase the dose to no more than four tablespoons a day, taken in divided doses. It is safe for long-term use.

Castor Oil Packs: The healing properties of castor oil packs were first popularized by the famed medium Edgar Cayce. The pack is formed by soaking a cotton cloth in castor oil (also known as Palma Christ oil). The cloth is then applied to the body, and covered and heated with a hot pad, typically for 20 to 30 minutes. In addition to helping detoxify when used on the abdomen of over the liver/gallbladder, the packs can boost immune function, release muscle tension, ease pain, reduce swell-ing and inflammation, and aid in reducing or eliminating PMS.

Oil Pulling: Oil pulling dates back to the time of ancient India and the origins of Ayurvedic medicine. It involves the rinsing of the mouth, gums, tongue, and teeth by swishing approximately one tablespoon of coconut, olive, sesame, or sunflower oil for 15 to 20 minutes in the mouth on an empty stomach (before eating/drinking—the ideal time to perform oil pulling is before breakfast). The swishing process mixes the oil with saliva, which in turn activates enzymes that draw toxins out of the body.

As the process continues, the oil gets thinner and white. If the oil is still yellow, it has not been pulled long enough. The oil must not be swallowed, for it has become toxic. Instead, when you finish the process spit the oil into the toilet (not the sink, because of the toxins it pulls out and contains), and then thoroughly wash your mouth, gums, tongue, and teeth with water. Daily use of oil pulling can help to remove bacteria, toxins, and other harmful agents that breed in the mouth and lymphatic system.

Zeolite: Zeolite is a naturally-occurring mineral compound that possesses a unique charge that attracts and binds heavy metals in the body, including cadmium, copper, lead, mercury, and uranium. Once bound, these toxins then safely pass out of the body via the urine. Research has found that the daily use of zeolite supplements for as little as one week resulted in a five- to sevenfold increase in the elimination of such toxins, while clinical studies with coal miners given zeolite found a 12- to 15-fold of toxin excretion. Zeolite is available as both a liquid and powder form at most health food stores and online. Use according to the directions on the label.

Chelation, Colon Hydrotherapy, and Sauna Therapy

You may find that you require medical assistance to most effectively detoxify and cleanse your body. The need for such assistance is not uncommon. If that is the case, I recommend you explore the following professional care therapies.

Chelation Therapy: The word *chelation* is derived from the Greek word *chele*, which means "to claw" or "to bind". Chelation therapy is a chemical process in which a substance is used to bind molecules, such as metals or minerals, and hold them tightly, so that they can be removed from the body. In medicine, chelation therapy has been scientifically proven to rid the body of excess or toxic metals. It is used by a growing network of physicians across the U.S. and abroad for that very purpose, as well as for improving the health of the arteries and overall cardio-vascular system, and as an adjunctive treatment for diabetes, bone loss, and osteoporosis. Because of the role heavy metals and toxins play in the onset of Alzheimer's and dementia, chelation also offers promise as helping to prevent such conditions.

Chelation therapy has been safely used in the U.S. for more than 60 years on well over one million patients. Originally, it was administered intravenously (IV), which is still the most common way for doctors to provide it to their patients. IV chelation is performed on an outpatient basis, is painless, and involves an IV solution of ethylenediaminetetraace-tic acid, or EDTA. An average course of treatment runs for 20 sessions.

EDTA is a synthetic amino acid related to vinegar, and is used as a food preservative in order to keep packaged food on the shelves lon-ger. Initially developed for intravenous use, EDTA was first used in the 1940's by the U.S. Navy for the treatment of lead poisoning. It was soon discovered that EDTA also removes other heavy metals and minerals from the body, such as mercury, iron, copper, and calcium. EDTA is approved by the U.S. Food and Drug Administration (FDA) for use in treating lead poisoning and toxicity from other heavy metals.

Prior to beginning chelation therapy it is recommended that patients receive blood and urine tests to determine their current health status as well as the degree of heavy metal toxicity they may be subject to. If you have an auto-immune disease, chelation may not be indicated, as the liberation of heavy metals may further stimulate the auto-immune reac-tion. Follow up tests during and after the course of the IV treatments are also recommended in order to monitor the patients' progress.

In addition to IV chelation, today there are oral EDTA/nutrient sup-plements, EDTA suppositories, and even EDTA chewing gum. EDTA can also be used in a bath so that you can actually get some of the ben-efits of chelation therapy while taking a bath. For most people, I rec-ommend a course of IV chelation treatments, followed by the ongoing use of either oral EDTA supplements or EDTA suppositories to protect against the ongoing exposure to heavy metals that we all face throughout our lifetimes. Both the use of oral and suppository chelation products should also be monitored by a physician.

The two leading advocacy and training groups for EDTA chelation therapy are the American College for the Advancement in Medicine (ACAM) and the American Board of Clinical Metal Toxicity (ABCMT). Both organizations can help you locate physicians in your area who are trained and skilled in the use of chelation therapy. Their websites are www.acam.org and www.abcmt.org, respectively.

Colon Hydrotherapy: Along with detoxifying your kidneys, lymph and liver, you also need to address the health of your bowels, or colon, which is where much of your body's toxins end up as they are broken down. The surface area of the intestines is more than 200 square yards. Within that expanse it is all too common that an accumulation of impacted feces, toxins, and other waste matter can occur. Thus, even though you may be having at least one daily bowel movement (at least two per day is ideal), your colon may not be healthy. The buildup of waste matter along the colon tract can result in a wide array of health problems, including diminished absorption of nutrients, suppressed immune function, inflammation, leaky gut syndrome and other gastrointestinal problems. This is why I often recommend that my patients consider having a few colon hydrotherapy sessions.

The principle behind colon hydrotherapy, also known as a colonic, dates back to the times of ancient Egypt. A colonic is one of the most effective ways to quickly rid the colon and large intestine of accumulated toxins and waste matter. In a session, a trained colon hydrotherapist gently inserts a speculum attached to tube from a colonic machine into the rectum. Filtered water, which can sometimes contain probiotics or oxygen, is then gradually run into and released from the colon via the colonic machine. This process helps to dislodge and eliminate impacted fecal and other waste matter from the folds, pockets, and lining of the colon. As this matter is eliminated, the body then begins to release other toxic residues from the blood and lymph, which pass into the colon to also be eliminated. A colonic session usually lasts for 30 to 45 minutes, and more than one session may be advised, depending on your degree of toxicity. You can find a trained colon hydrotherapist by contacting the International Association for Colon Therapy via their website, www.i-act.org.

Sauna Therapy: Sauna therapy, also known as hyperthermia, also dates back to ancient times, with its health benefits touted by the healing traditions of many of the world's cultures. The reason I recommend sauna therapy is because it is the only detoxification treatment that has been proven to release fat-stored toxins from the body. Fat tissues and cells are where much of the body's toxic overload occurs because, in order to protect itself, the body encapsulates toxins in fat as a means of quarantining toxins from other cells and tissues. Chronic toxin exposure and buildup soon defeats this purpose, however, enabling the encapsulated toxins to wreak their havoc.

Sauna therapy, properly administered, temporarily elevates the body's core temperature in much the same way that your body will generate a fever to kill invading bacteria and viruses. As this occurs, fat cells begin to release toxins, which can range from acidic wastes to heavy metals to pesticide and drug residues to chemicals such as dioxin and PCBs (polychlorinated biphenyls). The toxins are then eliminated through the sweat glands, which are very active at that time due to the intense perspiration that sauna therapy induces. Research has shown that regular sauna therapy can provide beneficial effects for a wide range of the body systems, including the cardiovascular, circulatory, endocrine (hormone), immune, neurological, muscular, and respiratory systems.

In the last few decades a new form of sauna therapy has been developed that has proven to be even more effective for eliminating toxins and improving overall health. Originally developed and tested in Japan and South Korea, this type of therapy is called far-infrared (FIR) therapy. Today, there are a range of far infrared devices people can use to obtain the benefits they provide, ranging from home FIR stationary and portable, tent-like sauna units, to FIR blankets and pads. Of these, the stationary and portable units provide the most benefit for most people.

FIR units emit a dry, radiant infrared heat, similar to one of the types of rays emitted by the sun. This radiant energy is able to penetrate deep inside the body to a depth of between 1.5 and 3 inches, depending on the unit. The sweat volume produced by the infrared radiant energy can exceed that produced by traditional saunas by 200 to 300 percent.

Studies have shown that the energy output from FIR units is closely tuned to the body's own radiant energy, enabling the body to absorb as much as 90 percent of the far infrared waves. By comparison, conventional saunas rely only on indirect means of heat: first, on convection (air currents) and then, conduction (direct contact of hot air with the skin) to produce its heating effect, resulting in far less absorption. In addition, the benefits that FIR units provide can be achieved in as little as 20 minutes inside the unit, whereas traditional sauna times are usually longer than that.

There is a growing body of research attesting to the benefits of far-infrared sauna therapy. Among the benefits FIR has been shown to provide are:

- Significant detoxification of heavy metals, chemicals, and other toxins
- Improved overall cardiovascular function
- Improved circulation and increased oxygenation of cells and tissues
- Improved metabolism and healthy weight loss
- Improved energy production
- Improved immune function
- Improved pulmonary (lung) function
- Improved skin tone and elasticity and reduction of cellulite.

Because of their health benefits, the use of FIR units has become increasingly popular in the U.S. over the last decade and today such units can be found in a growing number of doctors' offices and health clinics. Although the units are also available for home use, I recommend proper medical supervision, along with appropriate medical tests, before using FIR units, at least initially, especially since excessive use of FIR units can result in a too rapid release of toxins, which can have an adverse effect on various body organs, especially the kidneys and liver. Also, whenever employing any form of sauna therapy be sure to drink adequate amounts (at least 24 to 32 ounces) of pure, filtered water before, during or immediately after each sauna session to avoid dehydration. And once your session is finished, immediately take a shower in slightly cool water to rinse away toxic residue on your skin that is left as a result of your sweating.

Another effective way of removing toxins from the body involves the use of homeopathy. This will be discussed further in Chapter 9.

Now that you've read this far, you not only have a better understanding of why cleansing your body is the essential first step in your journey back to outstanding health, you, more importantly, know the many options available to you that you can do on your own, or with the assistance of your physician or health care provider to get started. I encourage you to do so as soon as you can, and to then commit to periodically undertaking additional drainage and detoxification measures throughout each year. By doing so, you will be helping your body eliminate much of the toxic load it will otherwise be forced to struggle to cope with.

Key Points To Remember

We live in a highly toxic world and you are being bombarded with exposures to toxins each and every day of your life. Because of this, it is important that you make the time to help your body and its organs detoxify.

There is a direct link between toxicity and tissue acidity in the body. When the body is in a state of chronic acidity, or acidosis, toxins are able to more easily take hold in the body's cells, tissues, and organs. Conversely, toxic load in the body causes and exacerbates tissue acidity. Therefore an effective detoxification program must also address the body's pH state.

You can assess your body's current level of acidity by performing a pH first morning urine test using pH strips that are available at most drug stores. After a week or two, you will have a good idea about your body's acidity level and can then use the test periodically to monitor your progress towards a healthier, more balanced pH state.

Among the most dangerous class of toxins are heavy metals, especially mercury, followed by arsenic, aluminum, cadmium, and lead. All heavy metals result in a wide range of health problems and diseases, including Alzheimer's and dementia, cancer, heart disease, and neurological conditions. Being tested to evaluate the levels of heavy metals in your body is therefore crucial with regard to developing an overall health plan.

A common source of mercury and other heavy metal toxicity is mercury dental amalgams.

There are two phases in the overall body-cleansing process: drainage and detoxification. The drainage process comes first and is primarily focused on aiding the kidneys, liver and lymphatic system in reducing their toxic load.

Your body's toxic load can be reduced through various techniques of drainage and detoxification. Many of these techniques lead themselves to self-care that you can undertake in the comfort of your own home.

Self-care drainage and detoxification methods include following a healthy, detoxification diet, drinking adequate amounts of pure, filtered water, skin brushing, performing a liver/gallbladder cleanse, undertaking the Master Cleanse fast (along with an enema or saltwater flush), the use of castor oil packs, oil pulling, and the use of detoxification aids such as bentonite clay and zeolite.

To further improve detoxification, professional medical assistance may be necessary. Three highly effective professional care methods of detoxification are chelation therapy, colon hydrotherapy (colonics), and sauna therapy, especially far-infrared sauna therapy.

You should always consult with your physician before undertaking any drainage and detoxification measures.

CHAPTER 7

Essential #3: Super Nutrition

The third essential key to outstanding health is to improve the health of your gastrointestinal tract (your gut), along with the quality of your diet. Though often ignored as such, the health of your gut is just as important as the health of your brain, heart, liver, and other organs. Moreover, when gut health becomes compromised it soon places a burden on these organs and can trigger a host of other health problems, as well. In this chapter you will learn why gut health is so important, what causes an unhealthy gut, and what you can do to restore your gut to optimal functioning.

The Significance of Your Gut to Health and Disease

The gastrointestinal system, begins with your mouth and includes your throat (pharynx and esophagus), stomach, small (duodenum, jejunum, and ileum) and large (cecum, ascending colon, transverse colon, and descending colon) intestines, rectum and anus. The GI tract is also supported by your liver, gallbladder, and pancreas, all of which play important roles in digestion. Energy Medicine sees the GI system as a triangle involving the liver, pancreas, and intestines. Each part of this triangle can affect the other parts, and consequently all three need to be treated.

Through the process of digestion, the GI tract provides you with the nourishment your body needs and is also responsible for eliminating many of your body's wastes and toxins. The digestion of food and drink begins in your mouth, and then continues in your stomach and small intestine. As the nutrients from food are separated out through the digestive process much of it is absorbed through the walls of the small intestine. In the colon, or large intestine, the remaining nutrients, along with water, are re-absorbed into the bloodstream, while undigested food, wastes and toxins are moved out of the body through elimination.

The digestive process begins as soon as food or drink enters your mouth to mix with saliva and various enzymes. Food is further digested as it enters the stomach, where the digestive compounds hydrochloric acid (HCl) and pepsin are secreted. It is also in your stomach where food is liquefied before passing onto the small intestine, where it is further broken down by other digestive enzymes produced by the pancreas (amylase to digest carbohydrates, lipase to digest fats, and protease to digest proteins).

As the digestive process unfolds, your liver produces bile, which is secreted into the small intestine and is essential for the proper absorption of healthy fats (lipids). The liver also stores fat soluble nutrients from food, such as vitamins A, D, E, and K.

When all of the steps of this process proceed as it is designed to run, food is digested efficiently and fully and, assuming one's diet provides a wide variety of nutrient-rich foods, the body obtains all of the nutrients it requires to stay healthy, produce and utilize energy, and perform its many functions. Any impairment to the health of the gut and the organs that support it interferes with this process, leading to incomplete digestion, nutritional imbalances, and the buildup of toxins and waste matter, especially within the colon. (It is because of this fact that many holistic practitioners today tell their patients that "death begins in the colon," a phrase that was first used as the title of a medical symposium held by the Royal Society of Medicine of Great Britain in 1913, at which more than 50 of England's most acclaimed physicians presented talks on the subject of disease in relation to toxins in the gut.) Unfortunately, less than optimal functioning of the GI tract is the norm, not the exception, in today's society, and, as we will discuss, is a major cause for many of the serious, chronic diseases that afflict our nation's populace, as well as many other people all around the world.

Your GI tract is also the home of your body's enteric nervous system. Known as the body's "second brain," it is located in the linings of the esophagus, stomach, small intestine, and colon. The enteric nervous system is brimming with neurotransmitter proteins that are produced by cells that are identical to neurotransmitter-producing cells in the brain. The complex collection of neurotransmitters in the "GI brain" enables it to act, learn, and remember in much the same way that the brain itself does. The GI brain is also responsible for producing "gut feelings." In addition, your GI tract comprises approximately 80 percent of your body's immune system (within the mucous membranes of the intestinal tract, there lies lymph follicles called Peyer's Patches).

The gut is by far the largest organ in the body. The small and large intestine have a combined length of 20 feet, and a surface area of 21,500 square feet. The inner wall of the small intestine can absorb food on the one hand, thus acting as a filter, and can also produce mucus (it secretes 20 quarts of mucus daily - most of it is reabsorbed in the large intestine), which will help detoxify the body. It is important that toxic substances are not also re-absorbed in the colon (large intestine). This is accomplished by the 100 trillion bacteria(also referred to as the intestinal flora) in the colon that retain these toxic substances, allowing them to pass out of the body via the stool.

In a healthy gut, the vast majority of these bacteria are beneficial, or "friendly," working not only to keep unhealthy bacteria in check, but also supporting numerous other processes in the body. Examples of friendly bacteria include *Lactobacillus* and *Bifidobacteria*, while examples of microbes that can cause harm in the body when they are unchecked are *Candida albicans*, *Clostridium*, and *Staphylococcus*. This ecosystem of bacteria in the gut is part of an overall population of microorganisms that coexist in your body known as the *microbiome*.

The microbiome comprises the collective genomes of these microorganisms (bacteria, fungi, protozoa, and viruses) that live inside and on the human body. Your body contains approximately ten times as many microbial cells as human cells. Researchers have also discovered that the genes of the microbial population in the intestines outnumber the genes in human cells by 1,000 times. More significantly, these microbial genes can and do influence the actions and functioning of human cells. The influences can either be positive or negative, depending on the health, or lack thereof, of the microbiome. This explains why upsets in your gut can frequently also result in diminished health elsewhere in your body.

Unfortunately, today more people than ever before suffer from some degree of impaired gastrointestinal functioning and, as a consequence, are burdened with a wide range of other health problems that either directly result from, or are exacerbated by, imbalances in the gut microbiome. Some of the more common conditions related to impaired gut health include chronic fatigue, depression, impaired brain function and cognitive ability, respiratory conditions, skin conditions, allergies, and various autoimmune diseases, including arthritis, Lupus, and multiple sclerosis. Poor gut health has also been linked to various types of cancer, as well as heart disease.

Causes of An Unhealthy Gut

There are a number of common causes of an unhealthy gut, including poor diet and nutrition, food allergies and sensitivities, infections and malabsorption, stomach acid (HCl) imbalances, heavy metal contamination, dysbiosis (abnormal intestinal bacteria), the overuse of pharmaceutical drugs, lack of exercise, and stress.

Poor Diet and Nutrition: Poor diet and nutritional deficiencies are epidemic in our society today due to the prevalence of the standard American diet (SAD), which is devoid of many essential vitamins, minerals, and other nutrients, and loaded with unhealthy fats, sugar and simple carbohydrates, artificial sweeteners, food additives, and preservatives. The SAD diet is also lacking in fiber, which is necessary for the proper elimination of food waste products and toxins, and naturally-occurring digestive enzymes that are necessary for proper digestion.

In recent decades, the typical American diet has also been negatively impacted by the widespread and heavy use of antibiotics, growth hormones, and other drugs, and food dyes used in factory farms to raise cows, pigs, chickens, and fish. Residues of these toxic substances enter the body when we consume foods harvested from such commercially raised animals. Gluten, a protein found in wheat, wheat products, and other grains, is another increasingly common threat to gut health, acting as a toxin to the intestinal mucous membranes, resulting in a wide range of GI problems, including "leaky gut," and celiac disease.

In the last decade or so we have also seen a dramatic increase in the use of genetically-modified organisms (GMOs) in our food supply, especially with soy and corn. While there have been no long-term human safety studies about GMOs, a growing number of animal studies show that GMOs can cause a variety of serious illnesses, including cancer. Despite these findings, GMO manufacturers such as Monsanto continue to resist calls for the labeling of all foods and drinks containing GMOs, so far with the full cooperation of the U.S. federal government. Recently, the state of Vermont passed the nation's first GMO labeling law for all foods and beverages sold within its borders, and other states may soon follow Vermont's example. In the meantime, the only way you can be certain that you aren't consuming GMOs is to obtain your foods and beverages from reputable organic farmers.

Food Sensitivities: Food sensitivities affect everyone to some degree these days. Therefore, they must be identified and addressed. When properly treated, patients will be much happier and healthier.

There are five major types of reactions caused by food sensitivities:

1. Chemical. Example: hyperactivity in children resulting from food additives.
2. Pharmacological. Example: insomnia and irritability due to excess caffeine in coffee.

3. Enzyme deficiency. Example: diarrhea after eating dairy products due to lactase deficiency.
4. Immunoglobulin E (IgE) reactions. IgE is an antibody found in the lungs, skin, and mucous membranes. It causes the body to immediately react to foreign substances such as pollen, fungus spores, and animal dander, and is also involved in allergic reactions to milk, some medicines, and some poisons. IgE antibody levels are often high in people with food sensitivities. Example: hives and asthma immediately after eating shrimp.
5. Food intolerance. This accounts for the majority of reactions, which most people refer to as a "food allergy".

Normally the protein portion of a food is broken down by the digestive enzymes of the pancreas into single amino acids, which are then absorbed from the small intestine into the bloodstream, and transferred to the cells for repair and regeneration of cellular proteins. In cases of food intolerance, incomplete protein digestion causes large amino acid complexes (instead of single amino acids) to be absorbed into the bloodstream. These large molecules are recognized by the immune system as foreign proteins, and antibodies are sent to bind to them.

These large amino acid-antibody complexes, once they enter the bloodstream, can travel to any number of distant sites in the body and set off an inflammatory reaction. Should they travel to the skin, acne will result; if they go to the joints, arthritis will occur. Other common reactions include sinus congestion, migraine, fatigue, depression, and irritability. Such reactions can occur anywhere from one to 72 hours after eating the offending food. The underlying cause of all these food reactions is weakness of the pancreas, with inadequate pancreatic enzyme production.

I recommend a blood test from Cyrex (www.cyrexlabs.com) to test for these food sensitivities. Electrodermal screening and applied kinesiology (see Chapter 9) can also be used to identify the offending foods.

To properly treat these food reactions:

- The patient must completely avoid eating the offending food for three months.
- Supplement the diet with pancreatic digestive enzymes.
- Toxins (the most common are pesticides) which affect the pancreas must be identified and removed from the body.
- Therapy should be given for contributing factors such as dysbiosis, stress, and electromagnetic stress. Immediate food reactions can be helped by taking 2,000 mg of vitamin C and 1 tbsp of baking soda.
- Initiate regeneration therapy for the pancreas. This may include acupuncture, herbs, homeopathic remedies, and other energy medicine techniques which will be discussed in Chapter 10.

The most common food reactions involve:

- Wheat and other gluten-containing foods.
- Soy, eggs, dairy, shellfish, citrus, peanuts, and corn.
- Nightshades: tomatoes, potatoes, eggplant (especially in cases of arthritis).

Infections and Malabsorption: Bacterial, fungal, and parasitic infections can all damage the gut and impair GI function. They primarily do so by causing the GI tract to become inflamed, and by releasing toxins into the gut. Gut inflammation makes it easier for infectious agents and toxins to penetrate beyond the intestinal wall, to enter the bloodstream. These harmful microorganisms can cause or worsen a wide variety of GI conditions, ranging from constipation and diarrhea, to colitis, Crohn's disease, irritable bowel syndrome (IBS), gastritis, pancreatitis, and ulcers.

People who suffer from GI tract infection often commonly suffer from malabsorption. Malabsorption can be caused by poor diet, a lack of digestive enzymes, and by a deficiency of immune antibodies, such as immunoglobulin A (IgA). Such antibodies in the gut help to protect against infections and toxins. Lack of these antibodies increases the risk of GI tract infection, and can increase the risk of autoimmune conditions such as ulcerative colitis (inflammation of the colon) and Crohn's disease (inflammation of the small intestine). In both of these conditions, immune cells react with and attack the cells the lining the intestinal walls.

GI infections and malabsorption, when left unchecked, will also lead to an overgrowth of unhealthy microorganisms in the gut, a condition known as *dysbiosis*. This sets up a vicious cycle, since dybiosis, in turn, further increases malabsorption, and is a major contributor to "leaky gut syndrome."

Stomach Acid Imbalances: Too little stomach acid (hypochlorhydria) is another factor that can cause digestive problems, malabsorption, and other gut disorders. The pharmaceutical industry, through its commercials, has led the public to believe that indigestion is always caused by too much stomach acid, leading to an explosion of antacid medications and proton inhibitor drugs, which in many cases can further reduce the amount of acid produced in the stomach (hydrochloric acid, or HCl). You need stomach acid for a variety of reasons, starting with proper digestion. Without it, your body is unable to extract and metabolize vitamins, minerals, and other nutrients from food.

HCl also plays an important role in protecting against harmful bacteria that could otherwise infect your body. A recent study that examined more than 800 hospitalized, critically ill patients on breathing machines who were also given stomach acid-reducing drugs to prevent ulcers from developing, found that the patients had a 300 percent higher than normal incidence of pneumonia. Why? In part because they lacked enough stomach acid to kill the bacteria that can cause pneumonia.

In addition to a higher risk of infectious conditions, chronically low levels of HCl have also been linked to other serious health problems, including asthma, allergies, depression, parasites, heart disease, osteoporosis, skin conditions, and immune disorders, such as type 1 diabetes and rheumatoid arthritis.

Even in healthy people, stomach production of HCl tends to diminish as we age. You can easily determine for yourself whether or not you are producing enough HCl using this simple at-home test. To perform it you will need to buy a betaine HCl supplement, which you can find at your local health food store.

In the morning, before you eat breakfast, take one HCl capsule and wait at least 20 minutes before you eat or drink anything. If your body's HCl production is adequate, you should feel a slight warmth or burning sensation in your stomach five to ten minutes after you take the capsule. This sensation is perfectly safe and will soon pass.

If you don't experience this sensation, repeat the test the next day, taking two capsules. Continue on each day, adding one more capsule per day, until you get to the sixth day and take six capsules. It is likely that you will experience the warmth/burning sensation before you get to the sixth day. If not, it is a sure sign that your body's HCl production is deficient. If that is the case, I recommend taking one capsule of HCl before each meal, along with a small sip of water (drinking at meals interferes with HCl, as well as other digestive compounds.) This is especially important when eating a protein-rich meal.

Over-production of acid by the stomach does occur as a consequence of increased tissue acidity (see below).

In addition to not drinking with meals (I recommend that you wait for one hour after you eat before drinking water), other helpful steps you can take include not overeating and avoiding big meals, chewing your food thoroughly before swallowing, and avoiding foods to which you know or suspect you have a sensitivity.

The Overuse of Pharmaceutical Drugs: Nearly all pharmaceutical drugs can indirectly impact GI function to some degree because of the burden they place on the liver, which, as mentioned above, plays a supportive role in digestion and is the primary organ involved in eliminating toxins. Certain types of drugs can more directly impair gut health. Among the primary offenders in this category are antibiotics, antacids and PPIs (proton pump inhibitors), and pain relief drugs (analgesics), especially nonsteroidal anti-inflammatory drugs (NSAIDs) such as Aleve, ibuprofen, and Motrin, along with Cox-2 inhibitor drugs such as

Celebrex, which have also been linked to a significantly increased risk of heart attack and stroke. Even plain, low-dose aspirin can be a problem if used regularly because of the risk it poses for causing gastritis and other GI problems.

Antibiotics, even used for only a short course of treatment, are widely used in the United States, both in humans and in the commercial raising of animals from which meats and poultry are derived. Antibiotics affect gut health because of how they destroy the good bacteria in the colon. In doing so, these drugs enable unhealthy bacteria to grow unchecked and throwing the gut's bacterial ecosystem completely out of balance. When this happens, unhealthy bacteria are able to migrate beyond the colon, and are able to spread to the small intestine, resulting in a condition called small intestine bacterial overgrowth, or SIBO.

Antacids, such as Tums and Rolaids, and proton pump inhibitor drugs, such as Nexium and Prilosec, both work to lower levels of gastric acid in the stomach. Antacids neutralize, or buffer, gastric acid and treat heartburn, while PPIs reduce gastric acid production and are primarily used to treat heartburn and gastroesophageal reflux disease (GERD). PPIs are also commonly prescribed to treat peptic ulcers. While both types of drugs can temporarily relieve symptoms related to gastric acid buildup, neither are intended for long-term use, yet are commonly used as such anyway. As a result, they interfere with the body's ability to produce adequate levels of HCl, thus impairing digestion and leading to malabsorption of nutrients. In addition, the chemicals that comprise both classes of drugs interfere with and alter normal biochemical processes in the body, both within and beyond the GI tract, including processes involved in immune and neurological function.

NSAID (I call them New Sorts Of Aspirin In Disguise) drugs are primarily used to relieve pain and chronic inflammation, and can also be prescribed for arthritis, fever, and headaches, among other conditions. The most common side effects associated with NSAIDs are GI tract problems. Like aspirin, regular use of NSAIDs can cause the stomach and intestinal lining to thin, resulting in bleeding. Other gut problems associated with NSAIDs include indigestion and malabsorption, and stomach ulcers. Additional side effects beyond the gut include anemia, heart attack, heart failure, and stroke.

For these and other reasons, I try to avoid or limit the use of pharmaceutical drugs in my patients whenever possible, choosing, instead, to directly address the underlying cause of their health complaints rather than merely reducing symptoms, which, at best, is all that most pharmaceutical drugs are able to do. Natural substances that I have used to help with symptoms of gastritis and heartburn are mastic gum and DGL (deglycirrhized licorice).

Lack of Exercise: While nearly all of us are aware of overall benefits that regular exercise provides, most people are less aware of its GI benefits. One of exercise's most immediate benefits in this regard in the prevention and relief of constipation. By regularly exercising you will stimulate your intestinal muscles to contract. This, in turn, causes the gut to more efficiently move food along the GI tract, a process known as peristalsis. Once food is digested, peristalsis also keeps the process of elimination regular and normalized. Even very gentle exercise can improve peristaltic function.

In addition to helping relieve constipation, regular exercise enhances the production of digestive enzymes and HCl, improves the assimilation of nutrients by the body, and can reduce the risk of certain types of cancer, including colon cancer. Exercise also helps prevent indigestion and diverticulosis, and helps gas to more quickly be expelled from the GI tract. Conversely, lack of exercise negates all of the above benefits, which is why daily regular physical activity is so important to gut and overall health. You should always avoid exercising right after eating, however,—allow at least two hours between exercising and meals—as doing so diverts energy away from your body's digestive processes.

Stress: The link between stress and impaired GI function is well-established, and you've doubtless experienced proof of that at various points in your own life. Stress reactions and the cascade of stress hormones they release have a direct effect on the GI tract. Common stress-induced gut problems include indigestion, excessive gastric acid production (heartburn and GERD), loss of appetite, and, in some cases, loose bowels or diarrhea. Research has shown that stress can also exacerbate pre-existing GI disorders, including colitis, constipation, Crohn's disease, and irritable bowel syndrome (IBS).

I have already discussed stress and its health-ravaging, premature aging effects in detail earlier in this book. Suffice it to say, if you are suffering from chronic stress, you need to apply the stress-busting techniques I have already shared with you, especially those in Chapter 6. The same holds true for any unresolved emotions or unhealthy beliefs you may be dealing with, as these can significantly impair gut health, as well.

The Pancreas And Digestion

Your pancreas is about six inches long, is a flat, oblong organ located deep in the middle of the abdomen and surrounded by the stomach, liver, spleen, gallbladder and small intestine. It plays a pivotal role in health and disease. As you learned in Chapter 3, one of the two primary functions of the pancreas is to produce the hormones insulin, glucagon, and somatostatin. Its other equally important function is to produce and release digestive fluids and pancreatic enzymes to digest protein, starch, and fat. After food enters the stomach, these enzymes pass through several small ducts to the main pancreatic duct and then to the small intestine, where they mix with bile from the gallbladder to aid in digestion.

The pancreas is the organ most affected by pesticides. Sugar, artificial sweeteners, and simple carbohydrates also take a serious toll on the pancreas, which, at least partly, explains the rising incidence of pancreatic cancer today. As a nation we are consuming too much sugar, and every one of us is affected by pesticides.

The pancreas is found to be the most stressed organ in the body a great deal of the time by practitioners of Energy Medicine. One of the first things I do with my patients is look at the energy of their pancreas when I test them in my office. A sluggish pancreas is frequently present.

Impaired pancreatic function is implicated in indigestion, gas, constipation, heart disease, arteriosclerosis, allergies, diabetes, immune dysfunction, prostate problems, susceptibility to infection, and many other illnesses. A sticky stool (adheres to the toilet bowl) indicates a weakness of the pancreas. If the stool floats on the water, this is a sign that fats in the diet are not sufficiently digested. Either one is eating bad fats, or there is a lack of healthy essential fatty acids, or fats are not being properly digested because of pancreatic weakness.

On a spiritual level, the pancreas is related to self-love, the breast is related to motherly love, and the heart is related to love of mankind. So having a healthy pancreas, will result in a healthy breast, and a healthy heart.

In traditional Chinese medicine (TCM) there are 12 organ systems and corresponding meridian pathways, each of which is related to two hours in the daily 24-hour cycle. The time for the pancreas (TCM refers to it as the spleen) and its optimal function is between 9 and 11 in the morning. That means the pancreas is working most effectively at that time. Twelve hours later the pancreas is designed to be in rest mode and therefore working least effectively.

Based on this TCM cycle, it's understandable that breakfast is the meal that most people are able to digest most efficiently. In the morning we have lots of naturally occurring pancreatic enzymes. However, most Americans eat very small breakfasts, or skip breakfast altogether, and instead have their biggest meal at dinner time, often late in the evening. It is in the evening when your pancreas is least able to produce digestive enzymes. Consequently, these people can't digest their food properly, go to bed with a full stomach, and then wake up feeling tired and lousy. When the pancreas is energetically weak, all foods should be heated, very little raw foods consumed, and water should be drank at room temperature (no ice water). An effective homeopathic remedy for the pancreas is *Leptandra*.

According to TCM, imbalances in the pancreas are also linked with compulsive behavior, obsessions, and worrying. Due to the role the pancreas plays in carbohydrate metabolism, such imbalances are further linked with depression, addiction, fatigue, and hyperactivity.

In addition to sugar and pesticide exposure, the following factors also cause the pancreas to be stressed, impairing its function:

> Alcohol, coffee, and packaged commercial teas and juices
>
> Emotional stress
>
> Eating too fast, not chewing your food
>
> Overeating. (Stop eating when you are no longer hungry, not when you are full.)
>
> Poor food combining
>
> Trace mineral deficiencies (especially chromium and zinc)
>
> Many prescriptions and over-the-counter medications.

People with allergies (food and/or environmental) have a poorly functioning pancreas, resulting in reduced production of digestive enzymes—amylase, lipase, and protease—which are needed to digest the starches, fats, and proteins that we consume. When pancreatic function is diminished, incompletely digested food can irritate the mucous lining of the intestines, resulting in the absorption of partially digested proteins, which will intensify allergic reactions. When the pancreas is stressed, taking pancreatic digestive enzymes with each meal (especially with dinner) can be extremely helpful.

Pancreatic enzymes also play an important role in helping the immune system in its battle against infection and malignancy. Taking pancreatic enzymes on an empty stomach before you go to sleep helps to "eat up" toxic debris and waste products, allowing your liver and blood, to more easily detoxify while we are sleeping.

Here are a few important guidelines for optimal digestion that will also spare your pancreas from stress:

> Practice proper food combining, such as eating fruits by themselves, and not combining proteins with starches.
>
> Avoid consuming fluids with meals, allowing at least one-half hour before a meal, and one hour after.
>
> Chew food carefully in order to optimally mix food with saliva.
>
> Chew at least 10 times per mouthful.

Do not eat very large meals.

Avoid late meals and refined foods as snacks.

Avoid excessive salt and sugar

Ensure a sufficient daily intake of fiber. It is not necessary to add extra fiber if you already eat plenty of fruits and vegetables. If you are usually constipated, check with your doctor for the most appropriate fiber supplement.

Perform physical exercise daily, on an empty stomach. Abdominal training and breathing exercises are very helpful for the digestive tract.

Read labels carefully. The fewer the chemical names, the better.

Avoid food colorings and unnecessary additives. The more natural, the better.

Eat organic food, as it is free of pesticides

Finally, make use of the drainage and detoxification techniques I shared with you in Chapter 6 to reduce your body's burden of pesticides and other toxins.

Dysbiosis: The Bacterial Imbalance That's Aging You Daily

As you learned earlier in this chapter, when you are healthy, the large intestine flora primarily consists of "friendly" bacteria that are essential to proper gut health, and which keep pathogenic bacteria and other microorganisms in check. When an overgrowth of these pathogenic or parasitic microorganisms occurs, it is called *dysbiosis*. Dysbiosis is widespread in the United States today. The end result of this condition is a wide range of health problems caused by the spread and overgrowth of these harmful microorganisms, including not just GI conditions, but also diseases such as chronic fatigue syndrome and cancer. Dysbiosis is also a contributing factor in many cases of obesity.

The primary causes of dysbiosis are the overuse of antibiotics and other drugs (including birth control pills and steroids such as cortisone), poor diet, excess consumption of alcohol, mercury toxicity, and exposure to pesticides and other environmental toxins. All of these factors disrupt the balance of microorganisms in the gut, causing damage to colonies of friendly bacteria, thus enabling the spread of other potentially harmful microorganisms. Left unchecked, this creates a chronic imbalance in the gut.

Compounding the problem of dysbiosis is what happens to the waste byproducts excreted by the microbial colonies when they become imbalanced. All microorganisms in the gut excrete wastes, just as all other living beings do. In a healthy gut, your body's elimination and detoxification mechanisms are able to easily handle and get rid of microbial waste. But when the number of unhealthy microorganisms grow beyond their normal boundaries, the amount of waste matter they excrete can over-tax the body's waste removal mechanisms, resulting in microbial waste build up. It is the combination of these two factors—microbial overgrowth and the excess waste matter the microorganisms excrete—that causes the health problems associated with dysbiosis.

Candidiasis: One of the common end results of dysbiosis is the unchecked growth and spread of *Candida albicans*, a naturally occurring yeast organism in the colon, leading to systemic yeast overgrowth throughout other areas of the body. This condition is known as *candidiasis* or, more simply, candida. Normally, friendly bacteria live in harmony with the candida yeast organism in your large intestine. Antibiotic drugs are one of the major offenders in disrupting this harmonic relationship—the good bacteria are destroyed and the candida proliferate. Mercury toxicity from silver-amalgam fillings is another major contributor to yeast overgrowth.

As this process proceeds, candida changes its anatomy and physiology from the yeast-like form to a mycelial, or fungal, form which can penetrate the mucous membranes of the large intestine and release toxins into the bloodstream. Resulting symptoms include flatulence, indigestion, depression, anxiety, irritability, PMS, migraine, mood swings, vaginal infections, and "brain fog".

Treatment of both dysbiosis and candidiasis should include the following:

- Eliminating all foods containing yeast (alcohol, salad dressings, vinegar, mayonnaise, mustard, ketchup, pickles, mushrooms, breads).
- Eliminating all refined sugar and other refined foods.
- Increasing dietary fiber—legumes, vegetables.
- Supplementing with lactobacillus acidophilus, bifidus, and other probiotics in order to reintroduce friendly bacteria into the large intestine.
- Eliminating the toxins from the digestive system and the body through stimulation (drainage) of the kidney, liver, and lymphatic circulation.
- Avoiding all poorly tolerated foods which may be depressing the immune system.
- Supplementing with digestive enzymes, and garlic
- Using only yeast-free nutritional supplements.
- Beginning specific therapies to strengthen the pancreas and the immune system.
- Practicing stress-reducing, relaxation therapies, such as yoga, meditation, etc.

Successful treatment of dysbiosis and candidiasis usually takes three to five months to achieve, but the rewards can last a lifetime. Some cases of candidiasis are more difficult to treat, however. This occurs when the patient is also allergic to the by-products of the yeast infection. The paradox is that even though patients are allergic to these toxins, they are also addicted to them. When this happens, anti-candida therapies can cause severe withdrawal-like reactions such as hyperactivity, extreme fatigue, hypoglycemia, mood swings, allergic reactions, etc. Most of these patients are also chemically hypersensitive, and are allergic to alcohol and sugar. In such cases, therapy should proceed extremely slowly and can last up to one year. With time, however, even these extreme cases can be treated successfully.

Leaky Gut Syndrome

Leaky gut syndrome is also increasingly prevalent in our society today. Its name is derived because of how it occurs. In a healthy gut, the lining of the small intestine, or mucosa, remains healthy and intact, preventing incompletely digested food, as well as toxins, from passing through the intestines into the bloodstream. Leaky gut occurs when the intestinal mucosa become damaged and inflamed. This allows the food molecules and toxins to enter the bloodstream.

Once in the bloodstream, the body produces antibodies against them. However, since the food molecules resemble other, normal components of the body the antibodies often cannot distinguish between the two, and end up attacking the body itself. This is known as an autoimmune reaction. As an example, gluten has a structural similarity to thyroid tissue and migrates to the thyroid (in the presence of a leaky gut), the body then sends antibodies to the thyroid, weakening the thyroid, and resulting in Hashimoto's thyroiditis. This same phenomenon can also occur with the gut bacteria and other microorganisms that enter the bloodstream, making leaky gut syndrome a significant factor in triggering and exacerbating a variety of autoimmune diseases. A blood test called ANA is indicative of an autoimmune state. The higher the titer (1:80 or higher) the more significant the condition.

Initial symptoms of leaky gut syndrome include bloating and gas, loose stools or diarrhea after meals, fatigue and headaches after certain meals, pressure in the upper abdomen, chronic viral problems, mood swings, and irritability, Once food molecules and gut microbes pass into the bloodstream producing auto-immune reactions, a wide variety of illnesses can occur, including rheumatoid arthritis, ankylosing spondylitis, Hashimoto's thyroiditis, asthma and other respiratory conditions, chronic fatigue syndrome, fibromyalgia, brain fog, cerebellar ataxia, multiple sclerosis (MS), and skin disorders.

Despite literally thousands of studies showing how widespread and serious leaky gut syndrome is, most doctors, especially conventional MDs, fail to consider leaky gut as a factor in their patients' health complaints.

Causes of Leaky Gut:

1. The Standard American Diet (SAD), which is inflammatory
2. Gluten
3. Other inflammatory foods such as dairy, processed foods, and fried foods
4. Chronic stress
5. Antibiotics, and NSAID medications

Cyrex also offers an excellent blood test for the diagnosis of Leaky Gut.

Gluten

Gluten is a protein found in wheat and other grains such as oats, rye, barley, spelt, and kamut, The wheat we are eating today is not the same wheat that we ate as kids, or that our parents ate. It has been both hybridized and deaminated. Hybridization refers to combining wheat with other grasses to create a new protein. This "new wheat" is triggering immune reactions within the small intestine and the rest of the body. Deamidation uses acids or enzymes to make gluten water soluble (it is normally only soluble in alcohol), so it mixes more easily with other foods. This also results in immune reactions within the small intestine.

Gluten toxicity results in some people having celiac disease. This occurs when the intestinal villi (little finger like projections on the surface of the small intestine, which is where fully digested food is normally absorbed) are destroyed. This is not very common. What is much more common is gluten sensitivity, which results in inflammation in the lining of the small intestine, and thus a leaky gut.

There are many foods that can cross react with gluten, and which can also contribute to a leaky gut. They include casein (dairy), corn, and instant coffee. This can also be identified with a Cyrex blood test.

Many people have written about the autoimmune epidemic in this country. *All autoimmune diseases are always accompanied by a leaky gut.*

Foods to Avoid If You Have "Leaky Gut"

- All sugars.
- All fruits that are high in sugars such as watermelon, mango, pineapple, raisins, canned fruits, and dried fruits.
- All products containing gluten mentioned above
- All dairy products
- Alcohol
- Instant coffee
- Lectins – they are found in nuts, beans, soy, tomato, eggplant, wheat, and wheat products.

Nutrients to Repair "Leaky Gut"

I have found the following nutrients and other supplements to be most effective for repairing leaky gut. Aloe vera gel is derived from the aloe vera plant and, in addition to helping to soothe and reduce inflammation in the gut, it also provides a variety of important immune-enhancing benefits. L-glutamine is an amino acid used as a source of energy by stomach and other GI tract cells, and helps to restore the lining of the stomach and intestines. It is also useful for GI conditions caused by chronic inflammation, such as colitis, Crohn's disease, and ulcers. Other helpful nutrients are MSM, tillandria, marshmallow extract, gamma oryzanol, slippery elm bark, marigold flower extract, omega 3 fatty acids, peppermint tea, DGL (deglycerrized licorice), and curcumin.

The most important nutrient is an antioxidant called glutathione. Glutathione is the major substance used by the body to help neutralize and eliminate toxins. People with long-standing autoimmune conditions never really heal their leaky gut because they have insufficient amounts of glutathione. This deficiency not only prevents their leaky gut from healing, but also makes them more susceptible to toxins that can disrupt not only their gut barrier, but also their barrier systems in the lungs and the brain (blood brain barrier) with resulting symptoms of chronic cough, poor concentration, and brain fog. Replenishing glutathione in these people is of utmost importance.

Parasites: An Often Overlooked Cause of Gut and Other Diseases

Though commonly thought to only be a concern in tropical, third world countries, parasitic infection affects tens of millions of Americans, many of whom are unaware that they are infected. Moreover, most physicians rarely consider the possibility that parasites might be a factor in their patients' disease symptoms. Yet, according to the Centers for Disease Control and Prevention (CDC) approximately one of every six Americans suffers from parasite infection.

The most common class of parasite infection is that of protozoa, which are microscopic organisms that, once in the body, rapidly reproduce in the gut and can then migrate to other organs, including the heart, liver, lungs, and pancreas. Parasites in this class include *Giardia*, which is primarily transmitted from contaminated food and water, *Cryptosporodium parvum*, which is primarily water-borne, *Entamoeba histolytica*, which is also found in contaminated food and water, *Toxoplasma gondii*, another food-borne parasite that can also be transmitted by cats and dogs, and *Trichomonas vaginalis*, which is primarily transmitted during unprotected, including oral, sex. Other, larger and less common classes of parasites include flukes and tape-, round-, and hookworms, all of which can be spread by contaminated water and food (particularly contaminated or undercooked meats and fish).

Once inside the body, parasites deplete the body of vital nutrients, impair immune function, and can cause a wide range of illnesses both within and outside of the gut. Common gut illnesses associated with parasites include colitis, Crohn's disease, diarrhea, and irritable bowel syndrome. Other conditions that can be caused or worsened by parasites include AIDS, allergies, arthritis, asthma, chronic fatigue syndrome, depression, immune disorders, impaired cognitive function, neurological conditions, skin conditions, and numerous other conditions.

Testing for parasites can be problematic because of parasites' complex life cycles. These cycles enable shed parasite matter during the life cycles to intermittently escape detection. Optimal testing involves taking stool samples at least 48 hours apart and collecting at least two to three samples.

Various blood tests can also indicate the possibility of, parasitic infection. An elevated eosinophil (a type of white blood cell) count can be seen in patients with parasites, as are the presence of antibodies to the parasites.

Common symptoms of parasite infection include bloating, a distended abdomen, dark circles under the eyes, unexplained allergies, unexplained constipation or diarrhea, unexplained fatigue, loss of appetite, sleep problems, sugar cravings, skin conditions, and anal itching. If you suspect you have parasites, seek the help of a physician who specializes in their treatment. Certain foods also provide anti-parasitic benefits. These include ground almonds, cabbage, garlic and onions, flax and pumpkin seeds, kelp, and pineapple and papaya. Various herbal remedies are also effective for preventing and eliminating parasites, especially Artemisia (wormwood), olive leaf extract, black walnut extract, garlic, berberine, and oregano extract.

The Link Between Gut Health and the Health of Your Skin

When people think about staying young and healthy, inevitably they also think of having youthful, healthy skin. Yet many people fail to connect the relationship the health of their skin has to the health of their gut. This connection is vitally important.

The reason the gut plays an essential role in the health of the skin is twofold. First, your skin is one of your body's organs for the elimination of toxins. This means that when your internal organs of drainage (liver, lymph, kidneys) are overburdened with toxins, these toxins are shunted outward by your body to the skin. As this happens, these toxins can clog skin pores and cause an unhealthy skin pallor, as well as skin blemishes such as acne. Additionally, liver spots on the skin, a common symptom of premature aging, are caused by the liver being unable to efficiently remove these toxins.

The second reason skin and gut health are interlinked has do with diet. A cleansing diet that is rich in vital nutrients, along with an adequate intake of pure, filtered water throughout the day, improves skin tone and appearance, along with preventing and alleviating skin wrinkles, baggy eyelids, and dark circles under the eyes. An unhealthy diet not only increases the amount of the toxins in your body, but also disrupts your body's acid-alkaline balance, turning it overly acidic. Chronic overacidity in the body is a primary cause of skin conditions such as dermatitis, eczema, and psoriasis. An unhealthy, acidifying diet also causes your body's lymphatic system to become impaired. This can result in sluggish lymph flow and the accumulation of fatty deposits and toxic debris in the body, along the neck, chin, and other areas of the face, leading to skin puffiness, a sagging, or double, chin line, and a wrinkled neck appearance, a condition sometimes referred to as "turkey neck."

Therefore, if you want to improve and preserve the health of your skin, in addition to properly cleansing it and using healthy skin creams to keep your skin vibrant, you must also address the health of your gut, as well as regularly engaging in skin brushing of your body and the other lymph-enhancing methods I shared with you in Chapter 7. (For more about your skin and how to keep it healthy, see Chapter 13.)

Reducing Acidity for a Healthier You

As we discussed in Chapter 6, proper acid-alkaline balance is absolutely essential for achieving and maintaining optimal health and ageless vitality. In healthy people, the pH inside the cells is slightly alkaline – between 7.28 and 7.45. In order to maintain this pH, we are always excreting acids through the urine, which is why the urine pH is always lower. An overlooked contributor to tissue acidity is fermentation in the gut, which is a result of eating too much sugar, and also due to eating fruit in the evening, when the amount of sugar digesting enzymes (saccharases) is low; thus the sugar released from the fruit is not absorbed, and is metabolized by the colon bacteria and fermented, resulting in the production of lactic acid.

Symptoms of Over-Acidity

When the tissues are acidic, we become more sensitive to pain. We neutralize pain by producing endorphins, but they only become active in an alkaline environment. The take home point is that in all cases of chronic pain, it is essential to treat tissue acidity.

In response to tissue acidity, the stomach secretes hydrochloric acid (HCl), resulting in symptoms such as heartburn. So the ideal treatment is to reduce tissue acidity, rather than giving antacids and acid blocking medication (which while neutralizing the stomach acids, will still allow the tissue acids to remain in the body). Patients with heartburn and GERD are best treated with a diet of no animal protein (which stimulates tissue acidity), and small amounts of either sea salt or Himalayan salt, which stimulates the pancreatic secretion of bicarbonate (which is alkaline and neutralizes acidity).

The skin reacts to hyper-acidity by increasing skin irritations, such as acne and eczema, along with increased sweating. Night sweats are frequently a sign of excessive tissue acidity.

Joints and muscles react to hyper-acidity with symptoms of arthritis and fibromyalgia.

Conditions such as chronic bladder infections, and chronic prostate infections are always a result of hyper-acidity.

And finally hyper-acidity will result in general symptoms of chronic fatigue, poor healing and accelerated aging.

Acid-alkaline balance also plays a vital role in the health of your gut. While a low pH (elevated acidic) level is important for proper digestion of foods in the stomach, overall, your health is best served by making sure that every meal you eat is comprised of foods, beverages, and condiments and spices that, once metabolized, have an alkalizing effect within your body. Such foods are not only nutrient-rich, they also help your body maintain its stores of alkalizing minerals, especially calcium, magnesium, and potassium, rather than having to deplete these stores in an attempt to buffer and neutralize acid buildup caused by meals comprised of foods and beverages that are primarily acidifying.

For most people, the ideal ratio of alkalizing foods to acidifying foods is 4:1, or 80 percent alkalizing foods to 20 percent acidifying foods. Achieving this ratio is much easier than you may think. And as you begin to notice the improvements to your health and energy levels as you shift your eating patterns in this way, you will soon have a strong incentive for continuing to do so. Moreover, shifting to eating primarily alkaline foods at every meal will quickly begin to improve the health and balance within your gut microbiome.

Alkalizing Foods and Beverages: Alkalizing foods and beverages are rich in alkaline minerals and contain little to no acidic substances. In addition, these foods produce no acidic ash when they are digested and metabolized, regardless of how many of them are consumed at any meal. Alkalizing foods include all green vegetables, most colored vegetables, and certain fruits, nuts, and seeds.

All vegetables are rich in vitamins, alkalizing minerals and salts, enzymes, phytonutrients (nutrients derived from plant foods), and fiber, and are particularly useful foods for restoring and maintaining acid-alkaline balance. Green (especially leafy green) vegetables are also rich in chlorophyll, which is what gives them their green color. Chlorophyll has the identical structure as hemoglobin in your red blood cells, except that it contains magnesium instead of iron.

Colored vegetables, though not as rich in chlorophyll, are also excellent sources of essential nutrients. Vegetables in this category that you can eat freely include beets, yellow cabbage, carrots, cauliflower, garlic, onions, potatoes, radishes, red and yellow peppers, scallions, turnips, and yellow squash. You should eat a certain amount of raw vegetables every day, while lightly steaming or sautéing the rest. This will ensure that the rich supply of enzymes that vegetables contain are not destroyed by overcooking.

Though fruits contain many essential nutrients, enzymes, and fiber, they are also abundant in natural sugars, making most fruits slightly acidifying when they are digested. Exceptions are bananas and avocados. Bananas and avocados are naturally alkaline, whereas citrus fruits and tomatoes are acidic by nature. It is best to eat fruits first thing in the morning, or as mid-morning or afternoon snack. Fruits are never a substitute for meals. Your low sugar fruits are the berries (strawberries, raspberries, blackberries, and blueberries).

A variety of nuts and seeds are also alkalizing, especially almonds, Brazil nuts, cashews, chestnuts, and macadamia nuts. Alkalizing seeds include celery seeds, cumin seeds, flaxseed, hemp seeds, pumpkin seeds, and sunflower seeds. All these seeds also make a healthy addition to salads. Both nuts and seeds are also packed with many important nutrients, making them an excellent choice for healthy snacks during the day. However, because of their high caloric content, nuts and seeds should be eaten sparingly, usually no more than one or two handfuls at a time.

Cold-pressed oils and certain herbs and spices are also alkalizing and can be freely used with your meals. along with alkaline water. Good sources of cold-pressed oils include coconut, flaxseed, and extra virgin (not pure) olive oil. Both coconut oil and olive oil can be used for cooking. The intestinal bacteria can convert olive oil into fat-soluble vitamins and other healthy fatty acids. In addition, research shows that coconut oil offers a variety of other important health benefits, including as a brain food that can help prevent the onset of dementia and Alzheimer's disease. Coconut oil also has strong anti-viral and anti-bacterial properties. Taking one or two tablespoons of coconut oil per day is therefore a good idea as part of your overall health maintenance program.

Flaxseed and olive oil can be added to foods after they have been prepared, and flaxseed oil can be a delicious complement to salads because of its rich, nutty flavor. For best results when using any of the above oils choose brands that are certified organic.

Most herbs and spices have an alkalizing effect on the body, as well. This includes herbal teas. Certain herbs, such as cayenne pepper, cinnamon, garlic, oregano, and sage, also function as spices that can add flavor to your meals. Unlike processed table salt, which should be avoided due to its acidifying effects, unprocessed sea salt and Celtic salt can also be used to spice up your meals. Both forms of these salts are alkalizing and are also rich in iodine, which is essential for healthy thyroid function.

Water: The ideal water should carry energy, and therefore should be as fresh as possible. Energetic water occurs when the water molecules are arranged in small clusters, which then can emit electrons. The more the water is processed (with chlorine and fluoride), the more acidic it is, the less energy it emits, and the less oxygen it contains. The best water should be from a spring, as opposed to today's municipal water which also contains high residues of pharmaceutical drugs.

Water should be as alkaline as possible, with an ideal pH of 7.2-7.6. I do not recommend distilled water as it contains no minerals. Distilled water is dead water, and our body needs minerals. On the other hand too many minerals in water may inhibit its detoxifying function. We should all drink at least 1 1/2 liters of water daily, and it should be ingested between meals, so as not to dilute the HCL and digestive enzymes.

All of the above foods and herbs and spices in the above categories should be a major part of each of your meals and snacks, while alkaline water, herbal teas, or pure, filtered water to which the fresh-squeezed juice of a lemon or lime is added, should be your primary beverage choices.

Acidifying Foods, Beverages and Additives: The foods, beverages and additives in this category all have an acidifying effect in the body once they are digested. They should be consumed sparingly or eliminated altogether. Acidifying foods are generally high in proteins, carbohydrates, and/or fats. They include:
- Breads
- Cheese
- Chocolate
- Eggs
- Fish
- Most grains and legumes
- Meats
- Milk and dairy products
- Poultry

I generally advise my patients to avoid all wheat, along with most milk and dairy products. All of the other types of foods listed above provide a variety of important health and nutritional benefits and should definitely be included in your daily diet. The key is to minimize their intake so that they comprise no more than 20-30 percent of each meal, with the rest of your meals given over to a wide variety of alkalizing foods, especially vegetables. In this way, you will still be getting all of the benefit these foods provide without burdening your body with excessive acidity.

In addition to eating in this way, I strongly advise you to eliminate most of the following food and beverages from your diet. Not only are they highly acidifying when consumed, the vast majority of them are also extremely unhealthy. They are:

- Alcohol (as for wine, please limit yourself to no more than 1 glass per day)
- Candy, cookies, donuts, etc.
- Coffee, commercial, non-herbal teas (1 cup of coffee per day is fine; substitute herbal teas for commercial tea)
- All refined and processed foods
- All simple carbohydrate foods (breads, pasta, white rice, etc.)
- Soda
- Sugar and all artificial sweeteners
- Tap water
- Yeast products (especially if you have or are susceptible to candida)

With the exception of wine, which can be consumed in limited amounts, you need to avoid all of the other items in the above list.

The Problem of Excess Animal Protein: A popular misconception about achieving acid-alkaline balance through diet is that protein-rich foods, especially animal-derived products such as meats, fish and poultry, are somehow unhealthy and should be avoided. Some proponents of acid-alkaline balance go so far as to insist that it can only be achieved through a vegetarian or vegan diet. This is not completely true.

Proteins are the building blocks of every tissue in your body and are needed for your body to be able to repair and maintain itself. Every cell in your body contains protein, and it is also a major component of the skin, bones, muscles, organs, and glands. Protein is also found in nearly all body fluids, including blood. Protein is essential for growth, for cell repair, the production of new cells, and even the buffering of acids. Without an adequate supply of dietary protein, none of these functions can be performed properly. That's because protein foods contain essential amino acids, which can only be supplied through diet since the body cannot manufacture them on its own.

When it comes to protein foods, the first thing to keep in mind is that only the intake of excessive protein ends up being acid-forming. The proteins your body uses, in its daily maintenance and repair, are fully used and do not leave an acid residue. So while it is true that excessive amounts of protein-rich foods can create an acid load in the body once they are metabolized, that does not mean that a healthy and balanced amount of protein should be avoided. While vegetarian and vegan diets have been shown to reduce the incidence of heart disease and cancer, many people feel better and have more energy when they eat healthy animal protein in prudent amounts.

On the other hand, eating excessive amounts of animal protein, especially without adequate alkalizing foods to counterbalance them, can indeed contribute to health problems over time, including heart disease, cancer, osteoporosis, and kidney disease. Many of my patients in their quest to feel better and maintain ideal weight reduce their intake of grains and carbohydrates, and wind up increasing their animal protein intake, thinking that that will allow them to increase their muscle mass. Excessive protein intake must be excreted (thus producing stress on the liver and the kidneys), broken down (in some cases raising uric acid levels and causing gout), or stored as protein deposited in the interstitial spaces between the cells. This will interfere with the transport of nutrients into the cells, and the excretion and transport of toxins away from the cells, thus inhibiting optimum cellular function.

Long-term ingestion of excess animal proteins will also result in loss of minerals from the bones, calcium deposits in tissues, thickening of the skin, redness of the face, and sun sensitivity. The key, as with all things related to health, is moderation and balance. Most people can obtain all of their protein needs by consuming around 50 grams of protein daily (adolescents and high performance athletes will need more).

Overall, moderate protein intake, along with following the overall acid-alkaline-balancing recommendations above, will supply you with all of the important health benefits protein foods provide, while neutralizing their acid load. But when choosing animal protein foods, be sure to select only free-range, grass-fed meats, poultry, and lamb, and wild-caught fish that are not high in mercury. For most people, the ideal serving size for animal protein foods is one that is equivalent to the size of their fist. Portions larger than that are usually excessive, while portions smaller than that usually will not provide you with all of the protein your body needs.

What to Eat, When to Eat, How Much to Eat

There is a vast amount of literature concerning nutrition, much of which is both confusing and conflicting. Poor lifestyle and nutritional habits contribute as much to the aging process as the passing of years. When it comes to your eating choices, the key concept is to view your body as a Ferrari, and to put high octane fuel (healthy foods and beverages) into it at all times. The following guidelines are very helpful in that regard.

1. Don't skip breakfast, and make breakfast and lunch your largest meals each day, as pancreatic enzyme production is at its peak in the morning hours.

2. Finish eating dinner no later than 8 PM and ideally hours earlier, and try to keep your dinner meals small, as pancreatic enzyme production is at its lowest in the evening.

3. Create meals that contain between 70 to 80 percent alkalizing foods and only 20 to 30 percent acidifying foods.

4. On average, limit your total protein intake each day to no more than 50 grams unless you regularly engage in rigorous exercise, in which case it can be higher. To prevent the acidifying effects

of excess protein, always eat a lot of alkalizing, non-starchy vegetables with protein foods.

5. For most people, a ratio of 40 percent protein, 20 to 40 percent complex carbohydrates, and 20 to 40 percent healthy fats for each meal is ideal.

6. As a rule, most people should increase their intake of fresh, organic fruits and vegetables, eat fish low in mercury at least three times per week, and eliminate all sugar, table salt (use sea or Celtic salt instead), canned and processed foods, bottled juices, milk, tap water, and unhealthy fats, especially hydrogenated fats, including margarine and other butter substitutes. (Such fats block the chemical pathways that are necessary for us to utilize the cholesterol manufactured by our bodies.)

7. Consume alcohol, and coffee sparingly.

8. Research has proven that the body requires certain essential fatty acids (now being removed from many foods) in order to manufacture certain hormone-like chemicals called prostaglandins, which are vital for proper immune function. Essential fatty acids in your diet can be increased by consuming cold-water fish. Examples include salmon, cod, mackerel, and sardines. Warm ocean fish such as snapper, flounder, and perch are second best. Fresh water fish (catfish, trout) contain the smallest amount of essential fatty acids.

9. To further ensure you are getting enough essential fatty acids, try to eat one tablespoon of extra virgin (not pure) olive or flaxseed oil daily on salads. Keep the flaxseed oil refrigerated after opening. As a snack food, walnuts are high in essential fatty acids. Supplements rich in essential fatty acids include fish oils containing EPA, evening primrose oil, and flax seed oil.

10. Avoid cooking food at high temperatures, as doing so destroys the enzymes that food contains. It is preferable to cook longer at lower temperatures, which also helps to preserve the nutrient content of foods. Stir-fried vegetables or wok crispy vegetables are healthier than those which have been over-cooked.

11. Fruits should be eaten by themselves, either one-half hour before a meal or two hours after. When fast-digesting fruits are held up in the digestive system longer than necessary by being combined with foods that digest more slowly, fermentation takes place and intestinal gas production is the result.

12. Proper food combining will also greatly improve digestion and assimilation of vital nutrients. Do not combine starches (pasta, rice, potatoes) with proteins (meat, chicken, fish). Unfortunately, this is the way meals are served in restaurants. The ideal way to eat is to combine non-starchy vegetables with proteins, or to combine non-starchy vegetables with starchy carbohydrates.

13. Avoid artificial sweeteners, such as saccharine, "Nutrasweet," and "Splenda." Stevia extract, an herb which is a natural sweetener, is an excellent substitute, and is healing to the pancreas.

14. Try to drink at least eight glasses of filtered or bottled water daily. Remember that at birth we are 97 percent water, and as adults we are 70 percent water. Premature aging is associated with a further loss of total body water. Don't drink water with your meals, however, as this dilutes the digestive juices necessary to digest your food. Never drink tap water unless you have a very good filtration system. You can energize water by leaving it in the sun for a short period of time.

15. Cut down on your total carbohydrate intake each day, limiting your carb consumption to no more than 40 percent of each meal, and ideally less. Also avoid simple carbohydrates. Americans by and large not only consume too many carbohydrates in their meals, they typically eat the wrong types of carbohydrate foods. The top carbohydrate foods in the standard American diet are cold breakfast cereals, bread, bagels, candy, commercial fruit juices and punch drinks, jams and jellies, muffins, potatoes (especially as French fries, white pasta, white rice, pizza, pancakes, soda, sweets (cakes, cookies, pies), and table sugar. When consumed regularly, these foods and beverages are guaranteed to produce fatigue, gas, bloating and other GI conditions, irritability

and mood swings, unhealthy weight gain, diabetes, poor sleep, and many other health conditions.

16. Take a moment before meals to give thanks for the food you are about to eat. Doing so fosters feelings of gratitude and contentment, which, as you learned in Chapter 6, can go a long way towards maintaining and improving your health. Giving thanks can also help trigger the relaxation response, making it easier for your body to most effectively digest the food you eat and make use of the nutrients it contains. You can enhance this experience by taking time to fully chew each bite of food, which not only aids your body's digestive processes, but also makes it easier for you to savor and enjoy the food you are eating.

Ideal Supplements for Lasting Gut Health

Though I have already shared a number of nutritional supplements with you in this chapter, I want to conclude it by sharing the two most essential classes of nutrients for lasting gut health, as well as a few herbs that can also help.

Enzymes: There are two primary types of enzymes that support gut health—digestive and proteolytic enzymes. Digestive enzymes include amalyse, cellulase, lactase, lipase, and protease, which help to digest carbohydrates, fibers, milk and dairy products, fats, and proteins, respectively. I recommend that you take digestive enzymes with each of your meals to enhance digestion. Most digestive enzyme formulas contain all of the above, as well as other enzymes. You can find such products at your local health food store and online. Use according to the directions on the label. For added benefit, consider also taking betaine HCl with your meals.

Proteolytic enzymes are primarily enzymes that are also produced by the pancreas (primarily protease, and they also contain chymotrypsin), as well as the enzymes bromelain, papain, lumbrokinase, nattokinase, and serrapeptase. When taken away from meals, proteolytic enzymes provide a number of important health benefits, including eliminating partially undigested food molecules, foreign proteins, infectious microorganisms, and other immune impairing substances. They may help combat cancer but stripping away the outer coating of cancer cells which helps such cells elude identification and targeting by the immune system. For this reason, the use of proteolytic enzymes has been used for decades by integrative cancer clinics in Europe and Mexico, and is also an essential component of the anticancer protocols of Nicholas Gonzalez, MD, a leading integrative cancer doctor and researcher in New York City.

Proteolytic enzymes also help to digest and eliminate fibrin, a blood-clotting protein which, in excess, can accumulate in the bloodstream, as well as in fractures, joints, and wounds. Because of this, proteolytic enzymes are often helpful in treating bone fractures, joint pain, and for preventing infections in wounds. They also act as potent anti-inflammatory agents, thus reducing the risk of developing the many conditions associated with chronic inflammation.

Although proteolytic enzymes can be taken with meals, to obtain the overall systemic health benefits they provide, they need to be taken away from food. Like digestive enzymes, they are available at health food stores and online. Again, use according to the directions on the label.

Probiotics: The term *probiotics* means "for life." Probiotic supplements support the literally trillions of the more than 400 species of life- and health-enhancing bacteria that live in the human gut. They include *L. acidophilus, bifidobacteria (bifidum* and *B. longum), L. bulgaricus, L. casei,* and *Streptococcus thermophilus.* Used as supplements, probiotics provide a variety of benefits, including helping to keep harmful bacteria and other microorganisms in check, protecting against food poisoning, mitigating the side effects of antibiotic drugs, improving immune function, aiding in the body's manufacture of various B vitamins, reducing high cholesterol, and improving the overall health and efficiency of the GI tract and its various functions.

While acidophilus remains the most commonly known and used probiotic supplement, research has established that a combination of multiple strains of probiotics provides a greater degree of these and other benefits. A recommended dose of a good, multiple strain formula is between one and 10 billion probiotic bacteria per day, and even higher dosages after a course of antibiotic treatment. As with enzymes, use according to the label's directions.

You can also aid and increase your body's own supply of gut probiotics by regularly consuming fermented foods, such as sauerkraut, kimchi, and miso soup, all of which can dramatically increase your body's supply of healthy gut bacteria over time.

Useful Herbs for Digestion: Herbs have been used for centuries in healing cultures around the world to maintain and restore gut health. Such herbs fall into a number of categories and include:

- Anti-inflammatory, such as chamomile, which aid in digestion and prevent and relieve inflammation of the GI tract.
- Astringents, such as meadowsweet, which help to prevent and heal bleeding in the GI tract.
- Bitters, such as gentian and yarrow root, which can help improve digestion.
- Carminatives, such as peppermint, spearmint, and valerian, which prevent and relieve gas and bloating.
- Demulcents, such as marshmallow and slippery elm, which soothe the lining of the GI tract.
- Nervines, such as hops, which prevent and ease stress.

Because of their medicinal qualities, I recommend that you first consult with an experienced herbalist or physician trained in herbal medicine before using any type of herbal remedy.

Key Points to Remember

Your gut is essential to your overall health. In addition to being where food and beverages are digested so that all of your cells, tissues, and organs, as well as your blood can obtain the nutrients they need, your GI tract is a primary way that waste matter and toxins are eliminated from the body.

Your gut also acts as your body's "second brain" because it is the home of the enteric nervous system, which is brimming with neurotransmitter proteins. These proteins are produced by cells that are identical to neurotransmitter-producing cells in the brain. The complex collection of neurotransmitters in the "GI brain" enables it to act, learn, and remember in much the same way that the brain itself does.

Your gut is also home to an estimated 100 trillion bacteria that co-exist in a delicate balance. This bacterial ecosystem is part of what is known as the human microbiome. There are more bacteria in our colon, than there are cells in our body.

Poor gut health is epidemic in the US today, and is primarily caused by poor diet and nutrition, food allergies and sensitivities, infections and malabsorption, stomach acid (HCl) imbalances, the overuse of pharmaceutical drugs, lack of exercise, and stress.

Parasite infections, which are far more widespread than commonly believed, pose another serious threat to your gut and overall health.

Other factors associated with poor gut health include an overworked and stressed pancreas, candida, dysbiosis, and leaky gut syndrome.

One of the primary ways you can improve the health of your gut is to follow a diet that consists primarily of alkalizing foods at each meal. For most people, this means meals that consist of 80 percent alkalizing foods and only 20 percent acidifying foods.

One of the easiest ways to increase the amount of alkalizing foods you eat is to include a rich supply of alkalizing vegetables with each meal, as well as regularly eating salads.

Proper food combining is also important for excellent digestion. This means eating fruits away from other foods (as snacks away from meals), not combining protein foods with starchy carbohydrates, eating non-starchy vegetables either with protein or with starchy carbohydrates, but not with both, and avoiding drinking with meals.

A variety of supplements can also significantly support gut health. Supplements in this class primarily fall into three categories—enzymes (both digestive and proteolytic), probiotics, and herbs that support the GI tract.

CHAPTER 8

Essential #4: Ignite Your Energy

T he fourth essential key to creating outstanding health has to do with developing a lifestyle that is not only healthy, but also energizing. The three hallmarks of an energizing lifestyle are greater energy at a level that is sustained throughout the day, a greater passion for living, and being aligned to your true life purpose. I've already discussed the latter two qualities in Chapter 5, where I also shared a variety of self-care tools and techniques you are hopefully already making use of to "live your life on purpose," with passion and enthusiasm.

In this chapter, you will gain additional tools and insights for creating more energy and better health. You will also learn about three very serious, yet often ignored, "energy sappers" that can negatively impact your health. Let's begin by exploring one of the most important essentials of an energetic lifestyle–regular exercise.

Exercise and Physical Activity

Regular exercise and physical activity can contribute more benefits to your health than almost any other health practice. And the benefits go far beyond physical health, resulting in greater emotional well-being, as well. This is not surprising when you consider that the word *emotion* contains the word *motion* within it. When we don't get our bodies in motion on a regular basis we don't feel well.

Regular exercise and physical activity increase blood flow. The more blood that flows, the more oxygen that gets delivered to your cells. More oxygen in your cells means your cells are able to generate more energy, because cells create energy from burning oxygen and glucose together. This occurs in the mitochondria, the cellular "energy factories" we've discussed previously.

The many health benefits that regular exercise provides are well-known. They include dissipation of tension, decreased incidences of the "fight or flight" response, reduction of anxiety and depression, increased self-esteem and positive emotions, increased muscular strength and flexibility, improved respiration and increased lung capacity (without regular exercise your lung capacity shrinks as you age), improved sleep, improved immunity, reduced risk of degenerative diseases such as cancer and heart disease, improved brain function and mental acuity, increased libido and improved overall sexual health, improved muscle to fat ratio (body mass index, or BMI), and improved longevity.

Research has repeatedly demonstrated that people who do not exercise regularly are far more likely to succumb to disease, become more pessimistic, experience poor sleep and chronic fatigue, and die younger than people who exercise. As a result of such research, many health experts now regard lack of exercise to be a more significant risk factor for illness and decreased life expectancy than the risks of high cholesterol, high blood pressure, being overweight, and cigarette smoking *combined*.

Even so, as a nation we are becoming increasingly sedentary. This is especially true of our children. Studies show that they are engaging in regular physical activity at a rate far below that of any previous generation. As a result, today's youth in America are becoming fatter, weaker, and slower than ever before. This trend, if not reversed, is setting our nation UP for a health crisis far beyond the one that is currently costing us over $3 trillion each year in health care costs.

Sad as our children's lack of, and aversion to, exercise is, I am not surprised that this is the case. After all, children model their habits based on the examples they see from their parents and other influential adults. And the examples they are being given are far from healthy. This fact was borne out by a recently published study conducted by researchers at the Mayo Clinic. Based on a representative survey of men and women between the ages of 20 and 74, the researchers found that, on average, the exercise habits of adult Americans are even worse than previously thought, with even men and women of normal weight being found to engage in fat-burning exercise and physical activities for a mere two minutes per day. Other research has found that adults who are obese, exercise for as little as 11 seconds per day.

The typical reasons most people give when asked why they fail to engage in regular exercise are either "I don't have enough time/I'm too busy," or "I'm too tired." These are not reasons; they are excuses, as the French proverb says, "He who excuses himself, accuses himself." But even if such excuses were valid, I have found that there is a deeper reason why people either don't exercise or do not continue to do so once they start: They don't experience the type of payoffs or immediate benefits they hope to achieve.

While it is certainly true that the physical health benefits regular exercise provides can take weeks, and even months, before becoming noticeable, that is not a valid reason for giving up too soon. Moreover, as mentioned above, exercise provides a host of mental and emotional benefits, as well, which can occur after even a single session of exercise. That's because exercise and physical activity trigger the release of "feel good" endorphins, and also provide immediate benefits related to brain function. As Harvard Medical School psychiatrist John Ratey, author of *Spark: The Revolutionary New Science of Exercise and the Brain,* has said, *"Exercise is the single best thing you can do for your brain in terms of mood, memory, and learning."* My advice to first-time exercisers, besides first discussing their exercise goals with their doctor and getting his or her clearance to begin, is to focus first on the gains you make mentally and emotionally after each exercise session, instead of focusing on the physical benefits that may take longer to become obvious to you. The key, as with all other aspects of health, is to be consistent.

However, there is another obstacle to obtaining the most benefits from exercise that many people do not realize. Put simply, what they know about how to exercise may be outdated and even wrong. This is especially true with regard to aerobic exercise, the type of exercise (walking, jogging, running, bicycling, exercising on stairmasters or treadmills, etc.) that most people who do exercise engage in.

Aerobic means "with oxygen," and aerobic exercise results in an increased intake of oxygen to fuel cells, tissues, and organs. For decades we were taught that, in order to obtain the most benefit from aerobic exercise, it was necessary to engage in it for at least 30 to 60 minutes at least three to five days a week. New research, though, is starting to disprove this recommendation, and in fact is finding that prolonged aerobic exercise may not only be ineffective for providing the health gains, but may actually be harmful due to the wear and tear aerobic exercises can cause to joints and the overall musculoskeletal system.

Daily prolonged aerobic exercise can also result in the breakdown and shrinkage of muscle, negatively impact the kidneys (due to dehydration), contribute to decreased insulin sensitivity, and accelerate the body's aging process. The good news is that there is a far more effective alternative to traditional aerobic exercise. Best of all, it offers superior results in a fraction of the time.

High Intensity Interval Training (HIIT): Imagine being able to achieve greater health benefits than aerobic exercise provides by exercising for only 20 minutes or less two to three times a week. That is exactly what high intensity interval training, or HIIT, can do for you. The reason why HIIT has become such a popular alternative to standard aerobic exercises has to do with the increasing number of its health benefits that ongoing research continues to discover. In large part, the benefits, which include stabilization of insulin levels, increased production of human growth hormone, more efficient burning of calories, and increased fat loss, are the result of how HIIT exercises activate what are known as fast-twitch muscle fibers.

It is the engagement, or stimulation, of this type of muscle fiber that is essential for the most effective intake of increased oxygen, and thus the energy that oxygen supplies inside the body. In addition, fast-twitch fibers are primarily *glycolytic*, meaning that they burn glucose quickly, which results in the increased production of ATP, or cellular fuel. When fast-twitch muscle fibers are activated, your body is also stimulated to grow muscle. At the same time, your body's insulin sensitivity is enhanced.

By contrast, standard aerobic exercise primarily only engages slow-twitch muscle fibers. Over time, this can cause both fast twitch muscle fibers to atrophy, thus resulting in a loss of muscle mass while simultaneously causing a loss of insulin sensitivity. This explains why so many practitioners of regular, prolonged aerobic exercise tend to experience health problems as they get older.

A leading researcher into the benefits and advantages of HIIT is Datis Kharrazian, DC, DHSc, MS. He has found that, compared to traditional aerobic exercise, HIIT is:

1. More effective for preventing and reversing the risk factors that can cause metabolic syndrome, also known as syndrome X.

2. More effective for improving overall cardiovascular function and reducing the risk of heart disease.

3. More effective for improving and maintaining optimal immune function.

4. Very effective for stimulating production of human growth hormone (standard aerobic exercise does not stimulate HGH).

5. More effective for triggering what is known as a nitric oxide (NO) response. (Nitric oxide is a form of nitrogen that has been shown to provide a range of health benefits, including improved immunity, improved cardiovascular function, and enhancement of sexual health in both men and women. NO is also involved in the body's neural development, thus aiding memory and other cognitive functions. It also helps control blood pressure, aids in the prevention of unhealthy blood clots, aids in tissue repair, and may play a role in helping the body defend itself from cancer.)

In addition to the above benefits, Dr. Kharrazian has found that HIIT, because of its stimulation of human growth hormone, helps maintain healthy bone density, blood glucose levels, and the health of brain synapses.

Another significant benefit of HIIT which Dr. Kharrazian has noted is its ability to significantly elevate levels of what is known as brain-derived neurotrophic factor, or BDNF. BDNF provides a number of important benefits to the brain and its neuron system, including helping nerves to grow, improving neuron synapse function and communication, supporting the branching network of neurons, and reducing the risk of neurodegeneration.

Given all of the above benefits, it is not surprising that a growing number of exercise experts and physical fitness trainers are now recommending a shift away from traditional aerobics to HIIT.

Getting Started With HIIT: As with any other type of exercise, when first beginning HIIT exercises, do so slowly and then work your way up to higher levels of intensity. There are many ways that you can begin HIIT, and all of them are variations of traditional aerobic exercises. The difference is that, instead of exercising as the same pace throughout, you will be varying your pace between a slow, relaxed, recovery phase, and shorter intervals of much greater intensity or exertion.

For those new to HIIT, especially those who are not used to exercising in general, one of the easiest ways to get started is by walking. Begin by warming up for three minutes, walking in a relaxed manner. Be sure to breathe deeply as you do so. Then walk as fast as you can without running for 30 seconds. During this time, also pump your arms back and forth as vigorously as you can. At the end of this 30 seconds, you should be short of breath and feel as if you can't go on any further at this rate. Then slow down and walk at a gentle, relaxed pace for 90 seconds. Then again go all out for 30 seconds, and continue shifting back and forth for a total of three all out and three relaxed, recovery phases. That's all there is to it.

As you become more accustomed to this HIIT approach to walking, increase the sequence until you are able to perform six to eight reps of each of the two phases. Once you reach this level, continue at that level each week, two to three times per week. (More than three times per week is not necessary for most people to achieve the benefits of HIIT.)

As mentioned, you can also adapt other aerobic exercises into HIIT approaches. This includes running, bicycling, working on a stationary bike, or, one of my favorite types of HIIT exercise, jumping on a re-bounder, or mini-trampoline. Spinning, a popular form of exercise at gyms, can also easily be adapted to provide an effective HIIT workout. Whichever type of exercise you choose, follow the same guidelines for HIIT walking above, always starting with a three minute warm up of gentle exercise, before shifting into the intensity and recovery phases. And once again, start out slowly, with no more than three reps of each phase per day, and then building up to six to eight reps each.

Caution: As with other types of exercise, HIIT is not without risk. The two most common risks of all types of exercise are what is known as metabolic overtraining syndrome, a condition characterized by oxidative stress placed on cells, tissues, and organs, and muscle injury due to added stress on the body.

Whereas muscle injury is obvious to anyone who experiences it, metabolic overtraining syndrome can escape one's awareness until more serious health problems arise. Therefore, it is important to know the early warning signs and symptoms of overtraining. They include an inability to complete or properly recover from your workouts, declines in your overall exercise performance, feelings of aggression and irrita-bility, depression, decreased muscle strength, impaired immunity, loss of libido, and, in women, a lack of menstruation. The risk of metabolic overtraining syndrome can also be made worse by pre-existing condi-tions, such as chronic inflammation, impaired immunity, nutritional deficiencies, hormone imbalances, and elevated or too low cortisol lev-els, as well as alcohol consumption, dehydration, and prescription drug use.

To prevent both muscle injury and metabolic overtraining syndrome always consult with your doctor before beginning, and during your exercise program, keep yourself hydrated by drinking plenty of pure, filtered water throughout the day, avoid saunas and prolonged hot showers on the days you engage in HIIT, don't overexert yourself, get adequate amounts of rest and recovery time between the days you exercise, and always replenish your body's nutrient supply after exercise by eating a variety of organic fruits and vegetables (especially non-starchy leafy greens), high quality protein foods, and healthy fats, while avoiding starchy carbohydrates, sugars (including commercial sports drinks), and all processed foods. (For more on healthy eating, see Chapter 7.) Finally, be sure to get enough good quality sleep each night (see below).

Completing Your Overall Exercise Program: The best type of overall exercise or physical fitness program is one that incorporates the benefits that aerobic and HIIT exercises provide with exercises that build strength, increase flexibility, and maintain your core (back, stomach and abdominal area, and pelvis). Building and maintaining muscle strength is important, particularly as you age. Strength training accomplishes this, and research shows that regularly engaging in strength training activities can significantly improve your body's ability to maintain healthy hormone levels and metabolism, increase its ability to efficiently burn calories, and reduce the risk of bone loss.

Stretching exercises also need to be part of your fitness regimen so that you can maintain your body's flexibility. Lack of flexibility can severely inhibit your physical performance, lead to poor posture, and increase your risk of injury. In addition, increased flexibility also leads to improved strength and function, allowing your body's muscle groups to operate at peak efficiency. Other benefits of flexibility include improved circulation and greater suppleness of your body's tendons, ligaments and connective tissues.

Maintaining the health and strength of your core is also important. Your body's core, which consists of 29 muscles, is the foundation for all movement throughout your body. Exercising and strengthening core muscles strengthens the back and reduces the risk of back and musculo-skeletal pain and injury, improves your balance, and helps to maintain and enhance overall GI function.

When most people think of strength training, they usually think of using free weights or weight machines. This approach can certainly work, yet is not necessary if you lack access to a gym in your area. More-over, not having to rely on weights and weight machines makes it far likelier that you will commit to your training routine.

You can use your own body weight to build up and strengthen your body. Examples of body weight exercises include pushups, which strengthen your arms, chest, and upper back; chin, or pull, ups, which also strengthen these same areas of the body; squat thrusts and lunges, which strengthen your glutes, thighs, hamstrings, quadriceps and calf muscles; and calf raises, which strengthen the calves, ankles, and toes. The advantage of these exercises is that you can perform them at home or while traveling.

If your prefer to use free weights or weight machines, that's fine too. Either way, for best results, perform one set of each exercise, one after the other, with brief (one minute) rests between exercises. Start by completing one circuit of all the exercises. As your strength and endur-ance increases, move on to doing two full circuits of all the exercises for a longer, more intense workout. As you do each exercise, focus your attention on the muscles you are working, and be sure to breathe. Most people can obtain the benefits of strength training in as little as two to three days per week, ideally on the days that you do not perform aero-bic or HIIT exercises, so that your body has enough time to rest and recover.

Stretching exercises can, and should be performed more regularly throughout the week. A full stretching routine can usually be done in as little as ten minutes per day, making them an ideal way to start or finish your day. A shorter stretching routine is also recommended before and after both aerobic and strength training exercises. Before beginning, however, take a few minutes to warm up your muscles, something you can easily accomplish by breathing deeply and walking about. This will enhance your circulation and make stretching easier.

When you stretch each area of your body, you should feel tension in the affected muscle or muscle group, but never to the point of pain. Breathe into each stretch to elongate and relax the muscle group, holding the stretch for at least 10 seconds or more. Repeat each stretch at least two more times. As you become accustomed to stretching, you should notice that your range of motion increases with each stretch, including with each successive repetition. Useful stretching exercises include neck bends, shoulder lifts, torso twists, overhead stretches, forward bends, and hamstring and quadriceps stretches.

A fairly new and innovative approach to stretching, known as active isolated stretching (AIS) was developed by stretching expert Aaron Mattes. To learn more about AIS, visit Aaron's website, www.stretchingusa.com.

When people think of core exercises, they usually think of sit ups or abdominal crunches. Although such exercises can certainly help strengthen the core, they are not without risk. More recently, a number of fitness experts and trainers have shifted their clients into an exercise called planking, which looks deceptively simple, yet can provide a very strenuous, core-shaping workout that also helps build strength throughout the rest of the body.

The standard planking pose is performed by lying face down on the floor or exercise mat, placing your hands palms down close to your neck and upper shoulders. From this position, rise up onto your forearms and toes and hold this position for as long as you can, taking care to breathe fully as you do so.

If you are not used to planking, don't be surprised if you can only hold the pose for 10 to 20 seconds. If that is the case, fine. Each day, try to add another five seconds to your time, gradually working up until you can successively hold this planking pose for at least three minutes, and ideally more. You may be surprised by the health benefits you start to achieve as your ability to hold the planking pose improves.

Two other popular and very effective forms of exercise that can be used to strengthen your core are pilates and yoga. Both of these exercise approaches not only effectively work all of the core muscles, they also provide both flexibility and strength training benefits. When beginning either pilates or yoga, I recommend you have a few sessions with a professional trainer in either modality. Such instructors can be found in most towns and cities across the U.S.

Nutrients That Can Enhance Your Exercise Program: In addition to following a healthy eating plan and not skipping meals while exercising, certain nutritional supplements can also be important when it comes to optimizing your exercise regimen. Among them are the minerals magnesium and potassium, both of which act as electrolytes in the body, and are therefore helpful in replacing lost electrolytes that occur during exercise. Vitamin C can also be helpful because of the important role it plays in the growth and repair of muscle tissue. Research has shown that vitamin C also helps to reduce fatigue and prevent inflammation caused by exercise, while enhancing cardiovascular function. Omega 3 oils also help protect against inflammation and protect the heart. Another nutrient with anti-inflammatory benefits is MSM, which is also useful for protecting joints and boosting metabolism.

In addition to the above nutrients, a number of other supplements are well-known for their specific exercise benefits. They are creatine monohydrate, whey protein, beta-alanine, conjugated linoleic acid (CLA), and branched-chain amino acids (BCAAs).

Creatine, which is available in pill, powder and liquid forms, is regarded by the International Society of Sports Nutrition (ISSN) as "the most effective" supplement for increasing high intensity exercise capacity and muscle growth. This is not surprising, since more than 95 percent of creatine in the body is stored in muscle tissue. Creatine increases the amount of energy available to the body via ATP, especially for short bursts of high intensity exercise, and replenishes ATP stores when taken after exercise. It also enhances cellular hydration. Research has shown that supplementing with creatine following high intensity exercise can result in greater gains in muscle strength and power, and faster, more complete recovery. Although elite athletes often take creatine at high doses, for most people a sufficient dose is between 1,000 to 2,000 mg once a day. To improve its absorption, it can be taken with a small glass of organic grape juice. *Caution:* People with, or who are at risk for, kidney disease should avoid creatine supplements.

Whey protein, which is available in powder form, is well-absorbed, and can be an important supplement after high intensity and strength training exercise because of its ability to help muscle repair by increasing protein synthesis in the body. Whey also improves levels of branched-chain amino acids (leucine, isoluceine, valine), cysteine, glutamine, and taurine in the body, and helps stimulate fat loss. Whey protein comes from cow milk. Look for brands that are organic, minimally processed, hormone-free, and derived from grass-fed cows, and use according to the label instructions.

Beta-alanine is a precursor of carnosine, a compound that is highly concentrated in skeletal muscles. Because of beta-alanine's ability to increase carnosine levels in the body, it can help to reduce muscle soreness after exercise because of its ability to buffer acid buildup in muscle tissue. This, in turn, helps to prevent and reduce inflammation of muscle tissue. Research has also found that supplementing with beta-alanine helps to reduce fatigue during exercise, optimizes hormonal responses to intense physical exertion, and can improve the body's muscle-to-fat ratio.

Conjugated linoleic acid (CLA) is a type of fatty acid found in meat, lamb and dairy products. CLA taken as a supplement has been shown to accelerate fat loss in the body, including belly fat, while helping to maintain lean muscle mass, especially when used in conjunction with strength training. Recent studies also indicate that CLA may help to increase testosterone levels. CLA supplements are available as both a capsule or a syrup at most health food stores. For best results, look for brands that contain at least 80 percent CLA and use according to the directions on the label.

Branched-chain amino acids (BCAAs) provide many of the same benefits as creatine and whey protein, helping to increase protein synthesis while decreasing the breakdown of muscle tissue and increasing recovery time. BCCAs have also been shown to help boost production of growth hormone in the body. Unlike most other amino acid supplements, as well as complete proteins, which must first be metabolized in the liver, BCCAs go directly to the muscles, where they can either be used as fuel during exercise, or for building and repair muscles afterward. For this reason, many elite athletes take BCCAs both before and after their workouts. A typical daily dose is between 5,000 to 10,000 mg.

Tips For Getting the Most Out of Your Exercise Program: When it comes to developing and benefiting from an exercise program none of us plan to fail. Yet, as my friend Suzanne Somers wrote in her Foreword to this book, when we fail to plan, failure often finds us. For this reason, I encourage you to have a plan in place before you begin to incorporate an exercise regimen in your life. Start by getting clear on both your short- and long-term goals. What do you want to achieve in each case? Write that down. Then create and write down the types of exercises in each of the categories above that you intend to perform, and on what schedule. I also recommend that you keep an exercise journal, so that you can track how much progress you are making week-to-week and month-to-month.

As you begin your exercise program, remember that it is important to not try to accomplish too much too soon. Slow and easy is the rule, not "No pain, no gain." One of the biggest reasons that people fail at, or stop, exercising is because they try to do too much too soon. So start off slowly, and stay at your beginning level for at least five to seven days before you increase your activity. This will help ensure that you progress in a safe and effective manner without over-exerting your body.

You may also find exercise becomes easier to commit to, and more enjoyable, if you do it with a friend or family member. To further help maintain your commitment to exercising, find healthy ways that you can reward yourself for staying on track.

To prevent boredom as you exercise, be sure to vary your routine and the types of exercises you perform in each exercise category. Not only will this help you maintain your enjoyment of exercise, but it will also help prevent your exercise gains from plateauing, which can happen as your body adjusts to exercise routines performed over and over again. This has been proven by research, which found that people who regularly change up their exercise routines are better able to maintain their health gains and become leaner and stronger than people who follow the same exercise routines.

And, finally, be sure to give yourself enough recovery time between your exercise sessions. Otherwise your body will not have the time it needs to properly rebuild and repair itself, especially after HIIT and strength training exercises. Lack of proper recovery time can also trigger a chronic stress response state, causing elevated cortisol levels that can lead to adrenal fatigue and "burnout". Over-exercising and lack of recovery can also cause chronic inflammation, and blood sugar and insulin imbalances. Proper recovery includes both spacing the days between both HIIT and strength training exercises, and also making sure that you are getting enough sleep each night and managing your stress levels.

Energizing Your Mind and Body With Breathwork and Meditation

As you learned in Chapter 5, cleansing and fortifying your mind is the essential first key to creating outstanding health. Cultivating greater awareness of, and better control over, the processes of your mind can also result in a greater energy. I have found that two of the most effective means for doing so are consciously working with the breath (breathwork) and meditation. Both of these methods dovetail into each other and, when practiced regularly, can provide you with significant health benefits. What follows is information you can use to immediately begin incorporating both of these energizing techniques into your daily life.

Breathwork: Proper breathing is vital for ensuring that your body is receiving all of the oxygen it needs, and for fully expelling carbon dioxide, as well as various waste matter when you exhale. As obvious as this may seem, in reality few people breathe fully and efficiently. In fact, although the lung capacity of oxygen in adult human beings is approximately two gallons, most people only inhale an average of 20 to 25 percent of that as they breathe. Such inefficient breathing results in a significant loss of potential energy, since most of the energy you need to live and function at an optimal state comes more from the oxygen you breathe, not your food.

To help determine how well you breathe, in terms of how much oxygen you are taking in, try this easy exercise: Breathe normally and then hold your breath at the end of your exhalation. If you can hold your breath for one minute or more, you are in good shape. Most people can only hold their breath for 15 seconds, a certain indication that they are not breathing efficiently.

Simply put, the more fully and efficiently you breathe, the more energy you will have and the healthier you will be. This fact has been recognized for thousands of years by spiritual seekers, yogis, tai chi masters, and healers, all of whom have used the powers of proper breathing to not only improve their health, but to also transform their consciousness and improve the quality of their thoughts. In modern times, research has confirmed that various breathing techniques can help bring about altered states of awareness and profound healing.

Learning to breathe fully and consciously is known as breathwork, the benefits of which go far beyond improved physical health. Proper breathing can also improve your mood, enhance mental alertness, and help you become more aware of deeply held and often painful, unhealed emotions and beliefs. By working with a breathwork therapist many people find they are able to heal such emotions and the unresolved traumas of the past more quickly and completely than they expected.

Researchers in the field of breathwork therapy consider that the primary root cause of shallow, inefficient breathing for most people occurred when they were born. The moment of birth is often traumatic for newborns, and is the time when they are first forced to breathe on their own. Very often this breath comes in response to the harsh shock of being outside of the womb, an event that can be both painful and confusing. In order to cope with and suppress such pain, newborns typically follow their first inhalation with a pause, momentarily holding their breath as they struggle to make sense of their new environment. This pause can trigger a lifetime of shallow, inefficient breathing, and condition the newborn to suppress pain and its related emotions instead of breathing into them so that they can heal.

You can observe this pattern in yourself the next time you experience shock, fear, pain, or worry. If you take a moment to observe yourself at the onset of such events, you will most likely find yourself holding your breath or breathing very shallowly. By practicing breathwork, you can begin to change such patterns to that you begin to breathe more fully, and with greater awareness.

There are many approaches to breathwork therapy, ranging from age-old practices such as yogic breathing (*pranayama*) and the breathing exercises of tai chi and qigong, to a variety of modern-day methods developed by breathwork pioneers such as Gay Hendricks, Leonard Orr, and Stanislav Grof. All modern versions of breathwork incorporate a conscious focus on the breath, along with learning how to move the energy of the breath through the body in order to connect with and resolve suppressed emotions and limiting beliefs. In addition, all of such methods utilize what Leonard Orr calls "conscious, connected breathing," meaning that there is no pause between each inhalation and exhalation. Breathwork is best learned under the guidance and supervision of a trained and experienced breathwork therapist. Typically, 10 to 20 sessions with such a therapist is enough to be able to then incorporate conscious breathing into your daily life.

There are a variety of energizing breathing exercises you can also do on your own, such as the three I shared with you in Chapter 2. What follows is another excellent technique you can use to become more energized. Try experimenting with this exercise three times a day (morning, evening and before bed). As you do so, you will most likely begin to experience a noticeable improvement in your energy, your mood, and your mental clarity. This form of breathing involves chanting of the vowel sounds as done by the Tibetans and the Greek monks. You inhale deeply and then chant the vowels while holding your breath—A-E-I-O-U. You will feel the energy moving from your chest to your abdomen. After two minutes your blood pressure and pulse will drop.

Meditation: Renowned mind/body medicine expert Deepak Chopra has stated, "If you were to ask me what the most important experience of my life has been, I would say it was learning to meditate. Meditation has been the key to my creativity, well-being, and happiness."

Dr. Chopra's experience with meditation is not unique. An extensive body of research has documented the many physical and mental/emotional health benefits regular daily meditation can provide. Physical health benefits include improved immune function; reduced stress, including decreased levels of the stress hormones adrenaline and cortisol; reduced free radical production; increased oxygenation of the blood and tissues; lowered blood pressure and heart rates; improved brain and cognitive function; improved sleep; reduced frequency of headache and migraine; and relief from chronic pain.

Recently, researchers from the U.S., France, and Spain, working together, made the remarkable discovery that meditation is able to create these and other physical health benefits by creating specific positive changes at the molecular level of the body. Their research found that meditators exhibit a range of positive genetic and molecular differences, including altered levels of gene-regulating processes and reduced levels of pro-inflammatory genes, which in turn correlate with faster physical recovery from a stressful situation.

The mental and emotional benefits of meditation have also been well-documented by scientific research. They include greater relaxation, improved mood, improved ability to focus on and enjoy the present moment, enhanced creativity and problem-solving ability. Studies also demonstrate that people who meditate regularly exhibit heightened levels of spiritual awareness, greater clarity and insights about life issues, and increased feelings of compassion, gratitude, and connectedness with all of Life.

Elements of meditation can be found in all of the world's spiritual and religious traditions. Though meditation can seem foreign or difficult for some people, as Dr. Chopra says, "Our body knows how to be still; we just have to give it opportunity." Providing that opportunity is what meditation does.

Meditation techniques fall into two primary categories: mantra meditation, which involves mentally repeating a specific word or phrase, and mindfulness meditation, which entails the practice of focusing on the moment during the course of everyday activities. All forms of meditation, especially mantra meditation techniques, involve some degree of conscious breathing techniques. The following is an example of such a meditation technique that incorporates breathing.

Find a quiet place and sit comfortably in a chair, with your back straight and your feet flat on the floor. Close your eyes and begin to breathe slowly and fully in and out through your nose, starting each inhalation and ending each exhalation in your lower abdomen. Keeping your eyes closed, stay focused on your breath, allowing whatever thoughts you may have to come and go without being absorbed by them. If your attention should wander, simply return it back to the natural rhythm of your breath. You can enhance this process by silently repeating a positive word or phrase with each inhalation and exhalation

In the beginning, try to perform this meditation for five minutes twice a day, once in the morning, after you wake up, and once in the evening before you go to bed. As you become more familiar and comfortable doing so, gradually work up to 20 minutes of meditation twice daily. Don't be discouraged if at first you find meditating difficult. For most people, sitting still and breathing without external stimulus can initially be challenging. With continued practice, however, you will begin to notice and better appreciate the benefits that daily meditation can provide.

In contrast to the above type of meditation, mindfulness meditation methods can be performed at any time as you go about your daily activities. The goal of mindfulness meditation is to become more conscious of our thoughts, emotions and actions. Although we often fail to recognize it, much of our daily activity tends to occur from unconscious, automatic, habitual behavior patterns. An excellent example of this is what usually occurs when we travel to work. We nearly always take the same route to work each day and upon arriving would be hard pressed to recall what we saw and passed along the way. Instead, our journey to work occurs mostly on automatic pilot as our thoughts and attention stray elsewhere.

By not paying attention to the present moment, our minds have a tendency to wander, and very often habit takes over without much conscious decision making. As Deepak Chopra points out, each of us has an average of 50,000 thoughts per day and almost all of them are the same thoughts we had the day before. This means that we are not only operating unconsciously most of the time, but we are very likely doing so from a foundation of unexamined, limiting thoughts and beliefs, causing us to *react* to life instead of consciously shaping our place within it.

The practice of mindfulness meditation can help you cease acting and reacting out of habit, dramatically enhance your awareness of all that is occurring in your life moment by moment, and afford you a much greater opportunity to recognize and change the habits that keep you from experiencing what is most important to you, including greater health and energy. As the spiritual teacher Thich Nhat Hanh, a leading proponent of mindfulness meditation, states, "Our true home is the present moment. If we really live in the moment, our worries and hardships will disappear and we will discover life with all its miracles."

In teaching mindfulness meditation, Thich Nhat Hanh often recommends we simply witness ourselves breathing. As he explains, "Our breathing is a stable solid ground that we can take refuge in. Regardless of our internal weather—our thoughts, emotions and perceptions—our breathing is always with us like a faithful friend. Whenever we feel carried away, or sunken in a deep emotion, or scattered in worries and projects, we return to our breathing to collect and anchor our mind. We feel the flow of air coming in and going out of our nose. We feel how light and natural, how calm and peaceful our breathing functions. At any time, while we are walking, gardening, or typing, we can return to this peaceful source of life. We may like to recite: 'Breathing in, I know that I am breathing in. Breathing out I know that I am breathing out.'

"We do not need to control our breath. Feel the breath as it actually is. It may be long or short, deep or shallow. With our awareness it will naturally become slower and deeper. Conscious breathing is the key to uniting body and mind and bringing the energy of mindfulness into each moment of our life."

Though it can prove difficult to remain mindfully aware at most times, by getting in the habit of practicing mindfulness for a few minutes periodically throughout the day you will soon find yourself becoming more aware of the continuously changing happenings, sensations, thoughts, and feelings in your life. This, in turn, will give you more control over your experiences, freeing you from negative, stress-inducing reactions that sap your energy and lead you astray from your goals.

Any moment in your day can be an opportunity to mindfully meditate, including driving to work, walking, waiting in line, and so forth. Mealtimes are also excellent times to cultivate your practice. All too often, most of us engage in other activities as we eat, barely noticing what we are doing. To practice mindful eating, begin by noticing yourself seated at the table, along with your surroundings. Then notice the food before you, including its colors, textures, and flavors. Then pay attention as you chew your food. Instead of "wolfing" it down, chew each bite fully and completely. Not only will this practice make you more aware and appreciative of the food you eat, it will also improve your digestion.

As you become more accustomed to being present and mindful of your experiences, you can apply the same principles of mindfulness as you interact with others. Doing so typically results in more effective communication with others, greater appreciation of them, improved relationships, less stress, and more energy.

Stress Management for a More Energized You

Mark Hyman, MD, describes stress as "the body's inability to produce energy for the mind to react to its environment." I agree.

The amount of stress you experience and how well you cope with it is largely due to your lifestyle choices. What follow are simple, yet highly effective, lifestyle tips you can use to both reduce stress in your life and manage it better. By incorporating the following guidelines into your daily routine you will soon begin to feel and be more stress-free.

Be sure to get enough sleep and try go to bed at the same time each night. (See below.)

Don't skip breakfast and be sure the foods you eat are healthy for you.

Exercise for at least 30 minutes for a minimum of three days each week.

Schedule your day so that you have free time to relax and spend with your loved ones.

Find a hobby you enjoy and commit to pursuing it on a regular basis.

Know what's most essential and important in your life and commit yourself to it instead of wasting time on matters that are unimportant.

Identify your fears and worries and examine them objectively. In most cases, you will find doing so will make them far less significant and much more manageable. (For more on this, see Chapter 5.)

Set up your daily schedule so that you have plenty of time to devote to your daily tasks, instead of having to hurry to meet your responsibilities.

Don't be afraid of compromising, especially about matters that aren't significant.

Once you decide to do something, act on it as soon as possible. Hesitations about taking action can dramatically ramp up your stress levels.

Cultivate laughter in your daily life and make a conscious effort to find the humor in things.

Regularly socialize with friends and family members, and make a commitment to be more loving.

Regularly engage in relaxation exercises and/or meditation.

Avoid the use of alcohol, caffeine, and comfort foods when you do feel stress. Such things are unhealthy for you and serve only to numb your problems temporarily, not resolve them.

Don't be afraid to discuss your situation with your family or friends, or to ask for help if you need it. Be assertive in the requests you make so that you are treated with respect and taken seriously by others. And keep in mind that everybody is stressed to some degree. Recognizing this fact makes it easier to realize that the stress you may be experiencing is far from unique. By sharing your issues with others you will likely discover answers to your problems from those who have also faced them. In turn, you may also be able to provide them with your own helpful insights. After all, we are all in this experience of life together.

From the above list of guidelines, choose at least one item that you can do today and put it into practice. Then, try to incorporate at least one more item into your daily lifestyle every few days. Do this at your own pace, *but be sure to do it.* As you do so, over time you will find that you are increasingly living a less stressful lifestyle without needing to work at it. All that is required to do so is making the commitment to try each of the above guidelines that have relevance to you and then repeat them on a regular basis.

Managing Stress with Diet and Nutrition: Poor diet can cause and worsen symptoms of stress. To combat stress, your diet needs to be free of all foods to which you may be allergic or sensitive, as well as food additives, sugar, sodas, and simple carbohydrates. Instead, emphasize the dietary recommendations I made in Chapter 7. Also be sure to eat a healthy breakfast, as skipping breakfast can add to stress levels by making you more tired and irritable.

During times of stress, also be sure to increase your intake of magnesium-rich foods, since magnesium is quickly depleted in times of stress and acts as a potent anti-stress nutrient. Such foods include nuts such as almonds, Brazil nuts, cashews, and walnuts; green leafy vegetables such as beet greens, kale, spinach, and Swiss chard; and grains such as brown rice, millet, quinoa, and rice. Seaweed, especially kelp, is also very rich in magnesium, and can be used as a seasoning. Most of these foods are also alkalizing when they are digested.

Also be sure to drink plenty of pure, filtered water throughout the day, and minimize your alcohol intake to no more than one glass of red wine or beer per day. You should also limit your caffeine intake, since too much caffeine can over-stimulate you, leaving you feeling "wired" and more susceptible to stress. If you drink coffee, try to keep your daily intake to one cup daily. Or you can try substituting green tea, instead. Green tea also contains caffeine, and is rich in healthy compounds, including L-theanine, an amino acid, and *epigallocatechin gallate*, an antioxidant, both of which can help lower stress hormones. Other useful tea choices for stress include chamomile, peppermint, and valerian root, which is also an excellent aid for a good night's sleep.

The following nutrients can further improve your ability to cope with stress: vitamin A, B-complex vitamins, vitamin B6, vitamin B12, vitamin C, vitamin E, and magnesium. Essential fatty acids (EFAs) are also important, especially omega-3 oils. If you suffer from hypoglycemia, add chromium, and the amino acid glutamine (1000 mg three times per day, half an hour before each meal).

Other Stress-Busting Tips: Physical exercise is another excellent means of reducing stress, so long as you do not overdo it. One of the easiest exercises you can use to release stress is to go for a walk. Besides being one of the most effective ways to exercise, walking can also be very relaxing. In addition, many people who regularly take walks find that it helps them to come up with new solutions to their challenges and problems.

You can also try laughing your troubles away. Studies have shown that genuine laughter reduces stress and the production of stress-related hormones while simultaneously boosting immune function. Laughter also provides us with what psychologists call "cognitive control," a term used to describe being able to influence how we respond to external events. Although the events themselves may be beyond your control, laughter enables you to shift the perspective from which you perceive such events so that they become less stressful and even humorous.

Another way of coping with stress is by keeping a journal. Research shows that regularly writing in a journal is a very effective way to become more aware of one's thoughts, emotions, and beliefs, as well as for providing insights and solutions to one's problems.

Conscious breathing is another one of the stress-release methods available to all of us. The next time you notice that you are stressed or feeling tension in your body, close your eyes for a few moments and allow yourself to take ten deep breaths. Learning to do this on a regular basis throughout the day can pay big dividends and keep stress at bay.

Numerous studies have shown that listening to music you enjoy can banish stressful feelings within minutes. Ideally, choose music of a relaxed tempo and listen to it while lying down with your eyes closed. The effect physiologically can be very similar to meditation. Music with a strong percussive beat can also be helpful, as it lends itself to dance movements. Don't be afraid to engage in such movements by yourself. Just a few minutes of doing so can often be all that is needed to jump-start a more positive, energized frame of mind. Listening to such music is an excellent way to boost your physical energy, as well.

Lastly, eliminate the word "stress" from your vocabulary. It too often is used as an excuse by people to explain their less than optimal behaviour. It is better to say, " I am challenged." and please re-read chapter 6 as often as you need to. Master that chapter and you master your life.

Sleep: The Most Important Hours for Revitalization

As Wayne Dyer states in his book, *Wishes Fulfilled*, "Sleep is the time when your conscious mind leaves the world of your five senses and joins in with your sub-conscious mind. Your sub-conscious mind responds to what has been programmed into it. We spend one-third of our life in this sleep state. This time can be viewed as a time that we receive instructions for how the other two-thirds of our life can unfold. We all want to run our lives smoothly. Therefore, a very important point is to maximally prepare ourselves to enter this natural sub-conscious state of sleep. How can we maximize the last five minutes of our day before we enter sleep? What should we think about? Do not review the day's frustrations and disappointments. Do not focus on how unhealthy you are, or on how you are not feeling as energetic as you used to be. Do not focus on thoughts that make you feel bad. This imprints your subconscious mind with thoughts of 'I am unhappy, I am frustrated, I am sick.' Your subconscious mind reacts with no desire to change your awakened state, so it will proceed to offer you experiences with what you have programmed it to do.

> "So you need to give it a different program, and you can do this best by starting with a new mindset in those precious five minutes before you fall asleep. Instead you need to program your subconscious mind with positive feelings and attitudes. Program it with how you would like your life to be. Think happy thoughts before you go to sleep. Think about your aspirations. Most importantly, you want to *assume the feeling* of what you want to occur in your life. You must tell yourself in those pre-sleep moments that your desires will manifest, and you must assume the feeling that they have already manifested. This begins the re-programming of your subconscious mind, which you can do every night before falling asleep."

Lack of, and poor, sleep is a big problem for so many people today. In fact, sleep problems rank with chronic fatigue and obesity as our nation's most common health complaints. Too many people either can't fall asleep or else they wake up in the middle of the night, or toss and turn, only to greet the morning feeling exhausted.

The importance of a good night's sleep cannot be overemphasized. Lack of sleep has been implicated in a wide range of health problems, including lowered immunity and a greater susceptibility to infections, increased stress and muscle tension, an increased risk of heart disease and certain types of cancer, increased weight gain, increased risk for developing type II diabetes, hormonal imbalances, high blood pressure, and impaired brain function. Lack of sleep also leads to a diminished ability to solve problems, decreased creativity, reduced productivity, and poor job performance.

In traditional Chinese medicine (TCM), sleep and its importance to health and regeneration is closely associated with the twelve major meridians and the organ systems that they correspond to. Each of these meridians is linked to two hours of the 24 hour cycle. The liver meridian, for example, is most active between 1 and 3 AM. In TCM, these hours are known as liver time, meaning it is then when the body's energy is most concentrated in the liver. If people tell me they wake up, or can't fall asleep between the hours of 1 and 3 then I know their liver energy is abnormal or imbalanced. Additionally, when people wake in the middle of the night and cannot get back to sleep, that is usually a sign of abnormal adrenal function.

A similar correspondence between optimum sleep and the body's natural 24-hour circadian rhythm has long been recognized by practitioners of Ayurvedic medicine. The term *circadian* is Latin and means "around a day." Circadian rhythms tend to follow the same cycles and patterns of the sun during a 24-hour period, and influence the times of day when you feel most awake and alert, as well as those times when you feel tired or sleepy.

The teachings of Ayurvedic medicine regarding sleep and circadian rhythm have been confirmed by modern science, which has found that many of the human body's neurological and endocrine functions follow this circadian rhythm, including the ideal sleep-wakefulness cycle. These findings show that for most people the ideal time for achieving the deepest, most restful levels of sleep and maintaining harmony with the circadian cycle begins between 9 and 10 PM. This finding substantiates the Ayurvedic teaching that eight hours of sleep beginning within that timeframe is much more restful than eight hours of sleep that begins after midnight.

Relatively few people today go to bed this early, however. If you suffer from sleep problems, though, I encourage you to try doing so. Going to bed earlier will eventually help you reset your biological clock and make it easier for you to wake up earlier feeling more restful, energized, and ready to be productive.

In addition to going to sleep earlier, in order to improve the quality of sleep, it is essential to know and address the various factors that can compromise healthy sleep. The most common contributing factors are:

- Poor diet and/or poor eating habits, such as eating late at night, can often cause or exacerbate sleeping problems. Excessive alcohol and caffeine intake can also cause sleep problems. Make sure to finish drinking alcohol four hours before going to sleep. Stop eating three hours before going to sleep.

- Legal medications, both prescription and over-the-counter, can similarly impair your ability to get a good night's sleep. These include beta- blockers, cold and cough medicines (they contain caffeine and synthetic stimulants such as ephedrine), oral contraceptives, synthetic hormones, and thyroid medicines. In addition, all drugs create a toxic burden on the liver and can impair other organ systems as well, making sleep more difficult.

- Food allergies and sensitivities can interfere with your ability to sleep peacefully and restfully and are a frequent cause of sleep disorders. Among the ways that food allergies and sensitivities can cause or worsen sleeping problems are the hypoglycemia (low blood sugar) they can cause, as well as increased histamine production. Sugar and carbohydrate foods are frequent triggers of food allergies that cause drops in blood sugar levels. This creates an adrenal stress reaction that puts the body in a state of stimulation characterized by jittery feelings and tension.

- Geopathic stress, refers to energy fields within the earth that are imbalanced and capable of disrupting the body's bio-electrical fields, and, therefore, the health of those who dwell near such areas. Manmade devices can also cause geopathic stress, as can power lines and power generators, due to the electromagnetic frequencies (EMFs) they emit. (For more about geopathic stress and EMF, see below.)

- Lack of regular exercise, which typically results in chronic muscle tension and the buildup of stress in the body, can make relaxing and falling asleep more difficult.

- Various psychological factors, including unresolved anxiety, depression, despair, stress, and grief, as well as positive emotions such as excitement and euphoria, can also interfere with your ability to get a good night's sleep. Such emotions can cause imbalances in your biochemistry, creating indigestion and other gastrointestinal problems, and interfering with the brain's ability to properly produce nerve signals and the production of hormones such as melatonin and serotonin that are necessary to restful sleep. Chronic stress can also cause depletion of the adrenal glands, further aggravating sleep disorders.

- Smoking, as well as secondhand exposure to cigarette smoke can interfere with healthy sleep because of the chemicals and nicotine cigarettes contain. Nicotine acts as a stimulant and can cause insomnia and other sleep disorders, while many of the other chemicals contained in cigarettes can create a toxic burden on the liver to further disturb healthy sleep patterns.

- Structural imbalances in your body, such as muscle tension and/or a misaligned spine, can contribute to sleep disorders due to how such imbalances interfere with the flow of nerve signals to and from the brain. They can also keep you awake at night due to the pain they cause in the muscles and joints. To help resolve structural imbalances, consider adding a few minutes of gentle stretching exercises to your daily routine (see above). For structural problems that you cannot resolve on your own, consider working with a massage therapist, bodyworker, chiropractor, or osteopathic physician. Yoga can also be very helpful.

- Over-stimulating yourself before you go to bed can make falling asleep more difficult. There are a variety of ways in which you can over-stimulate yourself, including late night exercise, watching television, or working on your computer, including checking your email. All of these activities serve to stimulate brain function by generating "busy mode" beta wave activity.

- The environment of your bedroom can also have a major influence on the quality of your sleep. Bedrooms that are excessively cold, hot, or humid, or which have poor indoor air quality and ventilation, can make healthy sleep difficult, as can sleeping in rooms that let in light from windows or other rooms, as well as sleeping on mattresses that are too hard, soft, or otherwise uncomfortable.

Guidelines For Achieving Healthy Sleep: The first step to improving the quality of your sleep each night is to create a healthy sleep environment in your bedroom. This means cleaning your bedroom at least once a week and washing blankets, sheets, pillow cases, etc., frequently as well, in order to prevent dust buildup and prevent mites. To further prevent dust build up consider using an air purifier in your home, and be sure that the filters on your heat ducts are professionally examined at least once a year and replaced as necessary.

Also be sure to allow for a flow of fresh air throughout your bedroom as you sleep. You can do this easily by keeping at least one window of your bedroom slightly open.

Sleep on a comfortable mattress, and be aware that you might be sensitive to the materials in your pillow, blankets, and sheets. As a general rule, cotton or wool blankets and sheets and feather pillows are healthier choices than the same items made from synthetic materials.

Make sure that the temperature in your bedroom is kept at a comfortable level. Temperatures that are too hot or cold can significantly interfere with your ability to get a good night's sleep.

Make your bedroom a place of sleep, not a place to watch television. Watching TV in bed keeps your brain in active mode, making falling asleep more difficult. In addition, keep your bedroom free of other electrical appliances, such as stereos, cell phones, computer, radios, etc.

Sleep in the dark. This means not only turning off your bedroom lights when you go to bed, but also making sure that curtains and shades are fully drawn as well to prevent outdoor light from entering your bedroom. Sleeping in complete darkness helps your body to produce the hormone melatonin, which is essential for healthy sleep, as well as many other functions in your body. The ideal position of your bed in the bedroom is so that you sleep with your head to the north.

In addition to creating a healthy sleep environment, other helpful steps you can take include not only going to bed earlier, but going to bed each night at the same time. By doing so, you will program your body to recognize that it is time for it to prepare for sleep and the restoration it provides.

Also, don't drink any fluids within two hours of going to bed. This will reduce the likelihood of needing to get up and go to the bathroom during the night.

Various herbal teas are also well-known for their ability to promote restful sleep. They include chamomile, hops, lemon balm, passionflower, skullcap, and valerian root, all of which can be prepared as teas. These herbs can also be used in combination to further enhance restful sleep.

A variety of nutrients are known to improve and restore sleep. These include B vitamins, magnesium, and an amino acid known as GABA (gamma-aminobutyric acid). GABA acts as a neurotransmitter and is widely distributed throughout your body's central nervous system. It is the most important and widespread inhibitory neurotransmitter in the brain, helping to prevent over-firing of nerve cells and decreasing overall neuron activities in the CNS. Over-firing can cause restlessness, spasmodic movements, irritability and anxiety.

GABA is also utilized by the brain to create tranquility and calmness through the brain's metabolic processes, supporting a relaxed state of mind, and therefore promoting healthy sleep when taken before bed-time. You can find GABA at your local health food store. A typical dosage ranges from 125 to 500 mg. Start at the lower level and work up to the higher level if necessary.

Another effective way to improve the quality of your sleep is to expose yourself to more outdoor sunlight. Researchers have established a definite relationship between sunlight exposure during the day and restful sleep at night. This is due to the interaction of sunlight with the brain's pineal gland, which is responsible for producing melatonin. Several studies have shown that melatonin production significantly drops, and in some cases can be completely inhibited, as a result of inadequate exposure to natural sunlight during the day.

Additional research has found that nighttime melatonin production is directly related to the amount of serotonin production produced during the day. Serotonin is sometimes referred to as the "feel good" hormone because of the sense of calm it produces in the body. Multiple studies have shown that people who spend most of their time indoors have lower levels of serotonin compared to people who regularly spend a bit of time outdoors. Less serotonin production during the day means less melatonin production at night, and therefore poorer quality sleep.

You can avoid this problem simply by making it a point to spend at least 30 minutes outdoors each day. Ideally, you should do so during the morning during the hours of 7 to 9 AM, as sunlight exposure during this time will trigger greater production of serotonin for the rest of the day, leading to greater nighttime melatonin production. Research has also shown that exposure to sunlight between 7 to 9 AM helps to maintain proper function of your body's circadian rhythms and biological clock. Finally, sunlight exposure helps your body to produce and maintain adequate levels of vitamin D.

If the above guidelines do not work, you may need to consider improving your sleep by supplementing with melatonin. Melatonin is secreted by your brain's pineal gland, with the highest levels of production occurring during sleep. Healthy sleepers produce adequate amounts of melatonin each night, while people who struggle to get a good night's sleep typically do not. For this reason, a growing number of physicians recommend melatonin supplementation on a temporary basis when sleep proves difficult to come by.

First, however, I recommend trying one of melatonin's precursors, L-tryptophan or 5-hydroxytryptophan (5-HTP). Both supplements can be taken an hour before you retire each night. L-tryptophan and 5-HTP are available at most health food stores. Use both according to label directions. For best results, combine either L-tryptophan or 5-HTP with vitamin B6.

Melatonin supplements are also available at your local health food store. I recommend they only be used under your doctor's supervision, Since it can promote sleep in as little as 30 minutes after it is consumed, you should only take melatonin at night, just before your bedtime. In addition, when you begin to use melatonin, your initial dose should be 1 MG. Most melatonin supplements come in a dose of between 1-3 mg per tablet. (**Note:** If you wake-up with a hangover after taking melatonin the night before, your liver needs further cleansing.)

Once you start to realize the benefits of melatonin, it is also advisable that you stop using it for at least two weeks, so that your body doesn't stop producing its own of melatonin. Then, if you still have trouble sleeping, you can start another cycle for another 2-4 weeks, still under your doctor's supervision.

Overlooked Threats to Your Energized Lifestyle

In concluding this chapter, I want to share with you three serious yet almost always overlooked threats to your health and energy—geopathic stress, electromagnetic frequencies (EMFs), and, the health of your teeth.

Geopathic Stress: As I wrote above, geopathic stress is caused by energy fields within the earth that are imbalanced, as well as various manmade devices and technologies, all of which can negatively impact the human energy field, and thus one's health. The term *geopathic* itself refers to pathologies, or diseases and energetic disruptions caused by being near areas of the earth that emit harmful radiation. Inner earth movements and earthquakes have brought about cracks and splits through which radiation escapes. The intensity of this radiation is increased at night, when there is a full moon, and when there is damp weather. Underground water under homes is another source of geopathic stress, and can undermine one's health.

As with much else to do with Energy Medicine, the underlying concept behind geopathic stress is not new. In fact, it has been recognized by many traditional cultures around the world for centuries, including in China, where the art of *feng shui* (the study of earth energies and their relation to health and overall human endeavor) was first developed. Feng shui practitioners are often called upon to select the most propitious places for new buildings, so that they are not built on or near land that emanates unhealthy energy.

Experts who study geopathic stress have found that it is caused by localized magnetic radiation from the earth, many of which are connected with geological fractures, large mineral deposits, and underwater passageways, especially such waterways that intersect with each other. Research dating back to the early 1970s has confirmed that areas of geopathic stress exhibit increased magnetic anomalies, and also increase electrical conductivity in the surrounding air and soil that can negatively interact with the body's energy field. Such negative impacts to human health can occur even when the magnetic anomalies are small.

One large-scale study conducted by the U.S. Department of Health, Education, and Welfare in 1979, found that geopathic stress is a contributing factor in between 40 to 50 percent of all cases of cancer in the U.S. Overall, between 30 to 50 percent of all people who are chronically ill are affected by geopathic stress to some degree.

Every organ system can potentially be impaired by exposure to geopathic stress. Common symptoms related to such exposures include chronic fatigue, lowered immunity, respiratory problems, an excessive need for sleep, headache, cold extremities, anxiety, depression, and otherwise unexplained mood swings. Sleeping above or near geopathic stress zones can also seriously interfere with healthy sleep. Cancer patients are particularly susceptible to geopathic stress and EMF's, and care must be taken to minimize these stressors.

As mentioned, various manmade devices are geopathic stressors. Common examples include electric clocks, electric blankets and heating pads, appliances in the bedroom (computers, TVs, radios, stereos), and heated waterbeds. For people who are particularly sensitive, even metal bed frames can be a factor, as can bedrooms situated above garages, steel girders, and fuel tanks. Household electrical current can be a factor, as well. The advent of smart meters and WiFi have also significantly increased the risk of geopathic stress. Because of this, it may be advisable to disconnect your home WiFi connection before going to bed. Some health experts even recommend turning off the home's circuit breaker before sleep for people who are ill.

You can use a gauss meter to determine if manmade geopathic stress is affecting you where you live, while natural causes of geopathic stress can often be determined by dowsing or feng shui practitioners. For more information about how you can create and maintain a healthy home environment, I recommend contacting the International Institute of Bau-Biologie and Ecology (IBE). *Bau-Biologie* means *"building biology"* or *"building for life,"* **and, like feng shui, explores the** relationship between buildings and the environment. You can locate someone trained in Bau-Biologie by visiting IBE's website: http://hbelc.org.

Finally, if you have pets, notice where dogs sleep in your home, as this is the area where the energy is optimal. We call this energy right spin or clockwise spin. Where cats sleep is the worst energy in the home (left spin or counter-clockwise spin).

Electromagnetic Frequencies (EMFs): The dangers of EMFs are closely related to geopathic stress and can greatly compound problems caused by it. Due to the advances in modern technology we live in a world burdened by a new kind of electromagnetic radiation pollution, which some health experts have termed *electrosmog*.

The advent of electrosmog first dawned in 1879, when Thomas Edison invented the first incandescent light bulb and went on to bring electric light to the world. Since that time, a wide array of new inventions that run on electromagnetic frequencies, ranging from radios and TVs and numerous other home appliances, to cell phone and WiFi devices and their networks that criss-cross the globe, have led to our entire planet being continuously bathed within an invisible array of energies that a growing body of research indicates can be potentially harmful. Moreover, with the increasing proliferation of wireless handheld and portable devices, it is literally impossible to escape EMF exposure in most towns and cities today.

The reason that EMFs pose a threat to your health stems from what you learned in Chapter 2—your body is first and foremost a system of energy, with all of your cells, tissues and organs dependent upon bioelectrical signaling for their communication with each other. Additionally, the adult human body is approximately 70 percent water and contains a high mineral content, making it highly conductive and susceptible to electrical impulses. External electric and magnetic currents that are not in harmony with the body's own energy field are capable of disrupting its coherence and healthy bioelectrical activities.

Olle Johansson, a neuroscientist at the Karolinska Institute in Sweden, has spent more than 30 years researching EMFs. As he explains, "If you put a radio near a source of EMFs you will get interference. The human brain has an electric field, so if you put sources of EMFs nearby it is not surprising that you get interference, interactions with [the body's] systems, and damage to cells and molecules."

People whose health is compromised by EMFs often suffer from what today is known as electrical hypersensitivity syndrome. This condition was first reported during World War II among radar operators in Russia. A decade later, in Australia, after television was introduced there, researchers reported a noticeable and rapid increase in cancer rates among people who lived near television transmission towers. Similar links to cancer and proximity to transmission towers, as well as electrical power lines, have since been reported by scientists all around the world. More recently, a similar increase in cancer rates, including brain cancers, has been shown as a result of regular cell phone use for five years or longer (talking on cell phones for 30 minutes or more each day), especially among children and young adults. (The manufacturers say their studies show that cell phones are not harmful; however the length of most studies is one year.)

Cell phones operate on microwave frequencies, a fact that many people do not know. Research dating back to the 1960s has proven that microwave radiation, such as that emitted by cell phones, causes a weakening and opening up of the blood-brain barrier. Moreover, the radiation from cell phone antennas has been shown to cause genetic damage.

Many of these initial findings about cell phone usage was discovered by George Carlo, Ph.D, M.S., J.D, a public health scientist, epidemiologist, lawyer, and the founder of the Science and Public Policy Institute. Between 1993 and 1999, Dr. Carlo headed a $28.5 million research program funded by the cell phone telecommunications industry. After he presented his research findings, the industry refused to heed them, and subsequently set about trying to discredit him. They also hired lobbyists, who played an initial role in crafting and getting Congress to pass the Telecommunications Act in 1996. This law prohibits citizens and municipalities from preventing the placement of cell phone towers near their populations based on their health concerns.

The full scope of the dangers posed by EMFs was brought home in 2007 with the publication of a 650 page report released by the Bioinitiative Work Group. The report cited more than 2,000 scientific studies that documented the effects of EMFs on human health, including DNA damage, immune system impairment, and an increased risk for cancer ranging from brain cancer to childhood leukemias. Exposure to high-intensity EMF radiation, such as from power lines (within 50 feet of your home or work), was also found to increase the risk of miscarriage.

As a result of these findings, the European Environmental Agency urged immediate action to reduce public exposure to EMF radiation from cell phone and cell phone towers, as well as from WiFi. Other countries have since followed suit to some degree, including Israel and

Canada. Here in the U.S., however, both the telecom industry and government health agencies continue to insist that further investigation is necessary to determine whether such actions need to be taken. For the most part, the US mainstream media and medical establishment concur with this.

Based on my own experience as a practitioner of Energy Medicine, I am unwilling to have my patients wait for a change in attitude by government and industry regarding EMFs. Instead, I encourage them to do all they can to proactively reduce the health risks linked to EMF exposure. This includes limiting themselves to talking on their cell phones to less than 30 minutes each day, to text or use headphones or the speaker phone option on their phones, and to avoid using their phones when the coverage signal is not strong. Weak signals with fewer signal bars means cell phones have to increase the amount of radiation they emit in order to broadcast their signals.

I also encourage my patients, and you, to consider using cell phones with a low specific absorption rate (SAR) rating. The higher the SAR rating, the more thermal energy cell phone emit. You can find a list of cell phone SAR ratings by obtaining a free report offered by the Environmental Working Group. It is available at www.ewg.org/cellphone-radiation.

Other helpful steps include considering replacing WiFi at home with Internet cable; getting rid of cordless phones in the home (the EMF risks of such phones come from their base, not their handset, as it is the base that emits the radiation), or to at least position the base away from bedrooms or near to where you spend most of the rest of your time at home; avoiding the use of microwave ovens; installing a kill switch in bedrooms to turn off the electricity that runs through bedroom walls; and keeping cell phones, as well as other devices that operate on and emit EMFs, out of the bedroom. Using a gauss meter to measure your home EMF levels is also advisable, as is turning off your home's circuit breaker before bed, especially if your utility company has installed a smart meter to monitor your home energy use. Working with a bau-biologist can also be helpful.

For people whose health is particularly affected by EMFs, other options include painting the interior of their homes with EMF shielding paint, placing EMF shielding film on windows and glass doors, and using shielding material to line drapes and curtains. You can find source for these and other products that product against EMF exposure at http://emfsafetystore.com.

Finally, to help counteract EMF exposures, try to regularly spend time outdoors, away from cell towers and power lines. Walking barefoot on grass or the beach for at least 15 minutes ("earthing") can go a long way toward being helpful in this regard, and also leave you feeling happier and more energized.

Your Teeth and Your Health: Perhaps the most surprising factor that can potentially impact people's energy and overall health is their teeth. Today, further confirmation of the relationship between dental and overall health can be found in the growing body of scientific evidence showing that bacterial plaque on teeth, and gum diseases such as gingivitis and periodontal disease, can significantly increase the risk of heart disease and various other health conditions.

The fact that the condition of one's teeth and oral health can, and often does, negatively impact health may seem strange until you accept that all parts of your body are interrelated. This fact was first recognized thousands of years ago by the originators of traditional Chinese medicine, who recognized that each tooth in the mouth corresponds to a specific organ in the body. The ancient tenants of TCM regarding teeth and the rest of the body were rediscovered by the late Dr. Reihard Voll, whose work I introduced you to in Chapter 2. In addition to developing the technique now known as electrodermal screening, Dr. Voll also used this method to prove that every tooth corresponds to a specific acupuncture meridian and its related organ system, and to joints and glands. Using Energy Medicine, he found that if a tooth became diseased or decayed, the organ it corresponds to could also become unhealthy. Conversely, he also found that weak organs can result in negative impacts on their corresponding teeth. I have long verified Dr. Voll's findings in my own practice of Energy Medicine with my patients.

We all know people who have had dental infections for many years, which have not triggered illnesses. Also many people have had mercury fillings for years, and have not gotten ill because of them. The explanation here is that these people are energetically strong enough to compensate for the toxic burden. However, if additional stressors occur (diet, trauma, emotional stress), or as these people get older with lessened ability to compensate for these stressors, illness will occur.

Other dental factors that can also have negative impact on your health include root canals, electrogalvanism, and TMJ (temporomandibular joint) syndrome. Root canals, like the use of dental mercury amalgam fillings, is a common practice in conventional dentistry today. Holistic, or biological, dentists, however, have long pointed out that 100 percent of root canal procedures result in the buildup of residual infections that enable bacteria to penetrate into the jawbone, as well as into the bloodstream, where they can affect other organs and tissues. Hal Huggins, DDS, one of the most acclaimed pioneers in the field of biological dentistry, points out that, because the environment of a root canal lacks oxygen, it allows bacteria to proliferate and undergo changes that can produce potent toxins that can cause further harm to other parts of the body.

Another pioneering dentist, the late Weston Price, former Director of Research for the American Dental Association, found that people with heart or kidney disease who also had root canals very often were cured of their conditions when the root canals were removed. Based on such findings, Dr. Huggins has stated that, "Extraction of root canal teeth should be the first thought when considering the health of the patient." He stresses, though, that when such teeth are removed, that the periodontal ligament that attaches the teeth to the underlying jaw bone also needs to be removed, in order to completely eliminate pockets of infection. Full removal of root canal teeth and ligament causes the old bone to begin producing new bone for healing. Once extracted, and the area is cleared of any infection, a bridge or an implant will be needed.

A Swiss study found that 93 percent of women with breast cancer had a root canal in the molar tooth on the same side as the breast cancer. This corresponds to the stomach meridian which also runs through the thyroid gland.

Electrogalvanism in the mouth occurs as a result of saliva interacting with any dental filling that contains metal. Saliva contains minerals, making it electrically conductive. Thus, as saliva interacts with metal fillings a type of battery effect is created, with the saliva acting as an electrical conductor. Over time, this can cause the fillings to erode, much like battery terminals, with the toxic material they contain leaking into the body. This is one more reason why I am opposed to the use of conventional dental amalgam fillings, and why I recommend that patients who have such fillings have them removed.

When I first started practicing energy medicine in 1987, I had a patient who complained of hearing radio stations all day (without listening to the radio). He could only sleep in a trailer by the beach. I thought he was crazy. When the dentist took out all of his mercury fillings, (the electrogalvanism was causing him to tune into radio stations) the music stopped. That was an eye-opener for me.

Electrogalvanism in the mouth can be detected with the use of Energy Medicine devices (for more about them, see Chapter 9), as well as by the use of a electrogalvanometer, a device that measures the electrical current and voltage generated by amalgams as they interact with saliva.

TMJ syndrome is another common health condition today. It is caused when the teeth, jaws, and muscles of the face become misaligned. Such misalignments typically occur as a result of tooth loss, teeth grinding (bruxism), and/or dental restoration procedures. Severe cases of TMJ syndrome can result in clicking sounds when the jaw moves, jaw pain, and difficulty opening and closing the mouth. But many other symptoms can also occur because of TMJ syndrome, many of which are not usually connected with the mouth and teeth, such as depression, lack of energy, back and neck pain, headache, insomnia, and impaired concentration and other cognitive functions.

To determine if your dental health is negatively impacting your overall health, and to address any dental issues you may have, I highly advise working with a dentist who specializes in holistic or biological dentistry. Ideally, your best option would be to work with a biological dentist who is also trained in the use of Energy Medicine tools and techniques. You can find such dentists in your area by contacting the International Academy of Biological Dentistry and Medicine (www.iabdm.org) or the Holistic Dental Association (www.holisticdental.org).

Having read this far, you can see that there is a lot that is involved when it comes to creating a truly natural, energized lifestyle. If most of what you have learned in this chapter is new to you, I advise that you don't try to implement it all at once. Instead, take your time and identify the areas above that may most require your attention. Start by addressing these areas first, taking care not to overwhelm yourself by doing too much at once. Then, as you make progress, continue to incorporate other of the above methods and tools that I have shared with you. Remember, it's the tortoise who won the race, not the hare. The slow play is the best play. By being consistent, you will create your own momentum, your health will continue to improve, and so will your energy.

Key Points To Remember

When it comes to creating an energized lifestyle, the essential first step is to engage in regular exercise and physical activity. Doing so can contribute more benefits to health than almost any other health practice, both physical and mentally/emotionally.

There are four elements that comprise an effective overall exercise program: aerobic exercise, strength training, stretching, and working with your core.

Conventional aerobic exercise has now been shown to offer less benefit than a new type of aerobic exercise known as high intensity interval training, or HIIT. Moreover, the superior benefits that HIIT can provide can be achieved in far less time than traditional aerobic exercise requires.

Proper diet and nutrition are also essential components of an effective exercise program.

In addition to exercising regularly, calming and working to focus the mind is also vital for becoming naturally energized. Two of the most effective methods for doing so are the daily practice of meditation, and the use of energizing breathing exercises performed periodically each day.

Adequate amounts of sleep is also essential. The most beneficial time for regenerative sleep begins between 9 and 10 PM. Sleep can also be enhanced by going to bed and rising out of bed at the same time each night and day.

A variety of foods, nutrients, and herbal remedies can also be used to promote deep, restful sleep, as can supplementing with melatonin under a doctor's supervision.

Learning how to manage and properly deal with stress is the final component needed for creating an energized lifestyle. Here, too, diet and nutrition can play important roles, as can regularly socializing with family and friends whose company you enjoy, spending time on your hobbies or other activities you enjoy, taking a walk, keeping a journal, and listening to music, as well as meditating, working with your breath, getting enough sleep, and exercising.

Even when all of the above elements of a healthy, energized lifestyle are adopted, other hidden factors can still sap your energy and health. Three of the most overlooked elements are geopathic stress, exposure to EMF radiation, and issues with your teeth, mouth, and jaw. Determining if any of these three factors are affecting you is therefore also vitally important.

CHAPTER 9

Essential #5: Regenerate With Energy Medicine

"In every culture and in every medical tradition before ours, healing was accomplished by moving energy."

~ Albert Szent-Gyorgi, MD, PhD, recipient of the 1937 Nobel Prize in Physiology or Medicine, and the discoverer of vitamin C

I have been practicing Energy Medicine since 1986. Having read this far, you know that I utilize many different treatment modalities in my medical practice, including nutrition, homeopathy, herbs, acupuncture, heavy metal detoxification, sensory resonance, low level laser, pulsed electromagnetic fields, photons, ionized oxygen, and natural hormone replacement therapy. Varied as these therapies may seem, from my perspective they all are forms of Energy Medicine because they all help to balance and maximize each patient's energy system.

I did not start out as a practitioner of Energy Medicine or anti-aging medicine. In fact, in 1986 I was a burnt out ER doctor. When I added all the hours of all the shifts that I worked in the ER, I had spent the equivalent of three full years living in a hospital! For most of my ER years, there were no trauma centers in L.A. The trauma cases went to the nearest ER. They used to call me Dr. Trauma, for I seemed to attract those cases, whenever I worked.

In that same year I came across an opportunity in Los Angeles, where a holistic clinic was looking for a medical doctor to do general practice and nutrition. I knew general practice from my time as a doctor in the emergency room, but didn't have a clue about nutrition. I set about learning nutrition, reading everything I could get my hands on. I took countless seminars, listened to numerous audiotapes, and hired a nutritionist to help me. I figured the best way to start was to obtain blood tests that showed the foods that people were allergic to. I reasoned that if I identified the allergic foods and had my patients avoid those foods, they would get better. But I was wrong. Nobody felt better, nobody lost weight, and their GI symptoms of gas, bloating, and constipation persisted.

In those days, I never asked why people were allergic to the foods their blood tests indicated. Could it be that they were allergic to those foods because of poor food combining choices? Were they eating those foods every day, even two to three times a day, because they were addicted to the body's reaction to those foods? Were they tired because they ate far too many carbohydrates? Did they gain weight because they ate too many carbohydrates, and not enough healthy fats? It was only later, as my self-initiated learning continued, that I came to recognize the importance of such questions.

I also thought that if you showed patients how to optimize nutrition, and encouraged them to regularly exercise, they would regain their health. One of my patients who followed that advice, yet did not improve, was my best friend, Bill. Concerned, I ran many new blood tests, and one of them showed that Bill had an elevated mercury level. His old amalgam fillings were leaking.

Back then, when I drew blood from the patient, I sent it to a lab in Colorado, and got a detailed report as to what metals were and were not compatible with the patient's blood, in order to replace the old fillings. I had heard an expert on mercury toxicity speak, and got a referral to a local biological dentist. When I met the dentist, I learned that he also practiced electro-acupuncture, meaning that he used a device that measured changes in skin resistance. This was new to me.

He explained that the principle behind electro-acupuncture was similar to technology that exists with the polygraph. When you lie on a polygraph test, your skin resistance changes and the needle squiggles. When a substance is not compatible with your body, your skin resistance also changes when tested using an electro-acupuncture device. In this case the dentist used it to determine which metals were and were not compatible with Bill. The results of his electro-acupuncture testing exactly matched the blood tests I had previously obtained for Bill. This was my first introduction to Energy Medicine and its benefits.

So impressed was I with the accuracy of the results of the Energy Medicine testing device the dentist used, as well as the ease by which he was able to obtain them, that I committed myself to becoming a practitioner of Energy Medicine, as well.

In this chapter, you will learn more about how and why Energy Medicine's tools and techniques can be so effective for not only evaluating, but also for treating, illness and energetic imbalances. Then you will be introduced to three very useful Energy Medicine therapies, as well as an effective Energy Medicine technique that is growing in popularity because of its effectiveness in measuring how well a person is responding to the various external stressors that can affect the nervous system, and in monitoring the effectiveness of any treatment.

My optimism about the future of Energy Medicine can best be explained by biophysicist James Oschman, PhD, a leading researcher in the field of Energy Medicine, who wrote that, Energy Medicine "includes techniques that are often capable of resolving medical issues that are difficult to diagnose or treat by other means. The public is attracted to Energy Medicine because the techniques provide excellent healing at all stages of disease, from pre-symptomatic to chronic and intractable. Moreover, the treatments are very cost-effective, are generally noninvasive, and have few if any lingering side effects." Dr. Oschman adds that, "the science behind energetic approaches is emerging as a rich and fascinating topic with major implications for prevention [of disease] and longevity." I agree.

Energy Medicine and the "Living Matrix"

Let me ask you a question.

Do you know what your body's most extensive organ is?

Most people, including many doctors, do not, and chances are you may not have even heard of it before. It is called *the connective tissue matrix* or, as Dr. Oschman has dubbed it, simply "the living matrix". It consists of both the body's connective tissue and fascial systems, as well their extensions into the nuclear matrix of all of the body's cells. Your skin, arteries, capillary and intestinal wall lining, immune cells, are all also part of the living matrix.

The connective tissue and fascial systems are closely interconnected. Connective tissue is found throughout the body and includes fat, cartilage, bone, and blood. The main functions of the connective tissue, depending on its type, include providing support for the musculoskeletal systems, protecting organs, and aiding in the transport of substances through the body. Connective tissue is composed of cells and protein fibers suspended in a gel-like material that is also called a matrix. Blood is a liquid connective tissue composed of a fluid matrix and blood cells. The fluid part of the blood, known as plasma, transports hormones, nutrients, and waste products, and plays a role in regulating body temperature.

The fascial system is a continuous structure that runs along the entire length of your body. In appearance it is similar to a spider's web. Fascia is very densely woven, covering and interpenetrating every muscle, bone, nerve, artery and vein, as well as, all of your internal organs including the heart, lungs, brain and spinal cord.

The cells within the living matrix (essentially your entire body), when they communicate with each other, do so under the control of "living light" particles known as biophotons. When heavy metals and other toxins become lodged in the matrix, Dr. Oschman and others have discovered, the biophoton-mediated process of cellular communication becomes impaired. This is because the toxins embedded within the living matrix create abnormal electromagnetic impulses that act as disruptive, inharmonious frequencies that negatively impact the ability of cells and tissues to function properly. Unless this disruptive process is halted and reversed via appropriate drainage and detoxification, using such methods as those you learned about in Chapter 7, before long the cells and tissues become overburdened, leading to biochemical changes that affect the body's organs and cause disease.

Using Energy Medicine to Evaluate Imbalances and Illness and Greatly Improve Treatment

Although few conventional physicians will admit it, even their most sophisticated diagnostic devices and tests can, and often do, fail to detect illness early enough in their patients until the cascade of disease has advanced to a state where it is much more difficult to treat. I touched on this fact in Chapter 2 when I discussed how many patients are told that they are healthy based on the results of conventional diagnostic tests, even though the patients, themselves, continue to experience symptoms that are not present when they are well.

As you also learned in Chapter 2, the primary reason for this disconnect between what a patient is experiencing and the results of his or her conventional diagnostic tests has to do with the fact that such tests only measure changes from a physical level (imaging studies) and chemical level (blood tests), not an energetic, or electrical level. All disease begins as a *dis-ease*, or imbalance in a person's energy field and flow of the life force in the body's energy pathways. This fact is something far too many physicians and other health experts today still fail to recognize or pay attention to. Most of the patients that I see come in complaining, "I don't feel well", even when the results of their imaging and blood tests are normal.

First, using a device called electrodermal screening (which you learned about in Chapter 2), I can quickly and accurately detect energetic imbalances in my patients' organs and acupuncture meridian systems.

By placing a noninvasive probe at the tip of a patient's finger, I can determine if there is a change in the skin resistance when various substances are introduced into the circuit. The substances can be dilutions of organs, specific toxins, foods, etc. If there is a change in the skin resistance, then I can conclude that energy in the organ is sluggish (I am not diagnosing a disease), or that there is a sensitivity to a food or a toxin. More importantly, it can alert me to when further testing, such as blood work, x-ray, CT-scan or MRI, is advisable. This is true preventive medicine, and is one of the reasons so few of my patients ever manifest serious illness.

The most important result of this kind of testing is that I am able to quickly and accurately determine which is the most effective treatment for the patient. I am always looking for two things - the treatment must be **effective**, and it must be **tolerated** (no side effects). Many treatments are effective, but not tolerated. One example is cancer chemotherapy. It is effective in killing cancer cells, but produces many side effects.

Here are some of the benefits of this type of energy testing:

Identification of a key toxin that is weakening the body.

Identification of allergies.

Detection of food sensitivities.

Determining which key negative emotion is preventing healing.

Finding the correct herbal, homeopathic, or nutritional supplements which will be most beneficial for the patient.

Finding which antibiotic is most effective and tolerated by the patient.

Finding which antidepressant is best to give the patient.

Finding which blood pressure medication has the least side effects.

The ability to test all supplements and pharmaceutical drugs that a patient is taking, to make sure that no side effects occur.

The result of these benefits is a healthier and happier patient!

By interacting with the body at its biophotonic, energetic level, Energy Medicine devices can quickly identify the specific toxins and other factors that are involved in this process, making it easier to treat them most effectively. In addition, these Energy Medicine tools can help neutralize the processes of chronic inflammation that toxins in the body typically cause.

Of equal, if not greater, importance, scientists now know that, when the body is in a state of good health, its cells and the elements they contain within them vibrate at a dynamic and complex harmonic rate. These cellular frequencies can be measured and analyzed using Energy Medicine devices, detecting when they become altered, which sets the stage for disease. Then, healing frequencies from various therapeutic Energy Medicine devices can be introduced to the body, helping to return these cellular frequencies to their healthy, dynamic state. In many ways, these devices achieve this result in much the same fashion that Star Trek's Dr. "Bones" McCoy tricoder device worked in the original 1960s TV series. If only Gene Roddenberry, Star Trek's creator, could still be with us to see how something he imagined so many years ago is now no longer science fiction, but science fact!

As you now understand, Energy Medicine devices offer a wide range of superior benefits, both in evaluating energy flow and helping to guide therapy, compared to many conventional medical approaches. Earlier detection of illness and imbalanced energy, ease-of-use, greater accuracy in choosing appropriate remedies and treatments for each individual patient—all of these and other benefits are available to physicians today should they be willing, as I was many years ago, to investigate and learn about Energy Medicine and how to use Energy Medicine devices. For now, that willingness is not common among the overall medical profession, yet I remain confident that, as science continues to confirm our primary nature as "beings of energy", not chemistry, that an increasing number of my peers will soon join me here on the frontiers of true, cutting-edge, noninvasive medicine.

Applied Kinesiology and Muscle Testing: Instant Energetic Feedback

Applied kinesiology (AK) was developed by the late Dr. George Goodheart, Jr, a chiropractor who, in 1964, discovered that testing specific muscles in the body enabled him to detect imbalances in his patients' organs and glands. By stimulating or relaxing muscles he was able to accurately diagnose and resolve many of their health problems. As a result, he began educating other chiropractors, and eventually other health professionals, and spent the rest of his life researching, refining, teaching, and writing about AK. Because of Dr. Goodheart's efforts, AK is used today by an estimated one-third of all chiropractors, as well as many physicians, including myself. Since its advent, AK has led to the development of other types of muscle testing, as well.

AK and all other forms of muscle testing work by assessing strength resistance of specific indicator muscles related to an organ, gland, or other part of the body. If the muscle tests strong, meaning that it can hold its resistance, this indicates that the corresponding body part is healthy, whereas if it tests weak it may indicate dysfunction, infection, the presence of toxins, or an energetic imbalance in the area of the body being assessed. Such testing provides practitioners of AK with immediate feedback from their patients' own bodies about their overall state of health.

One of the leading experts in, and educators about, applied kinesiology is Robert Blaich, DC. "Because of the close clinical relationship between specific muscle dysfunction and related organ or gland dysfunction," he explains, "applied kinesiology can be used to identify and treat a wide variety of health problems, whether the problem originates in a muscle, gland, or organ. In applied kinesiology, the muscle-gland-organ link can indicate the cause of the health problem and lead to further diagnostic tests for confirmation. Once the problem is identified, it can be treated by a variety of [AK] techniques to strengthen the muscles involved and restore health."

To better understand the relationship of your muscles to your health and body function, consider what happens when you bend your elbow. In order to do so, your bicep needs to "turn on," while your tricep must "turn off." If both of these muscles are turned on or off at the same time, you elbow either will not bend, or will not do so properly. This process of muscles turning on and off occurs with all normal physical activity. Sometimes, however, muscles become stuck on or off, leading to muscle weakness and stress. This, in turn, can impair the function of the organs or glands to which they correspond. Conversely, should an organ or gland weaken due to any cause, the muscle that corresponds to it will very often weaken or become stuck on and off, as well.

Muscles that are stuck on are tense, can spasm, and can often be painful. An example of a muscle stuck on is the calf muscle during a "charley horse." If you've ever experienced one, you know precisely what I mean. Frozen shoulder and tennis elbow are other examples of stuck muscles.

A number of factors can contribute to impaired muscle strength and function beyond physical injury and trauma. Such factors, all of which can be determined by AK, include spinal misalignment, nerve interference between the spine and muscles, lymph congestion and impaired lymphatic drainage, biochemical imbalances, heavy metals and other toxins, and organ or gland dysfunction. In some cases, abnormal pressure on cerebrospinal fluid can also affect proper nerve supply to muscles, as can blockages in the body's meridian system. If any of these conditions exist, muscles in the body will typically exhibit weakness or abnormal function when tested.

AK practitioners look to achieve a number of goals when working with their patients. First, they use AK to determine their patients' health status (including checking for the above-mentioned factors), correlating their findings with past patient history and any conventional diagnostic tests that AK testing may indicate are needed. Once this assessment is made, AK can then be employed to restore patients' posture and balance, range of motion, and gait. AK has also been shown to be effective for correcting organ, nerve, endocrine dysfunction, as well as improving digestion, respiratory function, and various other body functions.

AK is also effective for detecting food allergies and sensitivities, and for assessing the most nutritional and herbal supplements for each individual patient. For such testing, the patient may hold a sample of the food or supplement up near the chest or place it on his or her tongue. If muscles test strong when this occurs, then the foods and supplements that are tested are appropriate for that person. Muscle weakness during testing, by contrast, indicates that the foods and supplements should be avoided. A number of scientific studies have verified AK's accuracy for testing foods and supplements. One large-scale study published in the *International Journal of Neuroscience*, in 1998, for example, found that blood testing following AK testing for food allergies showed antibodies in the blood to the foods that AK testing had identified the test subjects were allergic to. (In response to an allergic substance, your body produces specific antibodies to neutralize and eliminate it.)

In many respects AK acts in much the same way as the Energy Medicine testing devices above do. The main differences are that AK is based on the interrelationship of muscles with organs, glands, or other body parts, instead of the body's energetic meridian pathways, and obviously AK does not require such devices. Though I find Energy Medicine devices offer a greater degree and range of diagnostic and treatment benefits than AK does, I make use of both methods in my practice, and recommend AK to others, especially those who do not have access to health practitioners trained in the use of Energy Medicine devices.

To locate an AK practitioner in your area, contact the International College of Applied Kinesiology (ICAK) at www.icakusa.com or, if you live outside the United States, www.icak.com.

Acupuncture: Smoothing Out the Body's Energy Flow

As you learned in Chapter 2, acupuncture is one of the oldest and most comprehensive forms of Energy Medicine. Given its widespread use around the world, it is also the most popular Energy Medicine technique today. Although its acceptance in the U.S. by the medical establishment did not begin until the 1970s, its use was endorsed nearly a century earlier by Sir William Osler, who is known as the father of American Medicine. In the edition of his book *The Principles and Practice of Medicine*, published in 1882, Osler wrote, "In lumbago, the treatment of preference is acupuncture."

Today, Western scientists have verified acupuncture's effectiveness as a treatment for a wide variety of health conditions. Based on this research, the World Health Organization (WHO) now recommends acupuncture as a helpful treatment for both acute and chronic symptoms of:

Respiratory Disorders, including asthma, emphysema, bronchitis, allergies, sinusitis, laryngitis, cough, common cold and flu.

Circulatory Disorders, including hypertension (high blood pressure), anemia, arteriosclerosis and angina pectoris.

Musculoskeletal and Neurological Disorders, including spasms, tendonitis, carpal tunnel, weakness, rheumatism, arthritis, low back, neck, and shoulder pain.

Gastrointestinal Disorders, including constipation, chronic diarrhea, gastrointestinal weakness, indigestion, anorexia, gastritis, colitis, Crohn's disease, bloating, vomiting, and food allergies.

Urogenital Disorders, including prostatitis, incontinence, urinary tract infections, and sexual dysfunctions.

Gynecological Disorders, including painful menstruation, infertility in both men and women, and menopause.

Eye, Ear, Nose and Throat Disorders, including decreased vision, glaucoma, tinnitus, and vertigo.

Post-operative problems, including nausea, mental fogginess, and depression.

Other disorders, including fatigue, adrenal "burn-out", headaches, insomnia, addiction, and skin problems.

Acupuncture has also been shown to be helpful for treating illnesses triggered by environmental factors such as environmental toxins, pesticide poisoning, and radiation. It can also be helpful for weight loss.

Two other notable areas for which acupuncture is increasingly being used is as a supportive treatment for cancer, and for treating soldiers injured on the battlefield. For cancer patients, acupuncture can significantly reduce the nausea and vomiting which are common side effects of patients undergoing chemotherapy, and/or using various other cancer drugs. For many patients these side effects can seem worse than cancer itself, and many oncologists can attest to the fact that the very thought of further chemotherapy treatments can cause some patients to vomit. Because of the growing number of studies confirming acupuncture's benefits in this area, a number of cancer treatment centers and hospital now routinely administer acupuncture before, after and in between chemotherapy treatment sessions to help control patient nausea and vomiting.

That acupuncture is a powerful tool for general pain control is also well-known. Less known, however, is the success it can have when used to alleviate cancer-related pain. This is another reason why acupuncture is now often recommended for cancer patients.

Because of acupuncture's pain-relieving benefits, the US military has recently begun using a specific type of acupuncture, known as Battlefield Acupuncture, to help alleviate soldiers' pains due to their injuries. According to Colonel (Ret.) Richard Niemtzow, MD, PhD, MPH, Director, United States Air Force Acupuncture Center, "The expanded use of acupuncture on the battlefield is being met with enthusiasm from physicians and patients because it works. Acupuncture may be used as a primary modality or as an adjunct to Western medicine. In either case, it is changing the face of military medicine as a force multiplier".

Col. Niemtzow was a co-author of a chapter entitled "Acupuncture in Military Medicine" in the book *Acupuncture in Modern Medicine.* The chapter reports, "On the front line, acupuncture has been used to treat PTSD and mild TBI [traumatic brain injury] at the Concussion Restoration Care Center (CRCC), Camp Leatherneck, Afghanistan...The former director of CRCC reported that, of the troops he personally treated, a majority of them experienced improvements in sleep and decreases in anxiety levels and frequency of headaches."

The chapter also highlights the effective use of acupuncture to treat military members for pain and pain-related ailments, including phantom limb pain, sleep problems, stress, and various psychological issues. Currently, acupuncture is being used at the Acupuncture Center at Joint Andrews Base, the National Intrepid Center of Excellence in Bethesda, Maryland, the Warrior Transition Brigade at Ft. Hood, in Killeen, Texas, the Integrative Medicine Center (IMC) at Ft. Bliss, in El Paso, Texas, the Naval Medical Center San Diego, California, and Wounded Warrior Program at Naval Hospital at Camp Pendleton, in Oceanside, California.

In light of the many important benefits that Western science has documented THAT acupuncture provides, what is sometimes lost when discussing it is something that bears emphasizing: The primary and original intent behind acupuncture is not the resolution of diseases and their symptoms, but, rather, *the maintenance and restoration of the proper flow of the body's vital energies.* Acupuncture, along with all other aspects of traditional Chinese medicine is based on the idea that no single part can be understood except in its relation to the whole. A symptom, therefore, is looked at as a part of a totality of the person and whatever factors may be affecting him or her, not as an isolated event. If a person has a complaint or symptom, acupuncturists seek to know how the symptom fits into the patient's entire being and behavior, as well as his or her past, and, most importantly, what energetic imbalances are present that need to be addressed.

Recapping what you learned about regulation in Chapter 3, too much and too little energy flow can result in poor health and disease. Examples of this fact can be found in a number of disease condition symptoms, such as high (too much) or low (too little) blood pressure or blood sugar levels, or hyper- and hypothyroidism, which are characterized by excessive or inadequate thyroid hormone production, respectively. Such imbalances tie into the ancient Chinese medicine theory of *yin* and *yang*, the twin aspects of vital life force energy known as *qi*. Health results when both of these aspects are balanced and in harmony with each other, which is what happens when qi is able to flow unobstructed through the body's meridians, or energy pathways.

A reflection of this healthy balance of energies can be found in pregnancy. In this example, yang, or male creative energy, can be likened to the sperm, while the receptive, female yin energy resides in the ovum (egg) and overall female reproductive system. Lack of yin energy can lead to a woman's inability to conceive, and low male yang energy will also result in infertility. An ideally healthy, fulfilling pregnancy occurs when both the male and female energies are in balance and in harmony with each other.

It is out of this philosophy of balance and health that ancient Chinese saying, such as "An ounce of prevention is worth a pound of cure," and "The best time to dig a well is before you are thirsty," arose. In the latter saying, digging a well represents addressing and maintaining one's health, while being thirsty equates to being sick. Unlike conventional Western medicine doctors, traditional Chinese doctors focus on prevention of disease, not its treatment. In the past, in fact, TCM doctors were only paid to keep their patients well; in cases where patients became sick, the doctors were expected to work for free until their patients' health was restored.

Because of acupuncture's ability to correct energetic imbalances before they become chronic and lead to disease, I recommend that you consider receiving regular preventive acupuncture treatments, just as I recommend the use of Energy Medicine testing preventively. By working with an acupuncturist whose focus is on prevention and the proper flow of qi, you will be taking a significant step forward along your road to outstanding health.

Today, acupuncturists, including physicians such as me who are trained in its use, can be found in most towns and cities across the U.S. When choosing an acupuncturist there are two factors I recommend you consider: How much training he or she received before beginning to practice, and, more importantly, how much experience he or she has.

Clinical Homeopathy: A Few Drops Can Make All the Difference

Homeopathy is a school of medicine founded by the German physician Samuel Hahnemann, M.D. (1755-1843). His experimental research and practical studies for homeopathy were carried out between the years of 1798 and 1818, culminating in the publication of Hahnemann's first major work, *The Organon*. The term *homeopathy* itself means "like suffering," whereas conventional medicine is often called *allopathy*, meaning "treatment with opposites".

Hahnemann's two fundamental propositions, which are unique to homeopathy, are:

1. The action of homeopathic preparations is determined by observing the objective and subjective symptoms which occur when they are administered to healthy human subjects in toxic doses.

2. The action of homeopathic preparations in the healthy subject constitutes their therapeutic potential with respect to the sick, meaning that the symptoms which they cause, they can also cure. When administered to sick people in order to cure symptoms, these homeopathic preparations are given in microdoses. This is known as the Law of Similars.

Let us rephrase the Law of Similars to: *Any substance which produces illness when administered in a strong dose to a healthy person can cause the disappearance of the same illness when administered in a weak dose to a sick person.* For example, a strong dose of Ipecac induces vomiting; in a homeopathic weak dose, it is a remedy for people with nausea and vomiting. Coffee prevents sleep in most people; in a homeopathic dose it is used to treat insomnia. Opium causes constipation; in a homeopathic dose it is used to treat constipation. Conventional medicine's methods of vaccination, immunization, and allergy desensitization act on similar principles, and thus are in accord with homeopathic law.

Homeopathy made great strides in the United States during the late nineteenth century. By 1900, 15 percent of American physicians were practicing homeopathic medicine. In large part, the popularity of homeopathy in the U.S. at that time was due to Dr. Constantine Hering, considered the father of American homeopathy. In the mid-19th century, Hering discovered that healing in homeopathy occurs in a set pattern:

1. Healing proceeds from the deepest levels (mental and emotional as well as vital organs) to more superficial sites (the skin and extremities); i.e., from the inside out.
2. Healing flows from the upper part of the body to the lower part.
3. Healing progresses in the reverse chronological order from the original presentation of symptoms.

According to the first part of Hering's discovery, a cure is generally in progress when the status of the emotional state and vital organs improve, even though skin symptoms may become worse. In the second part, or law, a patient is considered improved when arthritic pain in the neck has improved, even though there is no change in his knee pain. The third law states that patients will frequently re-experience old symptoms from their past during the healing process.

Homeopathic medicines are prepared in a very specific way. The initial or original substance is diluted in nine parts of water and then vigorously shaken 10-20 times. This is a 1/10 dilution, or 1X. To make a 2X dilution, one part of the 1/10 dilution is mixed with nine parts of water and again shaken 10-20 times. Other systems utilize a 1/100 dilution in lieu of the 1/10 dilution. This is known as centesimal dilution and is designated 1C (1/100), 2C (1/10,000), etc. Other dilutions such as LM and Korsakov are used less in the United States than in Europe.

The shaking process, called *succussion*, is vital in the preparation of homeopathic substances, for it seems to impart energy to the mixture. Homeopaths frequently use substances as dilute as 200X (or 200 dilutions of 1/10). It is believed that each succussion step imparts more energy to the mixture, so, although the 200X is extremely dilute, it is exceptionally potent. Because of their energetic nature, homeopathic remedies are intended to rebalance disturbances in the human energy field which are causing the physical symptoms. This is why they are so effective in not only eliminating the symptoms of a disorder, but bringing about lasting relief.

Critics of homeopathy usually dismiss it based on its Law of Similars ("like cures like"), as well the fact that many homeopathic remedies are so dilute that they no longer contain any physical trace of the original substances from which the remedies are derived. Such criticisms are usually levied by critics who lack a true understanding of the principles of Energy Medicine. In any case, mainstream scientific research is now confirming both the Law of Similars and the mechanisms of action that make homeopathy effective.

Some of the best research validating the Law of Similars has been conducted by Roeland van Wijk and Fred A. C. Wiegant. In one of their studies they investigated the recovery process of various cell cultures. In the study, the cell cultures were exposed to either the toxins arsenic or cadmium, or heated at damaging temperatures. Van Wijk and Wiegant measured the levels of stress proteins that the cell cultures produced in response to these exposures. They then demonstrated that the cell cultures, which had been damaged as a result of what they were exposed to, recovered more quickly when they were re-exposed to the same toxins in diluted form, or when they were very slightly reheated. The results of these experiments substantiate Hahnemann's original observations that "like cures like".

Various researchers have also offered a number of scientific models to explain homeopathy's mechanisms of action. The most recent, and for me most exciting, model is based on the biophoton research conducted by Fritz-Albert Popp, who discovered that coherent light energies (biophotons) are emitted by all living organisms, including cell systems. Based on Dr. Popp's discovery, biochemist and naturopathic physician Dr. Karin Lenger has theorized that homeopathic dilutions achieve their health effects because of the release of biophotons from the parent substances from which the remedies are made, whose strength increases with each increased dilution. According to Lenger, this results in a resonance (vibration amplification) phenomenon between the biophoton frequency of the original substance and the frequency in the body when it has been unbalanced by illness.

To test her theory, Dr. Lenger used magnetic resonance to place different high-potency (meaning more diluted or succussed) homeopathic remedies within a strong magnetic field. What she found was that each remedy resonated differently, and kept its own magnetic resonance, or energy signature. Based on her findings, Dr. Lenger states that homeopathic biophotons are bound to their carrier molecule (typically either water or sugar) by their magnetic poles, and, because these biophotons are magnetically bound with their characteristic properties, homeopathic remedies contain "information" that can bring about healing by regulating the electromagnetic field of the body based on the principle of resonance. Dr. Lenger's research has also proved that the highest energy of homeopathic remedies is found in those that are most highly succussed and highly diluted.

My own response to critics of homeopathy is simple: Information is a message. A message may tell a cell or organ to move into a regenerative mode. Frequencies and vibrations are also examples of information. Homeopathy is an example of how a different remedy can provide different information to the body. Conventional medicine, without realizing it, uses homeopathy every day in treating patients with angina. For this treatment, nitroglycerin 1/150, is given sublingually (under the tongue). This is an example of a drug prepared in a dilution that is really homeopathic.

Types of Homeopathy: Today, there are three main approaches to homeopathy: classical homeopathy, complex homeopathy, and clinical homeopathy. Classical homeopathy seeks to match the specific signs and symptoms of the patient (physical, emotional, and mental) with the known effects of a homeopathic remedy. In classical homeopathy, the practitioner prefers to use one remedy at a time in a high potency. After taking one dose, the patient waits four to eight weeks before the effects are clear to the practitioner. A second dose or a different remedy is prescribed only after the first dose has ceased its action (this may take several months). This type of practice is very difficult to master, requiring years of study and research before proficiency is attained. Classical homeopathy is intolerant of any other form of homeopathy, especially of clinical homeopathy.

Complex homeopathy frequently uses mixtures of low potency homeopathic remedies (1X to 20X) which are synergistic in action, meaning that they will work on specific organs or tissues; e.g., liver, pancreas, lymphatics, etc., simultaneously. Most practitioners of Energy Medicine use both classical and complex homeopathy in order to produce a more balanced effect.

Complex homeopathy attempts to approach the body from a physiological perspective (in a way similar to allopathic medicine), with one major difference. Whereas allopathic, or conventional, medicine seeks to treat symptoms by suppressing various physiological processes, complex homeopathy seeks to stimulate the natural healing symptoms of the body. Complex homeopathic formulas are composed of more than one ingredient (sometimes as many as 10 ingredients) in order to produce the most optimal synergistic effects to achieve the desired outcome.

Complex homeopathy acts to restore a patient's health through the following methods:

1. Stimulation of Drainage. Drainage refers to the process whereby blood flow to the organs of excretion (liver, lymph, kidney, lung, skin, colon) is increased by combining synergistically acting ingredients in low potency. The lower the dilution, the greater the chemical effects of the formula. Note we are talking about *chemical effects*, not energetic effects.

2. Stimulation of Detoxification. Detoxification seeks to remove toxins from their binding sites in the tissue into the blood, from where they can be excreted out of the body through the process of drainage. Detoxification can be accomplished with homeopathic dilutions of the specific toxins, or by homeopathic substances that have been found to neutralize the specific toxin.

3. Stimulation of Regeneration. Regeneration refers to the renewal of cells and tissues. It attempts to increase the length of the life

of the cell of the specific organ that is being regenerated, and increases the ability of the organs to regenerate themselves.

Complex homeopathy also attempts to balance the metabolism of a patient, not by giving hormones such as thyroid, estrogen, progesterone, prednisone, but by homeopathically stimulating the thyroid, adrenal, ovaries, etc. in order to maximize their function.

Clinical homeopathy involves using homeopathic substances for specific indications. One example is the use of *Arnica* for the treatment of bruising and trauma. Another example is the use of *Gelsemium* for stage fright. As for *Arnica*, it is very useful to stimulate healing from surgery when given as a 6X potency, twice a day for three days before surgery, and continuing for two weeks.

When it comes to regeneration, one might ask, Why not use nutritional supplements, herbs, vitamins, minerals, and foods to achieve it? Why use homeopathy? To answer this, we need to briefly review the biophysics of regeneration.

Each organ system, while connected to the essential life force of a person, is also a unique bioenergy system, vibrating at a certain resonant frequency. An imbalance in the organ's frequency represents a disturbance in its bioenergy, and slows the process of doing what the organ is intended to do on its own, to regenerate and renew itself. In order to stimulate regeneration, cells and organs need a specific input of energy of certain wave forms, which correlate to the weakened organ. They need the right amount of energy coupled with the right message.

The ideal regenerative remedy is a booster shot of subtle energy, which imprints the proper energy pattern into the matrix of that organ system, producing a message which ultimately returns that organ system to its natural resonant frequency. The best way to stimulate this process is through the use of homeopathy. We must remember that the concentrations of the key nutrients in the blood and in the intra-cellular fluid–which are necessary for cellular life to be sustained and renewed– exist in the range of micrograms, nanograms, and picograms.

Homeopathy also deals with micro-concentrations of substances which are necessary for cellular life to be sustained and renewed. By contrast, vitamins, minerals, foods and herbs first need to broken down, and thus require energy for their conversion to micro-nutrients before they can be used by the body. For many sick patients, these expenditures of energy for the processes of digestion and conversion to micro-concentrations, may further deplete their energy, thus impeding regeneration. Let us begin, therefore, with homeopathic microdoses and conserve energy.

Based on my personal experience proving homeopathy's effectiveness, I have made homeopathy a central part of my overall medical practice, and have developed my own product line of homeopathic remedies. Because of the ongoing research that continues to verify that homeopathy, in all of its varied forms, can be a very exciting modality to stimulate healing, I fully expect more doctors and other health professionals here in the U.S. will begin incorporating it into their practices in the near future. Eventually, my hope is that homeopathy will be taught in American medical schools and be officially included in our health care system, just as it is today in Britain, France, and other countries in Europe.

Heart Rate Variability: Tracking Energy Flow From the Heart

You are likely familiar with the use of electrocardiogram (EKG) by physicians to screen for heart problems. The EKG is a test that checks for problems in the heart's electrical activity and can be useful in detecting abnormally fast, slow and erratic heart rhythms, evidence of a prior heart attack, and impaired blood flow to the heart, which can be a sign of angina or an impending heart attack. Similarly, doctors often employ the electroencephalogram (EEG) to measure the electrical activity of the brain, and to screen for various brain disorders, including brain tumors, head injury, and dementia, as well as for epilepsy and signs of stroke. Both EKG and EEG are very useful tools.

In my practice, I also employ a different test, known as heart rate variability, or HRV. Heart rate variability refers to the pattern of your heart rhythms. HRV measures the subtle beat-to-beat changes in heart rate, with this measurement appearing on a graph as your heart rhythms. Since the late 1980's there has been increasing research into heart rate variability. HRV has become an important method of understanding the links between mind and body (behavior and biology).

Your heartbeat is constantly speeding up and slowing down. This is part of normal nervous system function and is what creates your heart rhythms. However, your heart's rhythmic pattern can be greatly affected by stress, as well as poor breathing habits, your thoughts, emotions and environment. Unlike your heartbeat rate, your heart rhythm pattern shows how stress, different emotions, and other factors are affecting your nervous system. This is important, because your nervous system controls and regulates all other systems in your body.

Essentially, the more variable your heart rhythm, the more each beat is slightly different in length from the preceding beat, the healthier your autonomic nervous system (ANS) is. The ANS is the subconscious part of your overall nervous system, acting as the autopilot of the body to control various physiological processes that we don't have to think about, like blood pressure, pulse, and breathing.

There are two parts, or branches, to the ANS—the sympathetic and parasympathetic nervous systems. Each branch has a different effect on your body's organs. The sympathetic nervous system (frequencies of 0.05-0.15 Hz) represents action and oversees your body's expenditure of energy, while the parasympathetic nervous system (frequencies of 0.15 – 0.5 Hz) is in charge of regulating your body's energy recovery, and is involved in rest, digestion, and healing.

When your body is at rest both the sympathetic and parasympathetic systems remain active. The actual balance between the two systems is constantly changing, however, as your body's regulatory processes work to maintain optimum functioning in response to all internal and external stressors. The test involves monitoring both the heart rate and its variability lying down for two minutes, and then standing up for two minutes. The standing up phase is the stress, as it is much easier for the heart to get blood to the brain lying down, than standing (because of gravity). The more often that each heart beat is slightly different in length from the preceding heart beat (both at rest and while standing), the greater the heart rate variability, and the healthier the parasympathetic nervous system (regeneration, relaxation, reserves).This test can detect how well my patients are able to adapt to stress, as well as show which treatment modalities will improve the health of patients (if a treatment improves heart rate variability, it is an effective treatment).

Research into HRV has shown that lowered HRV is associated with premature aging, decreased autonomic nerve activity, diminished hormone activity, and an increased risk of sudden cardiac death after acute heart attack. Other research has found that depression, panic disorders and anxiety are also associated with lowered HRV, and have a negative impact on autonomic function, especially the parasympathetic system.

HRV testing offers many benefits. It is noninvasive, very accurate and reliable, reproducible, and yet simple to do. As a result, I am confident that the use of HRV testing will continue to grow among conventional and integrative physicians alike. For more information, please go to www.intellewave.net and www.heartratevariabilityanalysis.com.

Key Points To Remember

Energy Medicine offers both diagnostic and therapeutic benefits that even the most sophisticated conventional medicine approaches simply cannot match.

By using Energy Medicine testing devices, physicians can not only detect the onset of disease much earlier than conventional medical testing can, they can also more accurately determine the causes of disease.

Energy Medicine testing also eliminates statistics-based "guesswork" when it comes to determining the proper remedy or remedies for each patient based on his or her unique needs. It can also determine the most effective types of other treatments that may be necessary for patient healing.

One of the primary reasons that explains Energy Medicine's effectiveness for both diagnosing and treating disease has to do with the body's largest organ, known as "the living matrix."

Connecting the body from head to toe, the living matrix and all of its trillions of cells is under the control of "living light" particles known as biophotons. By interacting with the body at its biophotonic, energetic level, Energy Medicine devices can quickly identify the specific toxins and other factors that impair cell function and communication, making it easier to treat the disease most effectively.

In addition to Energy Medicine devices, three primary Energy Medicine-based therapies that can provide major health benefits are applied kinesiology, acupuncture, and homeopathy.

Heart rate variability testing is another diagnostic tool based on the principles of Energy Medicine. Using HRV, physicians can quickly monitor and assess the status of a patient's autonomic (subconscious) nervous system and how stress, different emotions, and other factors may be affecting it, and also assess the effectiveness of any therapy.

CHAPTER 10

Essential #6: Hormonal Happiness

The sixth essential key to creating outstanding health is balancing your hormones and keeping your endocrine glands in a state of optimal health. Many people fail to recognize that there is a major distinction between the major hormones of the adrenal glands, thyroid gland, and pancreas (insulin) , and the minor hormones—the sex hormones. All of these hormones are important to your health, yet addressing what I call the major hormones is the first priority.

In Chapter 3, you learned about your body's endocrine system. In this chapter we are going to take a closer look at the most important endocrine glands, and the hormones that they produce and regulate. Then, I will cover what you need to know about balancing and maintaining healthy levels of your sex hormones, as well as human growth hormone. To begin, let's look at what hormones actually are.

A clue to the importance of hormones to your health can be found in the origination of the word *hormone* itself. It is derived from the Greek word *hormon*, which means "that which sets in motion," and from the name of the ancient Greek spirit *Horme*, who personified energetic activity, impulse and effort. Hippocrates spoke of *hormon* when describing vital principles of health and healing, while Carl Jung referred to *Horme* when he wrote and spoke about the mental energy that drives unconscious activities and instincts.

From the perspective of medicine, the word *hormone* means "to arouse or excite". That's because hormones are the chemical messengers in your body which, once they are secreted and enter the bloodstream, tell your cells what to do. Hormones oversee and regulate virtually all of the countless processes that your body performs each day, ranging from the cognitive functions of your brain to the pace and rhythm of your every heartbeat. They do this by binding with the appropriate receptor sites of the cell membranes of their target organs, in much the same way that a key fits into and turns a lock. Once this binding process occurs, hormones produce a wide range of health-enhancing effects on both the metabolism and the overall functioning of the target organs. As I tell my patients, hormones tell the body what to do with the information it receives from the outside (your external environment).

When it comes to staying young and healthy, the most important hormones are cortisol, DHEA, insulin, and the thyroid hormones, followed by the sex hormones estrogen, progesterone, and testosterone, along with human growth hormone. An imbalance or decline in these hormones plays a major role in the onset and acceleration of a host of both physical and mental/emotional illnesses and their symptoms. From my perspective, this is where conventional medicine has erred. In medical school, doctors are taught that hormone imbalances and declines in hormone production occur as an inevitable consequence of aging. This isn't so. Our hormones don't decline because we age. Rather, *we age because our hormones decline.* Understanding this difference is very important.

Researchers have long known that one of the primary mechanisms involved in the aging process is the decline in naturally occurring hormones in the body, first manifesting in our 30's, and then accelerating as we enter our 50's, 60's, and beyond. Since hormones affect virtually every bodily process, low levels of certain hormones and impaired communication within the endocrine system, create havoc with all other body systems, including the immune, cardiovascular, detoxification, and gastrointestinal systems. Chronic illness is also frequently associated with the body's decline in hormone production.

Similarly, in our society we often refer to people as they get older as "old and cranky," and, in many cases, with good reason, because so many people today as they reach their 40s and 50s *do* start to exhibit "cranky" behavior. Part of the reason—often the main reason—for this is a decline in hormone production. It is the endocrine, or hormonal, system of the body that most correlates to our mental and emotional make up. As an expert in hormone therapy who has been involved in this area of health care for many years, it is clear to me that our bodies' hormonal system responds to our outlook on the world *and also influences that outlook.*

Again, this is very important. By restoring my patients' hormone levels to optimal levels, they become much more positive, both mentally and emotionally. Their zest for life returns, and they become happier, more joyful, and more excited and passionate about the days and years ahead of them. So, how is it that hormones become imbalanced and decline? As with your body's energy levels and energy production, the answer lies with the same major culprits.

How Your Hormones Are Affected by Toxins and Stress

There are a variety of factors that negatively impact your body's endocrine system and its production of hormones. They include a sedentary, unhealthy lifestyle, poor diet, food allergies, poor sleep and sleep habits, the long-term use of prescription medications, exposure to electromagnetic fields (EMFs), lack of sunlight, and, of course, environmental toxins. All of the above factors fall into the two overriding categories of toxins and stress.

It is a sad fact of life for most people that the amount of stress they experience each year tends to increase, while all of us incur accumulating toxic exposure due to the amount of toxins in our air, water, soil and food supplies. As we've discussed, your body's primary internal organ charged with dealing with toxins is the liver. Your kidneys and lymphatic system also play significant detoxification roles, as well. In an ideal environment, these organs would have little difficulty in coping with and eliminating toxins.

None of us live in an ideal environment, however. Toxins are everywhere, even in the most seemingly pristine regions around the globe. A newborn baby has 200 chemicals in his/her blood. Breast milk contains over 200 chemicals. As a result, sooner or later, the body's organs of detoxification start to struggle and eventually become overwhelmed by the burden of toxicity. When they do so, they put out a call for help to the endocrine system. They say to the endocrine glands, "Come on, secrete more hormones and help us work a little harder." In response, the glands say, "Okay," and start secreting more adrenal hormones and thyroid hormones and so forth. But, since our exposure to toxins is an ongoing, daily occurrence, eventually the endocrine glands get tired`. Ultimately, what happens is you get a toxic body with very weak hormonal glands. And that's your setup for fatigue, a lowered sex drive, and chronic illness.

This same cascade of events occurs due to chronic stress, which is also rampant today. Most people are on the go all the time. Right now the goal in our society appears to be to work as hard as we can to be as successful as we can, regardless of the consequences and toll on our bodies. This creates huge amounts of stress, ultimately resulting in poor sleep and most likely fast foods. Travel takes its toll, as well, especially air travel, which exposes us to unhealthy, re-circulated air and ionizing radiation, jet lag, and so on (please take 1,000 mg of vitamin C every hour while travelling in an airplane to keep your immune system strong). The standard American diet (SAD), which is wholly lacking in vital nutrients and full of toxic additives, along with too much coffee and alcohol, too many soft drinks, and too much sugar, and not enough healthy water, further compounds matters. Add to this mix the fact that most people are not taking enough vitamins and other supplements and when you put it all together it's no wonder that, as a nation, we don't feel well, and that hormonal imbalances and deficiencies are so widespread.

Based on the above, you can see why addressing hormone deficiencies and improving hormone levels and hormone balance is such a vitally important key to restoring optimal health and putting the brakes on accelerating, premature aging. Doing so not only results in noticeable health gains in the near future, it also lays the foundation for continued health and vitality for many more years to come.

How the Health of Your Adrenal Glands, Pancreas and Thyroid Determine Your Health and Energy

Earlier in this book, you learned how important your liver is, both in terms of your health and also your energy levels. Now I want to show you why your pancreas, thyroid and adrenal glands are also important. Like your liver, they too are often overlooked by conventional medicine. Or, again like the liver, conventional medical testing may deem them to be functioning normally when, in fact, from the perspective of Energy Medicine, they may be woefully out of balance and in serious need of attention.

To better understand the importance that each of these glands play in your health, let's examine each of them in turn.

The Adrenal Glands

Your adrenal glands, which are triangular in shape and located above your kidneys, act as your body's energy reservoir. They play an integral role in both your energy levels, your ability to handle stressful situations, and your overall health. They also are essential for proper functioning of your immune system, proper production of white blood cells, and muscle strength and tone.

Your adrenals are composed of two parts, the inner region, which is known as the adrenal medulla, and the outer region, which is called the adrenal cortex. The adrenal medulla is responsible for producing and regulating a class of stress hormones known as *catecholamines*, which include adrenaline, noradrenaline, and dopamine. Catecholamines help your body respond to emotional upheavals, stress, low blood pressure, low blood sugar levels, exposure to extreme temperatures, lack of oxygen, and danger, all of which can activate the "fight or flight" response.

The hormones produced by the adrenal cortex are known as steroidal hormones. There are three classes of steroidal hormones: *mineralcorticoids*, which help regulate your body's fluid balance via regulation of the kidneys as they interact with sodium and potassium; *glucocorticoids*, which help metabolize carbohydrates, proteins, fats, and sugars, as well as helping to maintain proper blood pressure levels; and the sex hormones (androgens and estrogens), which oversee the health of your sex organs.

Today, one of the most common health conditions I find among my patients is adrenal fatigue, also known as adrenal burnout. Adrenal fatigue is epidemic in our country. In traditional medical practices adrenal failure is recognized as a disease called Addison's disease. In fact, President John F. Kennedy had Addison's disease and treated it with cortisone for years. We're not talking here about adrenal failure, but about adrenal fatigue which occurs when the adrenals are depleted. Yet it is definitely not being detected in most medical practices. Physicians don't look for it. They don't properly diagnose it, and they don't treat it correctly.

When patients come to me and complain about lethargy, fatigue, lack of energy or a reduced sex drive, or that they just don't have the same energy or the same sex drive, in almost all cases at the root of their problems, especially if they are past their thirties, can be traced back to impaired adrenal gland function. So working to restore and optimize their adrenal function is usually where I start. The reason for this is because, in the body, the adrenal glands and the hormones they produce represent survival, whereas the sex hormones basically represent reproduction. Survival is always more important than reproduction. So the body will do whatever it takes to maximize adrenal hormone output and survival. With that in mind, the body will convert the sex hormones into adrenal hormones to maintain survival at any cost, which is why when you are stressed and tired, your sex drive goes down. So you really can't go straight to the sex hormones (progesterone, testosterone, and estrogen) before you look at the adrenals. You've got to maximize adrenal function first.

If you have weak adrenals you are facing a serious health issue because, in many ways, the adrenal system is the key system to your overall health. For example, when a woman is pregnant and chronically stressed, she will start converting her own progesterone (of which she is producing high levels during pregnancy) into the adrenal hormones. By month seven of her pregnancy, the baby's adrenal glands kick in. At that point, if the woman's adrenal glands are operating at a subpar level, her body will start to draw upon the baby's adrenals. This causes the baby's adrenal glands to start revving up to supply the excess adrenal hormones that the mother needs.

Then, at birth, when the umbilical cord is cut, the mother is unable to continue to receive a boost of adrenal hormones from her baby. This is often the underlying cause of postpartum depression and fatigue. Compounding this problem, very often the newborn child may then become hyperactive, develop colic, or other health problems, all as a result of how his or her developing adrenal gland system was affected by the mother's stress, while the baby was in the womb.

Adrenal fatigue is caused primarily by chronic stress and poor lifestyle choices. Chronic stress can, and often does, overwhelm the adrenal glands' ability to generate and regulate stress hormones. When it comes to adrenal fatigue, or burnout, the two most important hormones produced by the adrenals which need attention are cortisol and DHEA. Initially, when you are stressed, your cortisol levels go up, and if you are the kind of person who takes stress home, you may have a hard time sleeping due to your cortisol levels remaining elevated at night, when they should be low. This, in turn, interferes with your body's ability to produce melatonin and growth hormone, both of which promote healthy, restorative sleep.

When we encounter a stressful situation, cortisol and DHEA are released as part of the regulation response. But during times of chronic stress the production and release of these stress hormones begins to slow down, ultimately leading to lower levels of these key hormones, and adrenal fatigue. When the adrenal glands are weak we no longer view stress as a challenge, we view it as a threat, which is why at that point we overreact to the little stressors. Then we can't differentiate between big stress and little stress. Ultimately the weakened adrenals set the stage for a move towards illness and disease.

Left unchecked, the effects of cumulative stress can become so great that the adrenals end up completely exhausted. At this point the adrenals are unable to respond to any stressor, and you will see low levels of cortisol and DHEA on a blood test. The end result is often feelings of deep fatigue in the morning and throughout the day, unhealthy blood sugar levels, carbohydrate cravings, irritability, and impaired mental functioning.

When the adrenals cannot produce sufficient cortisol to deal with stressful situations, the adrenals then produce adrenalin. Adrenaline is your body's last-ditch effort to cope with the ravages of chronic stress. As it continues to be produced, it can cause people to become anxious, trigger heart palpitations, cause shortness of breath, and other symptoms that occur when your body is in a crisis state due to stress overload. You can wake up in the middle of the night, wired, and unable to get back to sleep. Adrenaline also has an affinity for the joints, where it can cause weakness or stiffness. All of these symptoms are triggered by blown-out adrenal glands.

Poor diet (especially a diet high in sugar and simple carbohydrates), excessive coffee/caffeine consumption, skipped meals, and not getting enough sleep can also all negatively impact your adrenal health. Depending on which metabolic type a person is (see below), addressing adrenal exhaustion and restoring optimal adrenal health can range anywhere from a month to six months to a year.

If you are experiencing any of the above symptoms on a regular basis, your doctor can usually determine if your adrenal function is impaired by a fasting blood test that measures your cortisol and DHEA-S levels. A low white blood cell count on a blood test is another indication of adrenal fatigue. Many people with adrenal fatigue also present with pronated heels. Evidence of this can also be found on the soles of their shoes, with the outer edge of the heels of the soles being worn down.

To help protect the health of your adrenal glands, you need to learn how to manage stress more effectively. This includes not only effectively dealing with mental and emotional stress, but also stressors caused by chemical and environmental toxins, infections, physical trauma, inflammation, oxidative stress, and nutritional deficiencies. (For more on how to effectively manage stress, see Chapters 5 and 8.)

When the adrenals are fatigued, go slow with exercise. Any exercise that makes you feel tired, either two hours later, or the next morning, is too much for your body. Walking, slow jogging, and slow cycling are some of the best types of exercises for people with adrenal fatigue, while strenuous exercises such as circuit training, fast-paced jogging, and running on a treadmill should all be avoided.

Other adrenal-boosting tips include:

- Don't skip meals, especially breakfast, and include protein with every meal
- Have a mid-morning and mid-afternoon snack of nuts or seeds
- Avoid, or at least minimize. your intake of coffee and other caffeinated products
- Avoid alcohol, all fruit juices, sugar and other sweets
- Never eat high glycemic foods without protein (to determine the glycemic index of the foods you eat, visit www.glycemicindex.com)
- Eat at least five to seven servings of vegetables each day
- Use sea salt, Celtic salt, or Himalayan salt
- Eliminate the use of all unhealthy fats, especially all trans-fats and hydrogenated oils
- Do your best to go to bed at the same time each night (ideally no later than 11 pm), while getting at least seven to eight hours of sleep
- Try to obtain daily sun exposure each morning
- Look for opportunities to laugh throughout the day
- Meditate and practice deep, abdominal breathing
- Try not to overwork

- Avoid exposure to secondhand smoke (nicotine), and if you smoke, seek help so that you can stop.

The following nutritional supplements can also be helpful: Vitamin C (2,000 mg twice a day) B-complex vitamin once a day, along with vitamin B5 (1,000 mg once a day), vitamin E (400 IU once a day; look for a brand that contains a full array of tocopherols and tocotrienols), vitamin D3 5,000 IU daily, and magnesium (250 mg twice a day).

In addition, depending on the severity of their adrenal exhaustion, I give my patients B complex injections and 25,000 mg of vitamin C administered intravenously once a week. Adrenal glandular extracts can also help, as well as the herb licorice, which helps to boost cortisol, and is also a natural antiviral agent, and can help prevent and reverse respiratory infections that often afflict persons who have adrenal fatigue. Various adaptogenic herbs are also very useful for adrenal fatigue. Such herbs include ashwaganda, Siberian ginseng, cordyceps, and Rhodiola rosea.

The hormone pregnenolone can help improve adrenal function, as well. It is produced in the adrenal glands, as well as in the brain, is the precursor of all the adrenal hormones, and can also improve memory. (For more on pregnenolone and brain health, see Chapter 11.) Supplementing with DHEA may also be necessary. Lastly, the use of bio-identical progesterone cream can help strengthen the adrenal glands. In cases of extreme fatigue, it may be necessary to have cortisol, from a compound pharmacy, to be given at a dose of 5mg in the morning and again at noon.

The Pancreas

Your pancreas, which is located in the upper left-center region of your abdomen, behind your stomach and below your liver, oversees both hormonal and digestive functions, making it a part of both your endocrine and digestive systems. We discussed the digestive functions of your pancreas in Chapter 7. Here, I want to discuss the role your pancreas plays as part of your endocrine system.

As an endocrine gland, your pancreas is responsible for producing a number of important hormones, including insulin, glucagon, and somatostatin, among others. Of these, insulin is the hormone most people are familiar with. It is responsible for regulating the metabolism of carbohydrates and fats in the body, and plays a critical role in balancing and maintaining healthy blood sugar (glucose) levels in the body (without a sufficient supply of glucose to the cells, your cells would starve and die). Insulin attaches to a specific receptor on the membrane of a cell (like a key and a lock) in order to allow glucose to move into the cell.

When the body is too acidic, insulin will not be able to open the lock, blood sugar will increase, causing the pancreas to make even more insulin. This is what is called insulin resistance, and if it continues it will result in metabolic syndrome and type II diabetes. There is a very important blood test called Hemoglobin A1C, that measures your blood sugar over the past 90 days, and is a great indicator (when elevated at greater than 5.8) of insulin resistance. When Hemoglobin A1C is very low at 5.0, there is a 99 percent chance that you will be alive in ten years.

Glucagon has the opposite effect of insulin on blood glucose levels. Whereas insulin lowers blood glucose levels, glucagon raises them when they become too low. It does this by signaling the liver to convert stored glycogen into glucose and then release it into the bloodstream. Together, glucagon and insulin act as elements of a regulation system to keep blood sugar levels stable. Both of these pancreatic hormones are in turn regulated by somatostatin, which also plays a role in cell growth and nerve transmissions.

An important point to remember is that whenever you feel tired after eating a meal, you have eaten too many carbohydrates, which cause insulin to be secreted from the pancreas, causing blood sugar to be converted into fats. This requires a great deal of energy, and consequently you get tired. (For more on insulin resistance and how to prevent and reverse it, see Chapter 12.)

The Thyroid

Your thyroid is another important gland within your body's overall endocrine system. It is located in the lower part of the neck, below your Adam's apple, where it wraps around your windpipe (the trachea). Its shape resembles a butterfly, with two wing-like lobes attached to one another by a middle section called the isthmus. I tell my patients that their adrenal glands can be likened to the body's gas pedal. Extending that analogy, your thyroid gland acts like your body's carburetor, regulating how much gas will get to the engine.

The thyroid gland helps to regulate your body's internal temperature and overall metabolism, including how efficiently your body is able to convert food into energy. In addition, your thyroid gland also increases your cells' and tissues' ability to take in oxygen. It does this by increasing 2,3DPG, a substance made in red blood cells (RBCs) that controls the movement of oxygen from RBCs into the body's tissues. Your thyroid also stores various hormones that help regulate your body's growth, heart rate and contraction, and blood pressure. These thyroid hormones are essential for the healthy functioning of every cell in your body, and for helping to keep your body's immune system healthy. Other processes for which the thyroid plays important roles include cell growth and reproduction, circulation, nerve tissue sensitivity, regulation of sex hormones, regulation of both cholesterol and sugar metabolism in the liver, and hair, skin, and nail growth.

In order to produce its hormones, the thyroid requires iodine, a mineral found in certain foods (especially kelp and other seaweeds) and in iodized salt. The two most important thyroid hormones are *thyroxine* (T4) and *triiodothyronine* (T3). The thyroid gland also makes the hormone *calcitonin*, which is involved in calcium metabolism and stimulating bone cells to add calcium to bone.

The two most common types of thyroid problems are hyperthyroidism (overactive thyroid) and hypothyroidism (underactive thyroid). Hyperthyroidism results in excessive thyroid hormone production, and hypothyroidism leads to a deficiency in thyroid hormones. In either case, a wide range of health problems and symptoms can result.

Common conditions associated with hyperthyroidism include skin problems, fatigue, frequent allergic reactions, nervousness, gastrointestinal disorders, sleep disorders, losing weight, fever, and body pains. Hyperthyroidism can also be caused by taking too high a dose of prescription thyroid medication such as Synthroid or Armour Thyroid. Hypothyroidism, which is much more common, is characterized by symptoms of dry skin and hair, morning fatigue that improves after noon, unexplained weight gain, cold hands and feet, increased sensitivity to cold, and constipation. Other signs include thinning hair and/or thinning of the outside 1/3 of the eyebrows, teeth marks on the tongue, swelling or puffiness under the eyes (suborbital edema), and decreased Achilles reflex. Fibromyalgia and miscarriage can also be due, as least in part, to thyroid problems.

Many women complain of hair loss and hair thinning. As mentioned above, low thyroid function is often a cause of this. Other causes include increased toxicity, reduced levels of hydrochloric acid in the stomach, low iron levels, and mineral deficiency. Supplementing with a multi-mineral can also be helpful. Lastly, an essential amino acid formula may be necessary, as well.

80 percent of the hormone that the thyroid produces is T4 and 20 percent is T3. The body (primarily the liver and kidneys) converts T4 to T3. T3 is the metabolically active hormone which acts on the cells to improve metabolism. Many patients do not adequately convert T4 to T3 (resulting in a low Free T3 on the blood test). These patients frequently do better on a prescription medication that contains both T4 and T3 (Armour, Westhroid, Naturethroid, Compounded T4-T3), than on a pure T4 medication such as Synthroid. If that is the case and you are taking Synthroid (T4), your doctor may elect to add a medication called Cytomel (T3), or add a compounded T3 medication. Thyroid stimulating hormone (TSH), which is produced by the pituitary gland, acts to stimulate hormone production by the thyroid gland. If the TSH is greater than 3.0, most doctors will prescribe thyroid medication. However, many patients can still be clinically hypothyroid with a normal TSH, so it is important to have a complete thyroid blood panel drawn, as well as to carefully assess the patient's symptoms.

Hashimoto's thyroiditis is the cause of approximately 90 percent of all cases of hypothyroidism. This condition is an autoimmune disease in which the thyroid gland is attacked by one's antibodies. It was the first disease to be recognized as an autoimmune disease, having first been discovered by Hakaru Hashimoto in 1912. Hashimoto's disease is much more common in women than in men, and most commonly begins to develop in one's 30s, though it can also occur much earlier. All patients need to be screened for Hashimoto's Thyroiditis by a blood test called Thyroid Peroxidase Antibodies. Patients with Hashimoto's need higher amounts of vitamin D3.

A variety of factors can impair thyroid function, including poor diet, foods that act as natural suppressants of thyroid activity (see below), environmental toxins, and pharmaceutical medications, including antacids, antihistamines, anti-inflammatory drugs (NSAIDs), antibiotics, and some antidepressants. As with your liver, conventional medical tests can often indicate that your thyroid function is normal when in fact you may be experiencing a variety of symptoms stemming from underlying thyroid problems. By contrast, the Energy Medicine diagnostic tools that I use can quickly detect thyroid imbalances, and also indicate the underlying causes that are specific to each of my individual patients.

Years ago, a physician named Broda Barnes, MD developed a simple home test that can often be an accurate indicator of thyroid imbalances. To perform this test, you will need a thermometer that is placed under the armpit to measure body temperature. Set it beside your bed at room temperature before going to bed. Then, each morning for three days, as soon as you awake each morning, before getting out of bed, place the thermometer beneath your left armpit and keep it there for 15 minutes. Then write down the temperature reading. If your temperature remains below 97.5 degrees, low thyroid function may be a problem, with the degree of hypothyroidism directly related to how low your temperature is. (**Note:** The Broda Barnes testing method should not be used by women during the first few days and in the middle of their menstrual cycle.)

If you suspect your thyroid is out of balance, consult with a physician, ideally one trained in Energy Medicine or a holistically-oriented doctor who is skilled at diagnosing and treating thyroid issues. A complete thyroid blood panel should be ordered, including TSH, Free T4,

Free T3, and thyroid antibodies. It is important, when it comes to all of your body's hormonal systems, that you always consult with a doctor and that your treatment measures proceed under his or her supervision. If you are found to have low thyroid function and put on prescription medication, all of the above blood tests (not just the TSH), should be repeated in 60 days in order to arrive at the optimal dose. One very important fact is that if you have fatigue and go see your doctor and he feels that thyroid medication is warranted, he must make sure that you do not have adrenal fatigue. Giving thyroid medication to a fatigued person who is not first being treated for adrenal fatigue, will likely make the fatigue worse. So always treat the adrenals first. With that said, here are some self-care steps you can take to help protect your thyroid.

Diet: Eat a healthy, organic, whole foods diet and avoid eating dairy products, and especially wheat and wheat products, because of their gluten content, and of how widely bromine is used today in their production. Bromine competes with and displaces iodine in the thyroid gland. All other gluten foods should also be avoided, since gluten can significantly impair thyroid function.

If you suffer from low (hypo) thyroid function, also avoid foods such as broccoli, Brussels sprouts, cabbage, cauliflower (these four cruciferous vegetables can be eaten if cooked), kale, mustard greens, soybeans and soy products, spinach, and turnips, as well as pears and peaches, all of which naturally suppress thyroid hormone production. (If, however, you fall into the much rarer category of excessive (hyper) thyroid function, all of these otherwise healthy foods should be a part of your diet.) Foods rich in iodine, such as fish, kelp, and various root vegetables, along with iodized salt (the best options are Celtic, Himalayan, and sea salts) can also help boost low thyroid function.

Nutritional Supplementation: Useful nutrients for improving low thyroid function include vitamin A, B vitamin complex, vitamin B12, vitamin D3 (which is especially important for people with Hashimoto's disease), iodine, selenium, tyrosine (for hypothyroidism only), and zinc, as well as essential fatty acids (EFAs), which aid in hormone production.

(**Note:** The following nutrients can, in higher doses, interfere with thyroid function: soy and soy products, alpha-lipoic acid (in doses of 600 mg and above), and L-carnitine (in doses of 2,000 mg and above).

Dessicated Thyroid: Dessicated thyroid, also known as thyroid extract, refers to products derived from the thyroid glands of animals (primarily pigs) that have been dried (dessicated), powdered, and made safe for human consumption. Their use dates back to the 19th century. Dessicated thyroid products can be especially helpful for cases of hypothyroidism caused by Hashimoto's disease, since they contain T4 and T3.

The most common dessicated thyroid products used in the US today are Armour Thyroid, Westhroid, and Naturethroid. These products should only be used under a doctor's supervision.

For most people, starting at a dose of one-half grain once a day is most appropriate, staying at this level for two weeks, and then increasing by another one-half grain every two weeks until thyroid symptoms begin to reverse themselves. However, people who experience feelings of jitteriness from drinking coffee or other caffeine products should start at an even lower dose, and patients who have previously had a heart attack should delay using dessicated thyroid products for at least three months following their attack, and only after they are cleared to do so by their doctor. Should you begin using dessicated thyroid, it is also important that you have regular follow up blood tests every six months to a year, to better monitor your progress. During such tests, be sure to also ask your doctor to screen for your blood ferritin level. Ferritin is a protein in your body that binds to iron, storing it and releasing it in a controlled fashion, as needed. Ideally, it should be at least 70 ng/ml.

Metabolic Typing: Identifying Your Key Hormonal Gland

As an expert in the area of hormonal health, I have found that *it is far more effective to strengthen weak glands that produce hormones,* rather than simply seeking to boost their performance through the use of hormones themselves. This approach sets me apart from many in the field of hormone therapy who simply prescribe hormones when endocrine glands test weak. In order to restore hormonal glands to health, however, it is important to first identify the specific, or key, gland that has the most influence over each person.

One of the most significant problems with conventional medicine today—and it's a problem that also exists among many practitioners of so-called alternative therapies—is that treatment is approached from a "one-size fits all" perspective. That is, patients who present with the same condition will all be given the same medications, without any attention given to whether or not such drugs are actually appropriate for each patient based on their specific biochemical and bioenergetic needs. Such an approach to medicine is sometimes referred to as "cookie cutter" medicine, meaning that the same recipe of drugs and other treatments are prescribed for each patient regardless of whether they will be effective or not. Based on my many years of firsthand experience treating thousands of patients I can emphatically state that such a cookie cutter approach to medicine is a serious mistake, *and can seriously undermine one's health!*

The reason why one-size-fits-all medicine doesn't work should be obvious. It's simple, really: Each of us is unique, both in terms of our genetic makeup, biochemistry and so forth, and in terms of the tendencies we have as we go about our lives. Recognizing each patient's uniqueness and tailoring his or her treatment program accordingly is a major element in effectively and safely restoring optimal health as inexpensively and as quickly as possible.

This concept is not new. In fact, it corresponds to the concept of constitutional, or body, types. Thin, lanky people are known as *ectomorphs.*

Compact, muscular types, are known today as *mesomorphs,* and rounder, pear-shaped (heavy around the belly and thighs) people are known as *endomorphs.*

Interestingly, there are different personality traits associated with constitutional types. Ectomorphs tend to be thinkers who can be high strung, introverted, and reclusive, with a tendency to "live in their minds". Mesomorphs tend to be driven, action-oriented people with "type A" personalities, and endomorphs tend to be calm, deliberate people who are often characterized as having "type B", laid-back personalities. Given these differing characteristics and personality traits, it's only sensible to realize that what is appropriate for one constitutional type is not at all appropriate for another type.

This fact was recognized by the late Roy Williams, PhD, who helped pioneer many of the advances within the field of nutritional medicine in the 20th century. Dr. Williams, who also discovered vitamin B5 (pantothenic acid) in the 1930s, taught that each of us is genetically unique and that our nutritional needs can vary greatly in order for us to be able to experience optimal health and have an abundant supply of energy. He termed this principle *biochemical individuality.*

Since Dr. William's research, a number of researchers and physicians have built on his work, resulting in a concept known as *metabolic typing.* Much of the original research with regard to metabolic typing was conducted by a dentist named William Donald Kelley, DDS, who was able to cure himself of pancreatic cancer (one of the most difficult types of cancer to survive) by adopting a vegetarian diet and using a wide variety of nutritional supplements, along with various detoxification techniques. More than a decade later, however, the same approach that had restored his health failed to help his wife, who became extremely ill after being exposed to chemical toxins. Baffled when she didn't respond to his therapy, and in fact became even worse because of it, Kelley desperately decided to try adding beef broth and small amounts of meat to her diet. Within 24 hours of his doing so, his wife's condition began to improve, and soon she too was restored to full health.

This led Kelley to discover the relationship between a person's metabolic type, their biochemistry, and the type of diet and nutrients that were most appropriate for him or her. Eventually, he developed methods for determining each person's specific metabolic type and today is known as "the father of metabolic typing". For the rest of his life Kelley helped many people achieve remarkable, and documented, recoveries from illness using his methods, including many cases of cancer. For the most part, though, his work was ignored and he was attacked by the medical establishment as a fraud and worse. Before he died, however, he came to the attention of Nicholas Gonzalez, MD, and researcher William L. Wolcott. Dr. Gonzalez initially set out to debunk Kelley's claims, yet once he began to delve into Kelley's work and verified it for himself, he shifted his entire medical practice and today metabolic typing is a central component to the work he does as an integrative physician specializing in cancer care. Wolcott worked alongside Kelley for over a decade and is largely responsible for preserving and furthering what Kelley taught him, both through his company, Healthexcel, and in his book *The Metabolic Typing Diet.* (See *Resources* in the back of this book.)

Kelley recognized four major metabolic groups: Fast Oxidizers, Slow Oxidizers, Sympathetics, and Parasympathetics. Kelley grouped these four categories into one of two dominant systems. Both fast and slow oxidizers belong to what Kelley called the Oxidative system, whereas sympathetics and parasympathetics belong to the Autonomic system. He also recognized that each group corresponded to a specific endocrine, or hormone, type.

Since hormone therapy is one of my areas of specialization, I am most interested in the dominant gland, and their hormones, that most influences my patients. By determining which gland/ hormone type they are, I can more easily and effectively tailor make my treatments for each patient I see.

Although a basic determination of one's metabolic type can usually be found through a questionnaire, proper testing using Kelley's protocol involves analysis of a patient's saliva and urine samples and can be a bit complicated. Using Energy Medicine, I am able to greatly simplify this

292 | MICHAEL GALITZER, MD & LARRY TRIVIERI JR

process and effectively determine my patients' status quickly and easily. I do so by using a device known as the Vega, which is a more sophisticated version of the Dermatron that you learned about in Chapter 2.

One of the tests I conduct has to do with the body's response to sugar. I realized that I could use a sugar vial and test patients using electrodermal screening (EDS). To conduct this test I also developed the following homeopathic formulas: Growth Hormone (fast oxidizer), Pancreas (slow oxidizer – the endocrine pancreas), Thyroid (sympathetic), and Adrenal (parasympathetic).

The testing procedure is simple. Sugar will cause an increased skin resistance (or if using applied kinesiology, a weak muscle). Then I test patients by having them hold each of the vials containing the homeopathic formulas, one at a time. The formula that restores the skin resistance to normal indicates the patient's most important hormonal gland, and thus his or her metabolic type.

As an example, if the adrenal vial neutralizes the response to sugar, I would tell the patient that the adrenals were that person's key hormonal gland, and that the more optimal the adrenals become, the more energy they would feel, the better they could handle stress, and the more optimal their health would be (given all the other parameters, such as drainage, detoxification, exercise, and nutrition). Based on this finding, I am then able to tailor a treatment program for the patient that is specific for him or her, and that addresses and supports optimal adrenal gland function. This same approach works for the other three metabolic types and their key hormonal glands, as well. Most of the therapies in medicine are designed to treat lab values that are out of the "normal range." This form of metabolic typing that I employ states that even though the lab value for the specific gland/hormonal type is in the normal range, I want to continue to strengthen their key gland so as to optimize its function (instead of bringing a lab value from "out of the normal range to in the normal range").

Based on several thousand patients that I have tested and treated in this way I have found that 50 percent were Parasympathetics (adrenal), 25 percent were Sympathetic (thyroid), 20 percent were Slow Oxidizers (pancreas), and five percent were Fast Oxidizers (Growth Hormone). Interestingly, I find that I cannot get an accurate response using this test for children up to the age of 13, but after age 13 the test works well for everyone. I've concluded that these metabolic types were determined in childhood, and that there is an emotional connection to these organs, as follows:

- Adrenal – Fear
- Thyroid - Anger
- Pancreas – Love
- Growth Hormone – Anxiety

When I find that my patients are an adrenal type, and that their adrenal glands are exhausted, it usually takes six months to a year to get their adrenals back to health. If they are a pancreas or thyroid type, and their adrenals are exhausted, however, I can usually restore optimal adrenal function in as little as four weeks. What I have also found is that people with high blood pressure are usually pancreas or thyroid types. For pancreas types, the key mineral is potassium, while for thyroid types, the key mineral is magnesium.

Having treated thousands of patients with hormone-related health issues, I've found that each of the four metabolic, key hormone types generally have certain characteristics associated with them. Although these characteristics cannot provide as accurate an assessment of a person's key hormone gland as Energy Medicine testing does, it can provide you with clues to which key hormone gland is most involved in your own health. The characteristics for each metabolic, hormone gland type are as follows:

Parasympathetic (Adrenal)
- Slender Build
- Tend to have low blood pressure (especially women)
- Must eat breakfast
- Does not feel well if skips a meal
- Craves proteins
- Likes to snack between meals
- Meats will energize them

- Will gain weight by eating too many carbohydrates
- Constipation
- Frequently complain of fatigue
- Insomnia more likely
- Fear is the major issue

Slow Oxidizer (Pancreas)

- Blood Pressure is normal to high
- Tends to be a few pounds heavier than normal
- Does better on less protein and more healthy carbohydrates
- Feels okay if skips a meal
- Will gain weight when eating meats and fatty foods
- Healthy carbohydrates will give them more energy
- Sugar will have the most adverse effect of all the metabolic types
- Does not complain of fatigue
- Calm, laid back personality
- Sleeps well unless they (women) are in peri-menopause or menopause
- Love is the major issue

Sympathetic (Thyroid)

- Normal blood pressure
- Driven, action-oriented personality
- Does not need to eat breakfast
- Feels okay if skips a meal
- Does better on low protein, healthy carbohydrates
- Will gain weight when eating meats and fatty foods
- Can easily become deficient in magnesium, leading to anxiety and heart palpitations
- Does not usually complain of fatigue
- Does not like cold weather and cold rooms
- Sleeps well unless they (women) are in menopause or peri-menopause
- Anger is the major issue

Fast Oxidizer (Growth Hormone)

- Must eat breakfast
- Craves protein
- Usually physically fit and athletic
- Many overlaps with the Parasympathetic (Adrenals)
- Anxiety is the major issue

(As I mentioned above, I see very few of these people in my practice since only a small percentage of people overall fall into this category.)

Many doctors use blood and other tests to figure out which hormones are low and high and then make corrections. But my experience has shown me that you first have to figure out which hormone gland is the star player (metabolic type). Half the time it's the adrenal glands. Once I strengthen the adrenals, balancing their hormones becomes much easier. What I see is that these different metabolic types dictate our reactions to how we respond to treatment, both in terms of hormone therapy and also other treatments, including nutritional supplementation.

When it comes to improving your health, knowing your key hormonal gland and metabolic type is therefore very important. Once that determination has been made, it becomes much easier to know which hormonal gland to address first, rather than taking a "cookie-cutter" approach that proves ineffective in the majority of cases. If a patient comes to most physicians complaining of low libido or other sex-related issues, for instance, the physician will typically begin treatment by attempting to balance the sex hormones, perhaps with the use of estrogen, progesterone, or testosterone treatments.

But if adrenal exhaustion is the underlying cause of that problem, this approach will prove to be ineffective. The first and best course of action in such a case needs to be restoring proper adrenal function, beginning with strengthening the adrenal glands themselves.

The same holds true for the other key hormone glands. The best course of action in each case is to start to strengthen these glands. The beauty of the individualized approach to diagnosis and treatment of hormone related issues is that it allows me to quickly determine which key hormone gland is in need of attention. Once that gland begins to be strengthened, greater levels of health and energy soon follow.

Now that you understand the key hormone glands that influence your health, let's examine the hormones that are most often also in need of attention.

The Problem with High Levels of Cortisol

Earlier in this chapter you learned about the ill effects of adrenal fatigue associated with low levels of cortisol, and its consequences. If the adrenal glands are healthy, they initially respond to stress by producing increased amounts of cortisol. If high cortisol levels persist, metabolic and hormonal challenges will occur. High cortisol levels cause insulin resistance, and insulin resistance pushes cortisol levels even higher, resulting in a truly vicious cycle. When you have insulin resistance, you gain weight, crave sugar, and are constantly hungry. You also get fatigued after eating a high carbohydrate meal because of how much insulin has been secreted, while the cells are no longer responsive to insulin. The body converts carbohydrates into fat, which requires energy, and which accounts for the fatigue after meals.

High cortisol levels will result in symptoms of low thyroid function. When you have low thyroid function your hair falls out, you are constipated, your skin feels very dry, and you feel cold most of the time. Increased cortisol also contributes to high blood pressure.

For men, chronically high cortisol levels eventually cause a drop in testosterone because cortisol blocks testosterone from working at the cell receptor sites. A man will lose his sex drive and become overweight. He will frequently have high cholesterol and high triglycerides. It's a perfect set-up for a heart attack.

In women, the brain becomes less sensitive to estrogen when there is high cortisol, resulting in hot flashes in women who had previously been in perfect hormonal balance. Often, whenever a major stressor occurs in their lives, my female patients will call and ask me, "Why am I having hot flashes?" The reason is that the stressor causes cortisol levels to go up, which makes the cells less sensitive to estrogen.

Increased cortisol also occurs as a result of chronic inflammation, and chronic pain. The liver has a reduced ability to detoxify, promoting a leaky gut, which, in turn, can cause autoimmune reactions within the body. Increased cortisol can cause ulcers in both the stomach and small intestine, for example. Bone density can go also down. Additionally, high cortisol levels suppress the pituitary's ability to release luteinizing hormone, which is essential for ovulation. When cortisol suppresses ovulation it can result in infertility and diminished progesterone production.

If you have too much cortisol you will also have trouble falling and staying asleep. The reason you have a hard time sleeping is that your cortisol levels remain high at night, which is the opposite of what they should be. This can be helped by giving the supplement phosphatidylserine (PS), 100-300 mg at bedtime. Ideally, cortisol levels should be at their highest when you wake up in the morning, and be at the lowest while you are asleep. Chronic stress and toxin exposure inverts this process. The result is elevated cortisol when you need to be sleeping, and that turns off melatonin and growth hormone production. Melatonin is essential for restful sleep, while growth hormone is secreted in the first two hours of sleep so that your body can regenerate itself in the first half of your sleep cycle.

DHEA

DHEA (dehydroepiandrosterone) is the other key adrenal hormone needed to optimize our health. There is more DHEA in the human body than of any other hormone. The body can convert it into other hormones, such as estrogen and testosterone. In addition, DHEA is the only hormone that declines with age in *both* men and women, and its decline signals age-related disease. The higher the DHEA, the higher the pheromones, and the higher the sexual attraction.

Pheromones are chemicals that are secreted by us that result in smells that can have an effect on other people. The more stressed we are the less sexually desirable we are. By the way, pumpkin pie has the highest libido effect of any smell.

Signs of DHEA decline are varied, ranging from dry skin, dry eyes, and dry hair, to poor memory, anxiety, and irritability, to intolerance for noise, and poor sex drive, especially in women. Other indications of DHEA decline are decreased amounts of pubic and underarm hair.

The best means of testing DHEA levels is a DHEA Sulfate (DHEA-S) blood test.

In addition to the process of aging itself, declines in DHEA levels can be caused by chronic stress and elevated cortisol levels, poor diet (especially regular consumption of alcohol, caffeine, and sugar), lack of healthy fats, vegetarian diets low in dietary cholesterol, smoking and regular exposure to secondhand smoke, and various pharmaceutical drugs, such as prednisone, insulin, and opiates, It is important to note that whenever a person is prescribed prednisone, they must start taking DHEA.

Although DHEA supplements are available over-the-counter at both pharmacies and health food stores, as with other hormones, I do not recommend its use without being supervised by a physician who specializes in anti-aging and natural hormone replacement therapy. Ideally, such a physician, like me, will also be well-versed in the use of Energy Medicine. When properly prescribed and administered, DHEA can provide a host of health and anti-aging benefits. These include: improving overall performance, especially in people age 50 and beyond; immune system stimulation; regulating the body's interleukin-2 production; acting as a natural anti-diabetic agent; helping to protect against unhealthy weight gain and obesity; stimulating lean muscle mass; enhancing the body's ability to burn fat; improving memory, cognition, and learning skills; acting as a natural antidepressant; protecting against viral infections; improving libido, especially in women; improving the health of the ovaries in women; reducing the risk of coronary artery disease; and decreasing platelet aggregation.

It is best to take DHEA supplements (available as tablets, capsules, and creams) in the morning in order to mimic your body's natural circadian rhythm. Men should take 25-50 mg of DHEA per day, while women should limit their intake to 5-15 mg per day. Both men and women should also be screened for hypothyroidism before using DHEA, and men should first also have their PSA, DHEA-S, and testosterone levels checked. Men with an elevated PSA or who are at a higher risk for developing prostate cancer should be careful using DHEA supplements. Finally, because of how DHEA speeds up metabolic processes in the body, I recommend you use DHEA supplements with antioxidant nutrients, such as vitamins C and E (mixed tocopherols), beta carotene, CoQ10, and selenium.

Signs of excess DHEA use include greasy hair and skin, acne, excess body hair, unexplained hypertension (high blood pressure), insomnia, moodiness, and irritability. Should any of these symptoms occur when using DHEA, notify you physician and discontinue your use of DHEA supplements immediately.

In addition to supplementing with DHEA, you can maintain and help boost your body's supply of DHEA by following a healthy diet (see Chapter 8), emphasizing foods rich in essential fatty acids, and limiting your daily caloric intake each day. In addition to the nutrients mentioned above, magnesium and chromium supplements can also help, as can the herbs Panax and Siberian ginseng, both of which can strengthen the adrenal glands where DHEA is primarily produced. Managing stress, regular exercise, and getting enough restful sleep each night is also vitally important.

To reiterate, when your adrenal glands are off your whole body is out of tune. The adrenals are the body's response to stress, whereas the sex hormones (estrogen, testosterone, progesterone) represent reproduction. You can live without your sex hormones; you can't live without your adrenals. Survival is a much higher priority than reproduction. So when the body is under stress and the adrenals are tired, the body will convert estrogen to DHEA, testosterone to DHEA, and progesterone to cortisol. This is why the best thing you can do for a woman or man with burnt out adrenals is to first strengthen the adrenal glands, and then balance their sex hormones.

Balancing Your Sex and Human Growth Hormones

The ways that I and other anti-aging physicians work to balance and restore patients' sex hormone levels and human growth hormone (HGH) is often misunderstood, and considered by some to be controversial. Yet, it is also an important part of my complete outstanding health program, especially for people in their late 40s or older. Recent research confirms this, showing that this aspect of medicine holds great promise in slowing the aging process, and, as with balancing the major hormones discussed above, for helping to treat age-related diseases. I have been proving these findings in my medical practice for many years. *However, it is important to point out that hormone therapy is not a magic bullet, or a miracle cure, as some claims would have you believe. To be most effective, it must be part of the overall comprehensive approach to better health and vitality that I am sharing in this book. For best results when addressing your sex hormones and HGH, I encourage you to find and work with a physician with expertise in what is known as bio-identical hormone therapy.*

Also known as natural hormone therapy, bio-identical hormone replacement therapy (BHRT) involves the use of natural, nontoxic hormones to boost the body's production of sex hormones, and to then maintain them at the levels of healthy men and women in their 30s. This is a safer and more effective approach than relying on synthetic hormone drugs, which can cause harmful side effects. Before beginning any type of hormone therapy, though, proper clinical lab testing and evaluation, along with ongoing follow-up screening must be used. By working with a trained bio-identical hormone specialist and following my guidelines, you will be empowered to begin achieving the same kinds of results as my patients so that you, too, can experience the rejuvenation that occurs when your hormones are balanced.

Menopause vs. Peri-menopause

Menopause is defined as the absence of a woman's menses for one year. At this point women are usually deficient in both estrogen and progesterone, with symptoms that will be described below. Peri-menopause occurs in the 5-10 years before the loss of a women's period, and is associated with an imbalance of estrogen and progesterone. Progesterone levels are usually the first to decline, resulting in symptoms such as PMS, and menstrual cycles that can be either longer or shorter, while a woman's estrogen levels can fluctuate daily from very high to very low, resulting in a variety of symptoms.

Bio-Identical Hormones vs. Synthetic Hormones

Anti-aging physicians with an expertise in hormone therapy, including myself, prefer to use bio-identical hormones when treating patients because of how closely they mimic hormones that are naturally produced in the body. Doing so both increases the effectiveness of hormone therapy and greatly minimizes the risk of side effects.

Synthetic hormones are patented substances manufactured by drug companies and represent one of the most prescribed class of prescriptions by doctors. Such hormones are produced by altering the structure of the hormones in order that the drug companies can patent them. This change in structure, however, also alters how the hormones affect the body when they are used. In many cases, synthetic hormones are derived from the natural hormones and other substances of animals, and then structurally altered. One of the most common synthetic hormones, Premarin, for example, is derived from the urine of pregnant mares (its name is short for *pregnant mare urine*). Premarin is natural to a horse, but not to a woman.

Premarin is used to treat menopausal symptoms due to low estrogen. However, it is not the same as human estrogen, and, being a chemical, carries the risk of toxicity that all chemical drugs have. In addition, Premarin contains 50 different types of estrogen, whereas in humans there are only three naturally-occurring forms (see below).

All synthetic hormones are fraught with such risks because they are foreign substances and that is how the body responds to them.

It is for this reason that a growing body of studies continue to find that synthetic estrogen use increases the risk of breast and other cancers. Further research also links synthetic estrogen use to an increased risk of other health problems, including blood sugar imbalances, depression, edema, fibroids, headache, gastrointestinal conditions, low libido, osteoporosis, and unhealthy weight gain. To counteract such side effects, conventional physicians will often prescribe progestin hormones, which are synthetic versions of natural progesterone. But the use of progestins (e.g. Provera) can often complicate health problems, as their use has been linked to numerous other side effects, including breast pain and tenderness, insomnia, liver problems, water retention, and an increased risk of birth defects in women of child-bearing age. The Women's Health Initiative Study in 2002, found an increased risk of breast cancer and heart disease when women in their 50's and 60's were given Premarin together with Provera (PremPro).

By contrast, no studies have associated bio-identical hormone replacement therapy (BHRT) with increased risk of cancer. Bio-identical estrogen and progesterone are bio-engineered from natural plant products (wild yams), and contain the exact same chemical structure as natural female sex hormones. They most closely mimic natural human physiology.

This makes them much safer to use, in addition to increasing their effectiveness. Most importantly, bio-identical hormones are responsive to all of the body's enzymes and other co-factors that regulate their function and make them so efficient. There have been several studies in menstruating women that showed that the higher the progesterone level during her second half of the cycle (luteal phase), the lower the incidence of breast cancer. Unfortunately, many people, including most physicians, believe that estrogen and progesterone cause female cancers. In the 28 years that I have been using bio-identical hormones in thousands of my patients, I have only seen two cases of breast cancer. I have concluded that BHRT does not cause cancer, and, more importantly, helps you feel well, look well, and be well, by improving your sleep, energy, mood, and outlook on life.

Male and Female "Sex" Hormones: Why You Need Them Optimized

The major sex hormones are estrogen, progesterone, and testosterone. All three of these hormones are necessary for optimal health in both men and women. In women, sex hormones are primarily produced by the ovaries, while in men they are primarily produced by the testes (testicles). The adrenal glands are also capable of producing sex hormones. By the way, if your ring finger is longer than your index finger, men will have an increased testosterone level, and women will have an increased estrogen level.

Estrogen: Although estrogen levels naturally decline after menopause, today many women in their 40's are also deficient in estrogen, or have unbalanced estrogen levels, due to poor diet, environmental toxins, chronic stress, and the use of birth control pills. The main types of environmental toxins that affect estrogen levels are mercury and other heavy metals, plastics, pesticides, herbicides, and insecticides. Collectively, such toxins are known as *xenoestrogens*, so named because they are foreign to the body and compete with and disrupt natural estrogen. These same toxins can also cause estrogen levels to become unbalanced and elevated in men.

Signs of estrogen deficiency in women include menstrual problems, vaginal dryness, painful intercourse, low libido, sagging breasts and loss of breast fullness, insomnia, dry eyes, night sweats, hot flashes, bone loss, urinary tract infections, joint pain, hair loss, palpitations, migraines, mood swings, anxiety, depression, and impaired mental function ("brain fog").

For optimal health, estrogen levels needs to be kept in balance. Effective self-care steps you can take to help address estrogen deficiencies include eating enough protein and estrogenic foods, and, when appropriate, the use of natural bio-identical estrogen creams. Estrogenic foods are foods that help to raise estrogen levels in the body. Such foods include animal protein foods, apples, barley, brown rice, carrots, cherries, coconuts, peanuts, olives, plums, as well as nightshade vegetables (eggplant, tomatoes, potatoes, and sweet and hot peppers).

There are three main types of estrogen: *estriol*, which accounts for 80 percent of all estrogen, *estradiol* (the most potent form), and *estrone*, each of which accounts for approximately 10 percent of the remaining estrogen. The type of estrogen that I prescribe is called Biest Cream, which contains 80 percent estriol (the safest form of estrogen) and 20 percent estradiol. There are numerous studies that show the following beneficial effects of estriol: It offers breast cancer protection; it controls menopausal symptoms without causing growth of the lining of the uterus; it maintains a healthy vaginal flora; it maintains a healthy pH of the vagina, and it helps prevent urinary tract infections. Vaginal estriol also prevents vaginal dryness, helps treat pain on intercourse, and helps reduce incontinence.

Estradiol controls 400 functions in women. It acts as an anti-aging hormone in the body in a variety of ways. It maintains and improves healthy skin tone, helps to prevent bone loss (osteoporosis) and also reduces the risk of a heart attack. In addition, it reduces the risk of new onset diabetes.

Progesterone: Progesterone, like estrogen, is produced by the ovaries and adrenal glands in women. The word progesterone, means *for gestation* (pregnancy). If it were not for progesterone, pregnancy would be impossible, for it prepares the lining of the uterus for the implantation of the fertilized egg, and then helps to maintain it during pregnancy.

Progesterone plays a vital role in helping to keep estrogen levels in the body in check, and along with estrogen is involved in a woman's menstrual cycle. During the second week of this cycle, progesterone levels are at their lowest. They then start to rise during the third week, before significantly dropping again just before the onset of menstruation. In fact, it is the drop in progesterone that makes menstruation possible. Progesterone also helps to regulate blood sugar levels, and is a natural diuretic. It is an antidepressant, improves the function of the thyroid gland, normalizes blood clotting, stimulates bone growth, and helps restore normal sleep patterns. Progesterone decreases blood pressure, relaxes the coronary arteries, and is now being used to stabilize brain function after a traumatic injury. It is also essential for a healthy libido. Symptoms that can be caused by progesterone deficiency include anxiety and agitation, menstrual irregularities, sleep problems, loss of interest in sex, and water retention.

Both blood tests and saliva tests can be used to determine the relationship of progesterone to estrogen. A low progesterone to estrogen ratio results in estrogen dominance, an unbalanced condition that negatively impacts health. Conditions that can occur as a result of estrogen dominance include migraines, especially those that occur during the second half of the menstrual cycle or near the period, and premenstrual syndrome (PMS), which can be physical (fatigue, bloating, weight gain) emotional (fear, sadness, irritability), or both. Also, low levels of progesterone potentiate estrogen's ability to lower thyroid function.

Progesterone has the ability to transform itself to become other hormones, including cortisol. But this conversion ability also means that progesterone levels can easily become depleted, especially during times of chronic physical or psychological stress, when the adrenal glands might call on progesterone to supply more cortisol. Managing stress and minimizing your exposure to stressful situations is therefore very important when it comes to maintaining healthy progesterone levels.

Other steps you can take to help reduce the risk of progesterone deficiency include regular exercise, and avoiding the estrogenic foods discussed above. A number of nutritional supplements can also be helpful, including vitamin B6, vitamin C, magnesium, and zinc. The herb chasteberry, also known as vitex, can also be helpful, as research has shown that it can stimulate progesterone production while reducing excess estrogen.

Based on my clinical experience, however, the most effective way to boost progesterone, while also keeping estrogen levels in balance, is the use of natural progesterone cream, which can be applied topically. Such creams contain natural progesterone, made from yams, that is absorbed through the skin and is most easily utilized by the body, unlike synthetic progesterone drugs such as Provera, which can cause serious side effects.

Testosterone: Like estrogen and progesterone, testosterone is more than simply a sex hormone. It is a potent anti-aging hormone that plays important roles in regulating metabolism, stimulating red blood cell production, and helping to keep free radical production in check. It is also involved in protein synthesis and the building of muscle tissues, and helps prevent muscle from turning into fat. It prevents skin from sagging. Additionally, testosterone has been shown to protect against heart disease. In fact, research has shown that both men and women with the lowest testosterone levels have a 33 percent greater risk of premature dying from any cause, compared to people with healthy testosterone levels.

Testosterone is also a brain stimulant that elevates mood and protects against depression, and, most importantly, it helps generate excitement and passion. Diminished testosterone levels typically results in low libido in both men and women, as well as a loss of strength and physical endurance. In men, low testosterone can also cause erectile dysfunction (ED).

Although testosterone levels naturally decline as we age, today this decline is greatly accelerated by many of the same factors that cause estrogen imbalances, especially the increasing prevalence of heavy metals and other xenoestrogenic toxins in the environment. Poor diet and lack of exercise can also increase testosterone loss, as can chronic stress and many commonly used prescription drugs, including anticonvulsants, anti-fungals, birth control pills, calcium channel blockers, diuretics, glucocorticoids, narcotic painkillers, and statins. Illicit drugs, including marijuana, can also result in testosterone loss, as can smoking and excessive alcohol consumption. Testosterone can be very helpful for women, and should be given after a woman has first been balanced with natural estrogen and progesterone, and still complains of low libido.

I find that almost all men can benefit from testosterone replacement, usually beginning when they are in their 50s. When I measure men's testosterone levels, I pay most attention to their free testosterone, which represents the amount of testosterone available to the tissues. I almost always find it to be much lower than is healthy. To me, this is not surprising. After all, it's well-known that sperm counts today are 50 percent less than what they were 50 years ago. This being so, shouldn't we also expect to find that testosterone production in men has similarly declined?

I advise all of my male patients to take self-care steps to maintain and improve their testosterone levels. This includes eating a diet that avoids testosterone sapping foods and ingredients, such as sugar and simple carbohydrates, processed foods, foods laced with preservatives, unhealthy fats, and food in cans, most of which contain bisphenol A (BPA), a chemical compound that acts to disrupt hormonal balance, raising estrogen levels while simultaneously decreasing testosterone. BPA is also commonly found in plastic water bottles and other plastic food containers, so those should be avoided too.

Most men do well eating protein-rich and high-fiber foods, along with a wide array of fresh, organic, non-estrogenic foods. I advise minimizing carbohydrate foods, including complex carbohydrates, because of how they can spike insulin levels, which can have an adverse effect on testosterone. In addition, I advise men and women alike to regularly exercise, with an emphasis on strength training, and to learn how to more effectively cope with stress.

When addressing testosterone issues in men, I also find it is important to treat the prostate gland at the same time. Excessive red meat, dairy, coffee, and alcohol consumption irritates the prostate, so they should be minimized, while vegetables, and fruits like pomegranate help the prostate. Two herbal remedies that I also recommend for this purpose are saw palmetto and the extract of giant redwoods. Redwood trees live for a very long time, and redwood extract acts like a male tonic. Maca and tribulus are other helpful herbal remedies.

I also recommend vitamin C, vitamin E, fish oils, selenium, fish oils, zinc, GLA, lycopene, and pomegranate for prostate health. And, since we now know that testosterone can get converted to estrogen, especially in men who are overweight, or when testosterone is given by a weekly injection (by an enzyme called *aromatase*), I may also use chrysin in a cream form, and zinc, which act as aromatase inhibitors. Anastrozole is a prescription medication that is used 1-3x week by some physicians to also block aromatase. Kegel exercises, which involve squeezing your internal rectal muscles so that you are using your internal sphincter to massage the prostate, can also help. You can do 10 to 25 repetitions while sitting in your chair, or while driving, two or three times a day. By doing all of these steps we are maximizing testosterone and preventing its conversion to estrogen, while at the same time treating the prostate so that it stays healthy too.

Finally, I encourage both men and women to have more sex with their spouses or partners. Sex helps to keep the all of the sex organs healthy, as well as the prostate, and also helps to maintain, and even increase, testosterone levels. When it comes to testosterone, it really is a matter of "use it or lose it." If blood levels of testosterone are low in a man, I will prescribe either daily testosterone cream, or a weekly intra-muscular injection of testosterone, in order to restore testosterone levels to those of a healthy, younger man. In men in their 40's with low testosterone levels, I will prescribe HCG injections to stimulate testosterone production by the testicles.

Lab Tests Needed Before Prescribing BHRT For Women

Before beginning BHRT, women should have the following blood tests: If you are still menstruating, the blood should be drawn on day 20 or 21 of your cycle.

CBC

Chem profile

Insulin

Free T3, TSH,

Thyroid Peroxidase

Thyroglobulin Antibody

Estradiol

Progesterone

SHBG

IgF1, IGFBP3

Prolactin

Hs CRP

FSH

LH

Testosterone/Free Testosterone

DHEA-S

25 OH Vit D

Cortisol

HGB A1C

Your doctor will know what the above tests stand for. They can be obtained through blood tests in combination with the saliva panel assay that you learned about in Chapter 4. These tests will provide you and your physician with a comprehensive overview of your current health and hormone status, providing you both with a guide to what is necessary for you to optimize your hormones. Your doctor can order the saliva panel for you, or you can contact the following companies to order the test on your own:

Sabre Sciences (888) 490-7300 www.sabresciences.com

Diagnos-Techs (800) 878-3787 www.diagnostechs.com

ZRT Labs (866) 600-1636 www.zrtlab.com.

Other screening tests that need to be done first include a gynecological exam, pap smear, mammogram, and bone mineral density test.

The two bio-identical hormones most often in need of attention in women are estrogen and progesterone. Usually women will experience a variety of symptoms that can indicate imbalances of either of these interrelated hormones. Common indicators of estrogen deficiency include depression, dry eyes, fatigue, feelings of panic and anxiety, mood swings, insomnia, low libido, hot flashes, memory loss, migraine, loss of breast size and/or drooping breasts, night sweats, dry mucous membranes, dry vagina, and feeling uninspired.

Prescribing Bio-identical Estrogen: Should your doctor determine you can benefit from bio-identical estrogen or progesterone therapy, he or she will provide you a prescription for them. Estrogen is available in the form of creams, gels, drops, troches, patches, vaginal suppositories, and pellets (pellets are usually changed every three months). Progesterone delivery methods are creams, gels, drops, capsules, and vaginal suppositories. As mentioned, I use a formula called Biest Cream, which has an 80:20 ratio of estriol to estradiol. This is a very popular combination among practitioners of BHRT. Biest needs to be given every 12 hours in order to maintain a steady tissue level. The cream is applied to the forearm, and rubbed in with the other forearm. Other sites to apply the cream include the shoulders and thighs. Biest Cream takes about two hours to fully absorb. If you are worried about touching your husband, kids, or pets, and giving them a dose of estrogen, then you can rub the cream in behind your knees.

It is possible that the initial dose of Biest will not relieve hot flashes. If this is the case, I will increase the dose, or have my patients apply the cream to the labia. The labia is a mucous membrane and thus will absorb better. (**Note:** Do not apply Biest to your face or breasts.)

Some practitioners will prefer to prescribe estradiol, without the estriol, as a cream, or as a patch that is changed twice a week. The patch, which is bio-identical, can also be obtained from a regular pharmacy. Another mode of estrogen delivery is as a pellet, which is inserted into the skin (after a small incision), and replaced every three months. Estradiol should never be given as a pill or capsule, because it increases inflammation, increases triglycerides, and increases the tendency for the blood to clot.

If a woman complains of vaginal dryness or pain on intercourse, she can best be helped by compounded vaginal estriol cream or suppository, which is taken three times a week at sleep. Don't forget: happy wife, happy life.

Prescribing Bio-identical Progesterone: Bio-identical progesterone may be the only hormone needed for a woman in her 30's or 40's who has normal estrogen levels and low progesterone levels on a blood test, or exhibits symptoms of progesterone deficiency. Progesterone also needs to be prescribed to all women who are taking bio-identical estrogen. It must be emphasized that there are many gynecologists who refuse to give a women progesterone after a hysterectomy, with the reasoning that if there is no uterus, then there is no need for progesterone. This is a mistake, given all the positive effects that progesterone has in the body, as mentioned earlier.

During a woman's reproductive years, progesterone was always produced for the latter two week period of a woman's menstrual cycle. If a woman is still menstruating, I will prescribe progesterone from days 12-25 of her cycle (day 1 being the first day of her period), at bedtime, and usually as a cream. Some practitioners prefer days 14-28, and others prefer days 18-28. Some doctors will prescribe progesterone twice daily. If a woman has persistent insomnia, oral progesterone (whether as Prometrium or as compounded) can be given at night, because when given orally progesterone is metabolized to a compound that further potentiates sleep.

If a woman is in menopause, and has symptoms of hot flashes, night sweats, insomnia, etc., I will start her on estrogen first, and then add progesterone two to three weeks later. It can get confusing as to when to take progesterone, so the prescription may read take progesterone from the 1st through the 14th of every calendar month. Many menopausal women, upon starting BHRT, will experience a return of their menstruation. If bleeding occurs while they are taking the progesterone, they need to stop the progesterone on the first day of bleeding, and restart it two weeks later in order to respect their normal physiological cycles.

As there are many different dosing schedules for women in menopause, some doctors will prescribe progesterone daily, especially if women tell them that they sleep better during the two weeks that they take progesterone, or if women say that they feel much better when they take progesterone.

Prescribing Testosterone For Women: Many women whose menopausal symptoms have mostly been well treated with bio-identical estrogen and progesterone, will still complain of low energy (even after their adrenal fatigue has been addressed), depressed mood, decreased libido, and inability to achieve orgasm. These women need bio-identical testosterone, usually as a cream, in a dose of 1-5 mg daily, and given in the morning (testosterone like estrogen can also be given as implantable pellets). I also tell my patients that applying a small amount of testosterone cream to the clitoris 30 minutes before sex, can be very helpful.

Effects of Diet and Lifestyle When Taking BHRT

BHRT can be optimized by eating organic, taking amino acid supplements, and eating a Paleolithic diet consisting of fruits, vegetables, meat, poultry, eggs, and fish. Foods that will interfere with BHRT are caffeinated drinks, alcohol, dairy, sugar, sweets, bread, and pasta. Lifestyle issues that reduce the effect of BHRT include being overweight, tobacco use, alcohol, marijuana, and other recreational drugs.

Supplements That Promote Healthy Estrogen Metabolism: There still exists a big scare about estrogen causing breast cancer. Bio-identical estrogen will not cause breast cancer, especially when one follows all the health promoting advice that you have learned about in this book. Estrogen is metabolized in the liver, so the more optimal the liver, the easier it can break down estrogen into healthy estrogen metabolites. Please review the previously mentioned strategies for supporting liver health. Supplements that help the liver include, DIM, I3C, glutathione, methyl B12, methyl folate, taurine, Sam-E, N-acetyl cysteine, and calcium D glucarate. Probiotics and increasing dietary fiber are also very helpful.

Signs of Too High A Dose of BHRT: Excessive estrogen levels typically manifest as nervousness, irritability, salt and water retention, weight gain, bloating, blood clots, fibrocystic breasts, and fibroids getting larger, which may cause excessive menstrual bleeding. A blood test can show lowered levels of thyroid hormones.

Signs of excessive progesterone dosing include depression, fatigue, decreased libido, weight gain, bloating, back pain, carbohydrate cravings, and acne due to progesterone being converted to testosterone.

If testosterone is dosed too high, you will see irritability, oily skin, and acne (especially if testosterone is given with DHEA).

For Men Only

Before beginning BHRT, the following blood tests for men should be ordered:

CBC
Chem profile
Insulin
Free T3, TSH
Thyroid Peroxidase
Thyroglobulin Antibody
Estradiol
SHBG
IgF1 and IGFBP3
Prolactin
Hs CRP
LH
Testosterone/Free Testosterone
PSA and Free PSA
DHEA-S
25 OH Vit D
Cortisol
HGB A1C

If you are using a lab like Life Extension, where you can order your own blood tests, when you receive your results always discuss them with your physician.

In the majority of cases, the sex hormone most in need of attention in men is testosterone. Clues that men are suffering with testosterone deficiency, or "low-T," include emotional irritability, fatigue, memory and cognitive problems, low sex drive, erectile dysfunction, poor sleep, depression, lack of motivation, poor self-esteem, and an overall poor sense of well-being. Increased belly fat and a flabby chest ("man boobs") are also signs of low-T, as well as an excess of estrogen in one's system, which is why I recommend men be tested for estradiol.

Testosterone therapy can be administered via gels, creams, patches, or intramuscular injection. The most appropriate delivery method is something your physician can determine for you based on your lab results. When undergoing testosterone, it is important that men follow the dietary and nutritional recommendations I made above, and get regular exercise, especially strength-training exercises.

Again men also need to be aware of certain medications that can diminish testosterone levels. These include anticonvulsant drugs, antifungals, calcium channel blockers, statin drugs, diuretics, and steroids such as prednisone. Marijuana and heroin use can also lower testosterone levels, as can chemotherapy. All of the different forms of testosterone therapy mentioned above are bio-identical. The two modalities that I most often use are compounded testosterone cream and injectable testosterone cypionate.

The testosterone cream is applied to the skin once a day in the morning. In some men, an additional half dose is applied in the evening. The cream does not convert to estrogen, so overweight men, and men who have high estrogen levels on their original blood test would benefit from testosterone cream.

Injectable testosterone is given as an intra-muscular injection once a week, usually in a dose of 100 mg. Some physicians will give half the dose every 3-4 days. Injectable testosterone may convert to estrogen, so follow-up blood tests in 60 days will be needed.

Men in their 30's and 40's with low blood testosterone levels, should first be given HCG injections, three times a week, to stimulate testosterone production by the testicles.

Monitoring Therapy With BHRT

I prefer to see my patients every four weeks, for the first three months, looking for improvement in their presenting symptoms, and making sure that they do not exhibit any signs of overdosing, which rarely happens. I also run a bio-impedance test on every visit, looking at their "phase angle", which is a measure of cellular health. When the phase angle is increasing, I am reassured that BHRT is successful.

Many physicians will use blood tests and 24 hour urine tests to monitor therapy. When prescribing creams, the best time to get a blood test is three hours after applying the cream. There are many articles that suggest that blood tests are not the most reliable indicator of successful BHRT when creams are applied. When getting a blood test for a man on injectable testosterone, 2-3 days after the injection will be a good time to get a blood test. Blood tests are reliable if a patient is taking an estrogen patch, or if they are taking oral progesterone. Urine tests are quite reliable, but some patients find it too cumbersome to collect urine for 24 hours. Saliva test results often conflict with blood tests, and are most reliable to assess adrenal function.

Because testosterone increases red blood cell production by the bone marrow, men should also have a CBC to assess their Hematocrit levels. Too high a concentration of red blood cells might make the blood too thick. In such cases, men would then donate blood every six months if this persisted. Men should also have their PSA checked every six months for the first two years.

Women on BHRT should also have a gynecological exam yearly, combined with a trans-vaginal ultrasound to assess the uterine lining. Other tests would be done at the discretion of the gynecologist.

Testosterone Safety Issues: Given the increased popularity of testosterone therapy, a number of concerns have recently been expressed about the use of testosterone hormones having to do with safety issues. This includes a panel convened by the Food and Drug Administration (FDA)calling for the FDA to impose strict new limitations on testosterone use, and the FDA itself claiming that the benefits of testosterone treatments for healthy, aging men are unproven, and that the drugs could be risky. (To its credit, however, so far at least, the FDA has cautioned both patients and physicians not to stop testosterone therapy.)

In addition, some researchers have stated that men who receive testosterone therapy have been found to have higher rates of heart problems. These claims are primarily based on an observational study published in the *Journal of the American Medical Association (JAMA)*, which expressed concerns over an increased risk for heart disease following testosterone treatments. However, as more than 125 physicians and three medical associations made clear to JAMA when they petitioned JAMA to retract it, the study's conclusions are flawed and the study itself was very poorly designed, incorrectly leading to its negative results. Among the points laid out in the petition were the existence of "major errors" in the article's text and figures, and that the method of statistical analysis used was neither accurate nor appropriate. Moreover, the original numbers and data used for the statistical analysis, along with other statistical methods, actually demonstrated the opposite of what the study's authors claimed, namely that, instead of increasing the risk of heart attack, the raw numbers in the authors' tables actually showed that *testosterone therapy reduces heart attack risk, as well as the risk of death*. The petition was signed by the International Society for Sexual Medicine, the Sexual Medicine Society of North America, and the International Society for the Study of the Aging Male, and their member scientists and physicians.

The petitioners' findings that debunked this study are far from surprising to me, given how long and effectively I have used testosterone therapy to improve my patients' health. Moreover, there is at least 30 years of extensive research confirming testosterone therapy's health benefits, including as a protector against heart disease. Even so, as I pointed out above, neither testosterone nor any other type of hormone replacement therapy is a magic bullet. Nor is it appropriate for all men. In order to be both safe and effective, proper testing before and during treatment must be conducted to avoid the risk of unwanted complications.

Oxytocin

Oxytocin is produced in the pituitary gland, and comes from the Greek words meaning *swift childbirth*. It is released in large amounts during labor, and facilitates birth, maternal bonding with the baby, and breast feeding. It reduces anxiety, and promotes a woman's natural feelings of happiness, bonding, inner peace, and love. It can also promote a woman's ability to have an orgasm. The only caution is that if a woman has adrenal fatigue, it will make it worse. Oxytocin is available as an oral troche and as an oral solution, which need to be refrigerated.

Melatonin

Melatonin is produced in the brain's pineal gland. It induces sleep. It shortens the time to fall asleep. It relaxes one's muscles and nerves which improves the quality of sleep. It is an antioxidant, and therefore, neutralizes free radicals produced by toxins. Although not talked about, melatonin is very helpful to protect against radiation exposure from the excessive amounts of imaging studies that are given to patients. (By the way on the night after these tests, one can take a bath with 1 ½ cups of sea salt and 1 ½ cups of baking soda to help neutralize the radiation).

Melatonin helps to control circadian rhythms in the body such as sleep-wake cycles, and hormonal cycles. It helps to prevent jet lag. In Germany, high doses of melatonin are used at night in cancer patients getting chemotherapy. Its hormonal effects include increasing growth hormone, increasing thyroid hormone (T3), and lowering cortisol. It is also an aromatase inhibitor. Usual starting doses of melatonin are 1-3 mg at bedtime. Some people claim that melatonin has no effect on their insomnia. If a woman says that melatonin causes insomnia, then she is low in progesterone. If progesterone causes worse sleep, then she is low in melatonin.

Human Growth Hormone: Your Body's Turbocharger

Human growth hormone (HGH) is produced by the pituitary gland, which is located at the base of the brain, behind the bridge of the nose. This tiny gland (it's about the size of a pea), is sometimes referred to as the body's master gland because of its production of nine hormones, including HGH, that regulate homeostasis and various other processes, including, in the case of HGH, growth. HGH is released in episodic bursts every 4 hours. The biggest spike is in the first 2 hours of sleep, resulting in tissue repair and regeneration. HGH is necessary for building muscle and improving immune function. In addition, it helps keep your heart strong (remember, your heart is a muscle), aids in kidney function, and helps to protect against damage to the body caused by stress. It increases the body's production of all other hormones, except cortisol, which is why growth hormone should not be given until after a person's adrenal fatigue has been treated and resolved.

Signs of low growth hormone levels include poor self esteem, poor wound healing, increased body fat, reduced lean body mass, muscle weakness, reduced skin elasticity, and inability to stay awake after midnight.

Growth hormone scares people, because they think that it is going to cause cancer. Unfortunately growth hormone has been misrepresented because of its name. It's not really just about growth. Though it certainly plays a vital role in the growth of children, once we enter adulthood it primarily acts as a metabolic hormone. It stimulates protein synthesis, burns fats, and conserves carbohydrates.

Think of HGH as a turbocharger for your body. The key to its use is knowing when to apply the turbo charge. Just as you would not turbo charge your car's engine without first being sure that all four of its wheels were in place and properly aligned, it is inappropriate to use HGH until the four hormonal "wheels" of your body—the sex hormones, insulin, thyroid, and adrenals—are working optimally. You wouldn't want to turbo charge it in the beginning because it would be too much. First, you have to strengthen the endocrine glands and bring these other hormones into balance, while also reducing the body's toxic burden using the processes of drainage and detoxification we discussed in Chapter 2. Once all of that is accomplished, growth hormone can take you to the next level of health.

Before using HGH, however, it is important to determine its level in your body. I obtain information about my patients from blood, and saliva tests, where we look at the adrenal and thyroid hormones, insulin and Hemoglobin A1C to assess insulin resistance, then the sex hormones estrogen, progesterone and testosterone. Then we use a fasting blood test to measure a patient's IGF-1 (insulin-like growth factor) level (and also measure the IGFBP3). IGF-1 is produced in the liver under the influence of HGH. IGF-1 blood levels can indicate whether HGH level are sufficient, too low, or too high. But, since growth hormone declines with age, most people's IGF-1 levels are low. When IGF-1 levels are in a healthy range, they are usually between 200 and 300 ng/ml.

HGH is usually given as a daily subcutaneous injection. Women seem to need higher doses than men. If you are taking growth hormone you also need to exercise and have protein at each meal, both of which support HGH and maximize its benefits When you add growth hormone at the right phase of your body's overall restoration, when everything else is in balance and you are less toxic, you will get beneficial results. Side effects of people taking excessive amounts of HGH include paresthesias (tingling or burning in your skin), joint pain, elevated blood sugar, and edema. If any of these occur, stop HGH and consult your physician.

There are a number of self-care approaches you can take to boost HGH levels in your body, or at least slow its decline. These include managing stress so that it does not become chronic, losing weight if you are overweight, eating a healthy diet that is free of sugar and simple carbohydrates (sugar and simple carbohydrates cause a spike in insulin levels; when insulin levels rise, HGH levels decrease), avoiding alcohol, getting adequate sleep and going to bed earlier. Regular exercise has also been shown to boost HGH levels. For best results, be sure to include a mix of aerobic and strength-training exercises at least three times a week.

Additional Guidelines for the Use of BHRT

In addition to proper blood and saliva assay testing and my other recommendations above, when it comes to the use of bio-identical hormone replacement therapy, it is important to pay attention to each person's biochemical individuality, and metabolic type and key hormonal gland (see above). As my friend, colleague, and bio-identical hormone expert Michael Borkin, NMD, of San Diego states, "The key to successful bio-identical hormone replacement therapy lies in determining the proper priority of treatment. To accomplish this, the patient has to be approached as an individual. Everyone has a unique sequence of hormones that is the result of their own lifestyle. Once the dynamics of these hormones are analyzed, a treatment plan tailored to each person's specific needs can be developed to reestablish a healthy hormonal balance." This is where various tests, including Energy Medicine testing, must be conducted. Before beginning BHRT, be sure that the doctor you are going to be working with understands these points and takes the appropriate steps to determine the best course of action that will be most effective *for you.*

In addition, with the exception of oral progesterone such as Prometrium, bio-identical estrogen patches, Armour thyroid, and human growth hormone, I highly recommend that you obtain your hormone products through a compounding pharmacy. Compounding pharmacists produce their medications from scratch. This allows physicians like me to custom-tailor medications for our patients that may not otherwise be available from most drugstore pharmacies. Compounding is also necessary to allow pharmacists to prepare small quantities of hormone compounds more frequently, to ensure their greater stability. To locate a compounding pharmacy near you, visit: www.compounding-pharmacies.org/pharmacy-locations.

Rejuvenate Your Hormones Using Homeopathy

In addition to the use of bio-identical hormone replacement therapy and the various other approaches discussed in this chapter to balance and restore hormonal function, I will often use homeopathic formulas to regenerate glands that produce hormones. (For more about homeopathy, see Chapter 9.) The reason these formulas are so effective has to do with the biophysics of the body's regenerative process. As you learned in Chapter 2, each organ system of your body, including the endocrine (hormone) system, is connected to your vital life force, or *qi*. In addition, each organ system also possesses its own unique bioenergy system that vibrates at a specific resonant frequency.

Any imbalance in an organ's bioenergy impairs its innate processes of repair and renewal. In order to stimulate regeneration, cells and organs require a specific input of energy. The homeopathic formulas that I developed to help optimize hormone function provide this input of energy using certain wave-forms that correspond to specific endocrine glands. The formulas provide the glands with the right amount of energy, coupled with the right "message".

Unlike nutritional supplements, herbal remedies, and other forms of hormone therapies, homeopathic remedies do not first need to be broken down before they can be converted for use in the body. This conversion process requires expenditures of energy which. in patients who are already weak or sick, can further deplete them, thus impeding healing and regeneration. With homeopathy, this problem does not exist.

Based on years of clinical experience, I find that the homeopathic remedies I've developed work well and synergistically in conjunction with bio-identical hormone replacement therapy and the various other measures I employ to restore hormone balance and proper function. That's because the formulas provide the proper information, frequencies, and energies to the endocrine glands, enhancing their ability to remain more physiologically active while BHRT is also used. The formulas also enhance the receptivity of the cell hormone receptor sites to the bio-identical hormones.

Each of the formulas I've developed for this purpose contain homeopathic adenosine triphosphate (ATP) at a potency of 5X, which I found to be the essential energy frequency to assist regeneration of all tissues and organs, including the endocrine glands. Many of the formulas also have multiple potencies (both X and C dilutions). This makes them more effective because, when it comes to regeneration, energy by itself is not enough. There also needs to be a message that tells the cell to move into the regenerative mode. It is the combination of the X and C potencies that acts as the vehicle for delivering this message. In other words, the body is free to choose which of the potencies it needs at any one time. An additional advantage, of course, is that the homeopathic formulas are completely safe to use, making them an ideal treatment for hormone rejuvenation.

You can find out more about the homeopathic remedies I've developed, as well as how to obtain them, by visiting my website: www. DrGalitzer.com.

Conclusion

In concluding this chapter, I want to reiterate a point I made above. Before employing any type of hormone therapy for the sex hormones, it is most important that insufficiencies in the major hormone glands first be addressed, starting first with strengthening the adrenal and thyroid glands themselves, and then balancing the production of adrenal and thyroid hormones. As I mentioned, in the body the adrenals and the hormones they produce represent survival, whereas the sex glands and their hormones basically represent reproduction.

Survival is always more important than reproduction. This means the body will do whatever it takes to maximize survival first, especially with regard to adrenal hormone output. With that in mind, the body will convert the sex hormones into adrenal hormones to maintain survival at any cost, which is why when you are stressed and tired, your sex hormones and your sex drive goes down. So you really can't go straight to sex hormone therapy before you maximize adrenal function, as well as optimizing thyroid function and restoring adrenal and thyroid hormone balance.

Key Points to Remember

Hormones act as your body's chemical messengers and are responsible for overseeing and regulating a wide range of functions. When hormone levels decline or become imbalanced, poor health and lack of energy inevitably follow.

Hormone levels do not decline because we age, *we age because our hormone levels decline or become imbalanced.*

The most important hormones in terms of health and longevity are the major hormones: cortisol, DHEA, growth hormone, insulin, and the thyroid hormones. These are the hormones that represent survival. The minor, yet still important, sex hormones estrogen, progesterone, and testosterone primarily represent reproduction.

Two of the most significant causes of hormone imbalances and deficiencies are chronic stress and environmental toxins.

Poor diet, nutritional deficiencies, and unhealthy lifestyle choices are also contributing factors.

The adrenal glands, pancreas and thyroid gland all play important roles in maintaining proper hormone balance and overall good health.

Before treating hormone deficiencies and imbalances, it is important to first strengthen the hormone glands themselves.

Knowing the best approach to take when it comes to dealing with hormone issues lies in metabolic typing and determining each person's key hormone gland. This is something that can quickly, easily, and accurately be done using Energy Medicine.

Cortisol is commonly out of balance due to chronic stress. Chronic stress can ultimately lead to adrenal exhaustion and a wide range of health problems.

DHEA acts as your body's "mother hormone", meaning that your body can use it to produce other hormones. There is more DHEA in your body than any other hormone. Therefore, maintaining healthy DHEA levels is another key to creating outstanding health.

Human growth hormone (HGH) acts as a turbocharger for your body, but before growth hormone should be addressed, it is important that the "wheels" of your car be in place and in balance.

The sex hormones estrogen, progesterone, and testosterone offer far reaching health benefits beyond simply maintaining the health of your sex organs.

One of the most effective methods for optimizing hormonal function, especially of the sex hormones, is the use of bio-identical hormone replacement therapy (BHRT). Unlike synthetic hormones like Premarin that are structurally altered and can cause side effects, bio-identical hormones mimic hormones that are naturally produced in the body. Their use both increases the effectiveness of hormone therapy and greatly minimizes the risk of side effects.

Before men and women begin BHRT it is important that they have a comprehensive blood test along with a saliva panel assay to determine their current health status and specific needs. Follow up testing during the course of BHRT treatment is also necessary in order to monitor patient progress.

Bio-identical hormones are best obtained through a compounding pharmacy. Compounding pharmaceutical preparation methods offer many benefits over other pharmacies.

An excellent additional therapy for optimizing hormone function is the use of homeopathic formulas specifically developed to address hormone imbalances and weakness.

The sex organs represent reproduction in the body, whereas the adrenal glands represent survival. From the perspective of the body, survival is always more important than reproduction. When the adrenals are taxed, they will call upon the stress hormones to aid them. For this reason, it is essential that adrenal health be addressed first before treating sex hormone imbalances or deficiencies. Balancing thyroid function is also important.

CHAPTER 11

Awaken Your Brain

One of the saddest health-related trends in our nation today is the increasing incidence of Alzheimer's disease, dementia, and other brain-related health conditions. As with many other degenerative diseases, such types of brain disease were once rare; now, they are not only becoming commonplace, they are manifesting earlier than ever before. Where only a few short decades ago, afflictions such as Alzheimer's and dementia seemed to manifest only in old age, today they are afflicting otherwise seemingly healthy men and women in their 50s and, in some cases, even earlier. Currently:

One in eight Americans 65 and older has Alzheimer's disease.

45 percent of all Americans 85 and older have Alzheimer's.

Nearly 5 percent of all Americans below the age of 65 are also afflicted with Alzheimer's.

Alzheimer's disease is the sixth leading cause of death in the United States.

The statistics on dementia among Americans is equally grim, with the incidence of dementia projected to double every 20 years. ("Dementia" is an umbrella term describing a variety of diseases and conditions that develop when nerve cells in the brain die or no longer function normally. The death or malfunction of these nerve cells, called neurons, causes changes in one's memory, behavior, and ability to think clearly. In Alzheimer's disease, these brain changes eventually impair an individual's ability to carry out such basic bodily functions as walking and swallowing.)

It is commonly assumed that the rise in Alzheimer and dementia rates are primarily due to the fact that, overall, Americans are living longer than their ancestors. That assumption is erroneous. There are far more important factors involved, that take hold many years, and even decades, prior to symptoms of such conditions first becoming noticeable. Recognizing and addressing those factors before they become severe is the key to keeping your brain healthy and youthful.

Before we proceed further, here are some important questions to ask yourself:

Are you noticing that you are having memory problems?

Do you have difficulty focusing or concentrating?

Do you find it more difficult to learn new things, compared to when you were younger?

Do you experience moments of "brain fog", or mental confusion?

Do you tire easily, especially when engaged in mental activities such as reading, thinking, writing, etc.?

Are you experiencing a lack of motivation?

Are you less passionate about your life than you used to be?

Do you experience fatigue after eating certain foods?

A yes answer to any of the above questions can be an early indication that your brain is in need of attention.

Fortunately, your brain is one of the most adaptable and resilient organs in your body. When provided with what it needs to be healthy, it can exhibit remarkable powers of regeneration and renewal. The first step in providing for your brain lies with knowing what causes it harm.

Factors That Can Harm Your Brain

As I mentioned, aging, of itself, is *not* the cause of declining brain health. The actual causes are varied and usually interrelated. They include obvious causes such as poor diet and nutritional deficiencies and imbalances, environmental toxins, and chronic stress, to lesser known factors, such as blood sugar imbalances, brain inflammation, lack of oxygen, thyroid and other hormonal imbalances, gluten sensitivity and impaired gut health and related gastrointestinal problems, the overuse of pharmaceutical drugs, and lack of sleep. By understanding the roles that each of these factors play in damaging the brain, and then taking the necessary steps to prevent and manage them, there is much that you can do on your own to help ensure that your brain stays healthy.

Poor Diet and Lack of Nutrition: Poor diet and nutritional imbalances and deficiencies are a primary cause of brain degeneration. Deficiencies in various vitamins, minerals, essential fatty acids, and amino acids, especially B vitamins, vitamins C, D, and E, omega 3s, magnesium, selenium, and zinc, have all been linked to impaired brain function, as well as brain diseases, including Alzheimer's and dementia.

Nutritional deficiencies are compounded by unhealthy diets, which not only prevent your brain from getting all of the nutrients it needs, but also results in over-acidity and chronic inflammation, blood sugar imbalances, and the toxic effects of gluten (all covered below). As Dr. Datis Kharrazian, DHSc, DC, a leading researcher in brain health and brain regeneration states, "If you want your brain to work you have to change your diet." Doing so is absolutely vital.

One of the main reasons why a healthy diet and a daily supply of nutrients are so essential for proper brain function has to with how the brain operates. It does so primarily through the transmission of chemical messengers known as neurotransmitters, which are responsible for how the brain communicates with the rest of the body. For neurotransmitters to be able to transmit the brain's messages effectively, proper pH (acid-alkaline) balance is necessary, as well as an adequate supply of brain nutrients. When pH levels become too acidic as a result of poor diet, and nutrient supply is insufficient, the brain and its functions are adversely affected, eventually resulting in degeneration and symptoms of brain fog, memory loss, and dementia.

Environmental Toxins: It is well known that environmental toxins play a significant role in various neurological conditions, including autism, multiple sclerosis (MS), Parkinson's disease, in addition to other degenerative diseases, such as cancer, diabetes, and heart disease. Less well-known is the fact that these toxins can contribute to a wide variety of other brain conditions, ranging from attention deficit-hyperactivity disorder (ADD/ADHD), anxiety, and depression to learning disabilities, memory problems, and restless leg syndrome (RLS).

Environmental toxins harm the brain both directly, by crossing the blood-brain barrier, and indirectly, by compromising immune and liver function. Toxins that cross the blood-brain barrier deposit themselves within brain tissues, causing brain cells, tissues, and neurotransmitters to become impaired, and eventually leading to the buildup of brain plaque, which is a major contributing factor in the onset of Alzheimer's and dementia. This process is further exacerbated by the negative effects toxins have on the immune system and the liver.

Altered immune function caused by environmental toxins causes the blood-brain barrier to become more porous, or "leaky", in much the same way that toxins can cause leaky gut syndrome. The more porous the blood-brain barrier becomes, the easier it is for toxins to cross it and settle in brain tissue.

As you learned in earlier chapters of this book, your liver is your primary internal organ of detoxification, and can become overburdened and impaired by the buildup of toxins in the body. As this occurs, the liver's ability to make use of glutathione, an amino acid compound that is often referred to as the body's "master antioxidant" because of the primary role it plays in protecting the body's cells and tissues from free radical damage, becomes compromised. Though glutathione is found throughout the body, it is concentrated in the liver, where it plays a major role in the liver's ability to carry out its various detoxification processes. Simply put, lack of glutathione in the liver means impaired liver function, including detoxification, which in turn results in an increased buildup of toxins, both in the liver and throughout the rest of the body, including the brain.

Impaired liver function due to toxicity sets up a vicious circle between the brain and the liver. When brain function becomes impaired because of impaired liver function caused by toxins, it further impairs liver function, which, in turn, leads to further brain degeneration.

There are a wide range of environmental toxins that can negatively affect your brain. In addition to heavy metals, they include aflatoxins, benzene, bisphenol-A (BPA), formaldehyde, pesticides, polymers from plastics, and tetrachloroethylene, a chemical commonly found in upholstery products and also used during dry cleaning.

Chronic Stress: According to Dr. Kharrazian, "Nothing is more damaging to the brain than stress. Stress atrophies the entire brain, meaning it literally shrinks the brain." Research bears this out, and has also shown that chronic stress can impair brain and cognitive function, trigger brain inflammation, and negatively impact the blood-brain barrier, making the brain more susceptible to an influx of toxins and infectious agents.

No doubt you have experienced the effects of stress on your brain. Think back on a time when you found yourself working under stressful conditions, or to any other time in your life when you experienced significant stress. During such times you likely noticed a decline in your cognitive ability, perhaps forgetting an appointment or temporarily having difficulty remembering something. Once the stress passed, your memory may have returned to normal yet, over time, the accumulation of additional stressful experiences can begin to take a toll on your brain.

Unfortunately, stress is unavoidable. In our typically fast-paced society, your brain is regularly forced to juggle and prioritize the events of the day, while simultaneously processing and remembering often highly complex, detailed information in ways past generations could not begin to imagine, let alone cope with. Nearly all of us, to some extent at least, have become multitaskers who are regularly on the go. On top of that, in order to meet the demands of the day, many people skip meals, subsist on coffee or unhealthy "energy drinks," and, when they do take time to eat, consume fast-food or otherwise nutritionally deficient meals in order to keep themselves going. Such behaviors act as further serious stressors to the brain. Thus, it's hardly surprising that so many people today complain of "brain fog" or mental fatigue.

Stress harms the brain and its functions in a number of ways. The first way involves the brain's neural networks. These web-like pathways are composed of neurons. Combined, these neural networks consist of an estimated 100 billion neurons that "light up" or "fire" in response to external stimuli, such as sights, sounds, smells, tastes, or touch, as well as during the brain's many processes, including learning and memory.

Until recently, most people were accustomed to thinking about learning and memory as being akin to storing information and experiences in a filing system, where they could be retrieved as needed. Ongoing research into the brain and how it functions has disproven this analogy. In fact, learning, memory, and mental perception all depend on a far more complex process in which the brain's neurons and neural networks play vital roles. Put simply, each time you learn, perceive, or otherwise experience something, what you are experiencing causes neurons to light up, and your experience—including everything you see, hear, smell, touch, and taste—gets encoded into your brain as a memory.

As an example of how this process works, let's say a few years ago you attended a concert by one of your favorite bands. If you should be asked tomorrow if you had ever seen the band, that question would act as a verbal trigger that would instantaneously light up the part of your brain's neural network where the memories of the concert you attended are encoded. As this occurs, you most likely will be able to recall the concert in clear detail, even including the people next to you in the audience, the songs that were played, and the emotions you felt as the band performed. Yet, although the memories of the concert may seem like actual snapshots or moving images of that time, what is actually occurring is that your brain is reactivating the specific pattern of neural network firing that first occurred as you enjoyed the concert.

There are countless specific neural network patterns that are stored in your brain, many of which have been reactivated so often that you don't even notice the reactivations when they occur, such as when you return home each day from work, or drive to your local gas station, or recall the names of friends, family members, and co-workers. All of these activities happen automatically, without you needing to pay attention to them, because of how frequently the neural network patterns associated with them have been stimulated in your past.

By contrast, when you need to recall something that is not a regular part of your life, such as the directions to a place you've only been to a few times in the past, more mental effort is usually required to "light up" the neural network pattern linked to that memory. In both examples, however, memory retrieval is an active, dynamic process that depends on a high level of interaction of brain neurons. When this interactivity is interfered with, memory can become impaired, as well. This is precisely what happens as a result of stress. Studies have shown that the release of stress hormones, such as adrenaline and, especially, cortisol, interferes with the brain's ability to process memory, as well as other brain functions. Moreover, research has also demonstrated that excessive levels of cortisol caused by chronic stress can directly impair neuron function, as well as neuron growth and development.

Other studies have also found that high cortisol levels can cause the part of the brain known as the hippocampus, which is considered the seat of both learning and memory, to become over-activated. Over time, this impairs the various functions that the hippocampus controls, including the ability to learn and remember. It's important to note that the hippocampus is the part of the brain that is first affected at the onset of neurological conditions such as Alzheimer's and dementia.

Chronic stress also takes a toll on the brain's ability to oversee the autonomic nervous system (ANS), which is responsible for regulating all physiological functions that occur without conscious thought, including breathing, digestion, and the functioning of your heart and other body organs. This does much to explain why chronic stress takes such a toll on overall health.

Blood Sugar Imbalances: Stable blood sugar (glucose) levels are essential for healthy brain function. Blood sugar levels that are too high (hyperglycemia), too low (hypoglycemia), or which regularly fluctuate between levels that are high and low, can all impair your brain's ability to perform its many tasks.

The reason blood sugar levels are such vital factors in brain health is because glucose is the brain's primary source of fuel. Optimal blood sugar levels help ensure that overall brain chemistry remains balanced, and also prevent damage to, or loss of, neuron structure and function, as well as the death of neurons. Balanced blood sugar levels are also required for proper production of neurotransmitters, as well as healthy neurotransmitter metabolism and function.

Imbalanced, or unstable, blood sugar levels either deprive the brain of enough glucose or flood it with too much glucose. Either way, brain health is negatively impacted. Brain symptoms caused or made worse by low blood sugar include excess production of the adrenal hormones epinephrine and norepinephrine, as a result of low levels of the adrenal hormone cortisol. Cortisol, as mentioned earlier, prevents low blood sugar. Other symptoms caused by low blood sugar include mood swings, anxiety, irritability, forgetfulness, and feelings of lightheadedness.

High blood sugar levels result in insulin resistance, as the pancreas continues to produce insulin in an effort to force glucose into the cells. However, the excess glucose gets converted into fat, increasing total body fat. The conversion of glucose into fat requires energy, which creates fatigue. High insulin levels cause chronic inflammation, disruption of other hormones, and impaired neurotransmitter function, all of which, in turn, can cause degeneration of the brain and its functions. In addition, elevated blood sugar and insulin resistance also causes excessive production of cortisol.

Common symptoms and indications of high blood sugar and insulin resistance include fatigue and sleepiness after meals, cravings for sugar and sweets, over-dependence on coffee or other stimulant drinks for energy, frequent urination, increased sensations of hunger and thirst, unhealthy weight gain (especially around the belly and thighs) and difficulty losing weight. According to Dr. Kharrazian, all of these symptoms are "red flags that the brain is under attack and rapidly aging". As Dr.

Kharrazian also points out, fluctuating blood sugar levels in combination with insulin resistance are quite common.

The primary cause of blood sugar imbalances and insulin resistance is poor diets that contain high levels of sugars and excess carbohydrates, and insufficient levels of quality proteins and healthy fats. Skipping meals and food sensitivities can also be contributing factors.

Brain Inflammation: Another significant cause of impaired brain function is brain inflammation, also known as neuroinflammation. Just as chronic inflammation in the rest of your body can cause a wide range of health problems, it can also trigger brain and cognitive problems. In fact, inflammation in the brain and elsewhere in the body creates a vicious circle. As inflammation occurs in the body it causes the release of a class of proteins known as cytokines, especially within the immune system. "These cytokines send messages across the blood-brain barrier that activate inflammation in the brain, which alters brain function and destroys brain tissue," Dr. Kharrazian explains. "Likewise, inflammation or degeneration in the brain can trigger systemic inflammation that results in such issues as joint pain, gut pain, skin disorders, or more."

A growing body of research is confirming a correlation between impaired brain health, chronic inflammation, and autoimmune responses in which the body's immune system attacks healthy tissues and organs. Studies have also linked brain inflammation to chronic depression. When inflammation in the brain occurs, the rate at which neurons fire slows down. This, in turn, can lead to brain fog and impaired memory. Brain inflammation also reduces energy production in brain cells. Chronic brain inflammation can lead to neuron death and the onset of neurodegenerative diseases.

The primary cells of the brain that are affected by inflammation are called *microglia*, which act as the first and main type of active immune defense in the brain and central nervous system. Under healthy conditions, microglia perform and maintain numerous important functions that help ensure healthy function and protect the brain from inflammation and premature aging. But when they interact with toxins, bacteria, or other foreign matter that penetrate into the brain due to a leaky blood-brain barrier, they trigger an inflammatory immune response. Because microglia have no "off switch", once they become activated they will continue to promote brain inflammation for the rest of their lifespan, causing the destruction of brain tissue and increasing the risk of brain degeneration. Additionally, once activated, microglia typically activate other surrounding microglia, creating a domino effect of ever worsening inflammation in the brain.   In addition to the invasion of foreign toxins and microorganisms into the brain, a number of other factors can cause brain inflammation. Among the most common causes are nutritional deficiencies, a high-carbohydrate diet, wheat and other gluten foods, regular alcohol consumption, poor circulation, and elevated homocysteine levels (see Chapter 13). Health conditions such as diabetes and gastrointestinal disorders can also play a major role.

Oxygen Supply: A sufficient supply of oxygen to the brain is one of the most important requirements for healthy brain function. In fact, oxygen deprivation lasting more than five minutes is all that is usually necessary to cause permanent brain damage. Signs of a lack of brain oxygen include poor focus and concentration, cold extremities (hands and feet), poor finger- and toenail health, and fungal growth on the toes.

Most of us typically believe we are getting all of the oxygen we need simply because we are still breathing. But, as you learned earlier in this book, most people are habitually shallow breathers, and are thus deprived of an adequate supply of oxygen on a daily basis. While it is true that you are obtaining enough oxygen to survive, it is very likely you are not getting enough oxygen to *thrive*, thus putting your brain at risk for deterioration.

Oxygen is carried to your brain by your blood, which also transports the nutrients, hormones, and neurotransmitters that your brain requires. Poor blood flow, or circulation, is the primary cause of lack of oxygen in the brain, and also the cause of vascular dementia, which is the second most common form of dementia after Alzheimer's disease. Lack of oxygen also prevents brain neurons from producing all of the energy they need to survive and carry out their many functions. In short, poor circulation and lack of oxygen to the brain go hand and hand.

A number of factors can cause poor circulation and diminish the brain's oxygen supply. Perhaps the biggest factor is stress. As you've learned, when under stress, your body initiates the "fight or flight" response. During this response, breathing becomes shallow, often with prolonged pauses between inhalation and exhalation (notice how you hold your breath when you are frightened).

Other primary factors that can deprive your brain of sufficient oxygen include both high and low blood pressure, anemia, poor lung function and respiratory conditions, smoking, and lack of a specific form of nitric oxide known as endothelial nitric oxide, or eNOS, which is found in blood vessel walls (the endothelium) and plays an important role in healthy circulation and helps dissolve plaque buildup in the arteries. Various diseases can also inhibit oxygen flow to the brain, such as heart disease and diabetes.

Hormone Imbalances: Healthy hormone function is also essential for a healthy, optimally-functioning brain. Both brain neurons and microglia cells have receptor sites for hormones, and research has shown that healthy hormone balance plays important roles in preventing brain inflammation and degeneration, as well as in helping neural networks to grow and branch out, and in maintaining optimal neuroplasticity (the ability of neurons, and hence the brain, to adapt its neural pathways in response to changes in the environment, as well as changes in behavior, learning, memory, and emotions, and changes occurring as a result of bodily injury). Hormones also help to maintain the shape and structure of the brain.

Hormone imbalances can seriously impair all of the above functions, as well as accelerate premature aging of the brain. Because of how dependent neurotransmitter activity is on hormone balance, any hormonal imbalance can also negatively affect your thoughts, attitudes, perception of life, and how your body functions. These include the sex hormones (estrogen, progesterone, and testosterone), and thyroid hormone.

Estrogen and testosterone provide brain benefits for both men and women, particularly with regard to cognitive and memory function. Both of these hormones also help prevent the buildup of beta-amyloid deposits that are associated with both Alzheimer's and dementia. Thyroid hormone also helps maintain memory, as does DHEA. On average, people with Alzheimer's disease have 48 percent less DHEA than healthy people of their same age group. Imbalanced levels of cortisol can also affect memory.

Three other hormones that play important roles in brain health are pregnenolone, progesterone, and melatonin. Pregnenolone is sometimes referred to as "the hormone of memory" because of the many roles it plays. In addition to helping to produce DHEA, estrogen, progesterone, and testosterone, pregnenolone helps to regulate and balance the nervous system, improves stress resistance, improves both physical and mental energy levels, enhances nerve transmission, enhances memory, promotes nerve growth factor, blocks the production of acid-forming compounds, and reduces pain and inflammation. It also directly influences acetylcholine release. The body's production of pregnenolone declines with age. On average, both men and women at age 75 have 65 percent less pregnenolone than they did when they were 36.

Progesterone, which is produced in the brain, spinal cord, and peripheral nerves from pregnenolone, has a significant positive impact on GABA receptor sites in the brains of both men and women. In women, it also helps maintain proper dopamine activity and dopamine receptor sites. Studies have also shown that progesterone helps to regulate the activity of the brain's microglia cells. It also plays an important role for protecting and repairing myelin sheaths, which act as protective coatings of the nerves, and in protecting against brain inflammation.

Melatonin is both an antioxidant and a neurotransmitter. In addition to promoting healthy sleep and enhancing immune function, melatonin helps to protect nerve cells from damage caused by heavy metals. It is especially effective in this regard as a protector against cobalt damage. This is of particular significance for Alzheimer's patients, who typically have high cobalt levels and low levels of melatonin.

Evaluating hormone levels is therefore very important when it comes to protecting brain health. To learn much more about hormones, and how to balance them, refer back to Chapter 11.

Gluten Sensitivity and the Brain-Gut Connection: As you learned in Chapter 7, your gastrointestinal (GI) tract acts as your body's "second brain". Both the brain and the GI tract act synergistically with each other. Imbalances in the GI tract can negatively impact the brain, while GI function can be compromised by impaired brain function. The sensitive relationship between the brain and the GI tract is known to physicians as the "brain-gut axis".

The importance of the brain-gut axis to health is evident from the moment of conception. As soon as the female egg is fertilized by sperm, both the brain and gut begin developing at the same time, doing so from the same cluster of tissue. From out of this tissue evolves the central nervous system of the brain, and a corresponding system known as the enteric nervous system of the GI tract. Both of these systems in the human body are connected by the vagus nerve, the longest of all the cranial nerves. The vagus nerve, which originates in the region of the brain known as the medulla oblongata, travels to every major organ in the body, sending nerve impulses, or messages, to and from the brain. It is also the primary nerve that regulates the parasympathetic nervous system, which is responsible for promoting calm and easing the effects of stress. In addition to how the vagus nerve links the brain and GI tract, many of the same neurotransmitters, hormones and other biochemicals that are found in the brain are also found in the gut. Due to research about this linkage of the brain-gut axis, we now know that a healthy gut helps to support the brain and maintain mental and emotional health.

Symptoms of imbalances in the brain-gut axis include both GI disturbances and symptoms of impaired brain function, such as "brain fog," mood swings, behavioral disorders such as ADD/ADHD, and cognitive and memory problems. Research has established that poor gut health can cause or worsen a range of brain-related issues, including anxiety and depression, memory loss, schizophrenia, and neurological conditions such as Parkinson's disease.

I have already discussed the roles that poor diet and nutritional imbalances play in impairing brain function. Now I want to focus on gluten, a dietary protein found in wheat and wheat foods such as bread and pasta, as well as various other foods, including barley, rye, spelt, and most brands of oats, along with beer, processed condiments, deli meats, soy sauce, and many food additives. I am in complete agreement with Dr. Kharrazian's statement about gluten: "No single dietary protein is a more potent trigger of neurological dysfunction and neurological autoimmunity than gluten." Simply put, though most people believe they do not have a problem with it, *gluten acts as a poison in your body.*

When I point this fact out to my patients, some of them object to my recommendation that they avoid all gluten-containing foods, saying, "But, Dr. Galitzer, people have been eating wheat for thousands of years." That's true. Yet the wheat they consumed then is no longer the wheat that is available to us today, and that includes the gluten the wheat contains. Because of various food production methods used in the past few decades to create larger and faster yields of wheat and other gluten crops, wheat and other gluten foods that were once healthy for humans are healthy no longer.

The two main production methods that turned gluten into a poisonous substance are hybridization and deamidation. The process of hybridization with regard to wheat involves the combination of different wheat strains to create a new, so-called hardier protein. This alteration process can change the protein sequence in wheat by as much as five percent, which may not seem significant, yet which results in a wheat that is quite different from the original wheat strains used to make it. And science is proving this fact, having found that this "new wheat" is far more likely to trigger autoimmune reactions, particularly in the brain and nervous system, compared to the wheat of our ancestors. Similar unhealthy changes occur when barley, rye, and other gluten-foods are also hybridized.

This problem is made worse by the process of deamidation, which makes use of acids and enzymes to make gluten water soluble, so that it is able to be added and more readily mixed with other foods and food products. (Gluten found in wheat grown decades ago was usually only soluble in alcohol.) Researchers have found that deamidation causes gluten to further trigger autoimmune reactions, and to act as a major, yet often hidden or misdiagnosed, cause of inflammation and degeneration of tissues, again especially in the brain and nervous system.

The fact that gluten is more of a brain issue than an issue of the GI tract is not well-known to most people, including doctors, and may seem surprising. One reason for that is because many people, when they think of gluten, immediately also think of celiac disease, a serious autoimmune condition that targets and damages the gut. However, there are far more people who are affected by gluten without developing celiac disease, than there are people who do develop the disease. In addition, many people develop what is known as silent celiac disease, a condition that does not target the GI tract, but rather the thyroid gland, joints, and other parts of the body, and most especially the brain and central nervous system.

This fact was confirmed by research which found that only one-third of people with gluten-related brain symptoms also suffered from GI problems. Additional research has shown that gluten can cause a wide range of brain-related conditions, including cognitive impairment and memory loss, dementia, psychiatric disorders, neuropathy and overall impairment of the nervous system, headache and migraine, movement disorders, and various other problems. Based on such research, Dr. Kharrazian says, "We are now learning that gluten sensitivity destroys the brain and nervous tissue more than any other tissue of the body, including that of the gastrointestinal tract."

There are three main ways that gluten attacks the brain and nervous system. First, it provokes an autoimmune reaction in the brain or nerve tissue because the immune system mistakes such tissues for gluten, since the protein structure of gluten is similar to the protein structures of these tissues. This similarity can cause the immune system to mistakenly produce antibodies to the brain and nervous system whenever gluten-foods are eaten.

Secondly, gluten can trigger an immune reaction to an enzyme in the brain known as *transglutaminase-6*, resulting in an autoimmune response that can destroy brain neurons in much the same way that celiac disease damages the GI tract. Finally, the autoimmune reactions to gluten can damage the blood-brain barrier, resulting in a condition known as "leaky brain" syndrome, which is very similar to the leaky gut syndrome you learned about in Chapter 7.

The problem of gluten sensitivity can be compounded by food proteins that cross-react with gluten. Cross-reactions occur because certain proteins in other foods resemble gluten enough to provoke the same type of reactions that gluten provokes. They include oats, yeast, sesame, certain brands of instant coffee, and casein, a protein found in milk, cheese, and other dairy products.

Despite how widespread gluten sensitivity is today, many doctors, including both gastroenterologists and neurologists, continue to ignore or underestimate the ways in which is can be harming their patients. Moreover, the most common medical tests used to test for gluten sensitivity are not up to the task for truly making an accurate diagnosis. For this reason, I recommend the use of tests available exclusively from Cyrex Labs. The first test is called the Wheat/Gluten Proteome Sensitivity and Autoimmunity Panel, which screens for gluten sensitivity. The second test is called the Gluten-Associated Sensitivity and Cross Reactive Foods Array, which, as its name suggests, screens foods that most often cross-react with gluten. For more information about these and other tests available from Cyrex, visit www.cyrexlabs.com.

Pharmaceutical Drugs: The ongoing use of pharmaceutical drugs is one of the primary causes of dementia and other brain conditions, including delirium, in the elderly. This is especially true of people who have been prescribed more than one drug at a time. This is known as drug-induced cognitive impairment.

Given how widespread the use of pharmaceutical drugs has become in our society, drug-induced brain problems no longer affect just the elderly. This is not surprising, given that all pharmaceutical drugs carry some risk of side effects. Common side effects related to the brain that can be caused by regular drug use also include anxiety, "brain fog", depression, erratic behavior patterns, and suicidal thoughts. In certain cases, drugs, either alone or used in combination can even cause brain damage.

Many drugs can also interfere with the brain's ability to produce energy because of how they impair mitochondria function. As you learned early in this book, mitochondria act as your cells' energy plants. Among the highest concentrations of mitochondria in the body are those within the brain and the heart. Many pharmaceutical drugs contain fluoride derivatives. Fluoride negates magnesium's many roles in the body, one of which is activating ATP within the mitochondria.

Another area of concern regarding brain health is the potentially harmful role that statin drugs may play. Statins, which act to lower cholesterol levels in the body, represent the most widely prescribed class of drugs in the U.S. today. As you will learn in more detail in Chapter 12, despite the insistence of the medical establishment otherwise, cholesterol of itself is not a risk factor for heart disease. Cholesterol plays many important roles in helping the body to maintain its health, including within the brain and the nervous system.

One of the most important roles cholesterol plays is in the formation of synapses, or connections between neurons. Synapse formation is directly dependent on cholesterol, and without enough cholesterol proper learning and memory function cannot take place. In fact, one of the reasons that healthy sleep is beneficial to learning and memory is because it enables the brain to make more cholesterol. Because of how statins inhibit cholesterol levels, a number of health experts speculate that the rising rates of Alzheimer's and dementia over the past few decades may, at least indirectly, be related to the corresponding increase in statin use over that same time period.

Another class of drugs that can significantly increase the risk of impaired brain function are the benzodiazepines. Benzodiazepines include many anti-anxiety drugs, sleeping pills, and tranquillizers. A 2014 study published in the *British Medical Journal* found that the use of benzodiazepine drugs for as little as three months can increase the risk of Alzheimer's by as much as 51 percent, and that the risk increases the longer such drugs are used.

Overall, the primary classes of drugs that have been directly linked to impaired brain function are:

Analgesics (pain medications).

Anti-arrhythmia drugs.

Antibiotics.

Anticonvulsant drugs.

Antidepressants.

Antiepileptic drugs.

Antihistamines and decongestants.

Benzodiazepines (anti-anxiety drugs, sleeping pills, tranquilizers).

Beta blockers.

Bismuth (a common ingredient in drugs used to treat diarrhea, heartburn, upset stomach, and other gastrointestinal complaints).

Blood pressure medications.

Cancer chemotherapy

Cholesterol-lowering drugs (statins).

Corticosteroids.

Ibuprofen.

Narcotic drugs (opiates).

If you are currently using prescription drugs and suspect they may be affecting your brain function, speak with your doctor. In almost all cases normal brain function can be reversed or returned to its pre-drug state by stopping the use of the offending drug. The weaning off process needs to be supervised by a physician.

Lack of Sleep: As it is for the rest of your body, sleep is the time of repair for your brain. During sleep, your brain also consolidates the memories of what you learned and experienced during the day. Sleep also aids your brain in ridding itself of wastes.

Lack of sleep not only impairs healthy brain function because of how sleeplessness and fitful sleep act as a stressor on the brain, it can also cause the brain itself to atrophy, or shrink. This fact was confirmed by a recent study published in the medical journal *Neurology*.

In that study, which involved 147 adults between the ages of 20 and 84, researchers used MRI scans to examine the link between sleep problems like insomnia and the study participants' brain size. The MRI scans were done approximately three and a half years apart, with the first scans done at the onset of the study. After the first scan, the study participants completed a questionnaire related to their sleep habits. Based on the questionnaire, 35 percent of the study group were found to regularly experience insomnia or other types of sleep problems and overall lack of sleep.

The second MRI scans were given at the end of the study. The results of these scans showed that those who were poor sleepers exhibited a significantly more rapid decline in the size of their brains over the course of the study than those who slept well, with the most atrophy occurring in the frontal, temporal, and parietal regions of the brain. The frontal lobes help oversee and regulate motor functions (movement), planning, reasoning, judgment, and impulse control, and are also responsible for personality expression. The temporal lobes play an important role in organizing sensory input (especially seeing and hearing), language and speech production, as well as memory association and formation, and emotional responses. The parietal regions of the brain play a vital role in the brain's processing of information (including touch and pain sensations), visual perception, speech, and spatial orientation. The reduced size of these brain areas among poor sleepers was most pronounced in study participants over the age of 60.

Numerous previous studies have also demonstrated how important healthy sleep is for brain health, and how lack of, or fitful, sleep can negatively impact the brain and its many functions. Lack of sleep has also been found to be a contributing factor in the development of Alzheimer's and dementia. Therefore, ensuring that you obtain adequate amounts of quality sleep each night is vitally important for maintaining the optimal brain health.

Given the importance of sleep for proper brain function, as well as overall health, many people turn to sleeping pills to obtain the sleep they need. I do not recommend this option unless it is absolutely necessary, which is rarely the case. Especially because, as you read in the section on pharmaceutical drugs above, sleeping pills are among the many medications can harm the brain, and significantly increase the risk for developing Alzheimer's disease. Rather than resorting to the use of such drugs, if you suffer from sleep problems, I highly advise that you follow the sleep-promoting strategies and recommendations in Chapter 10.

Managing the Factors That Can Harm Your Brain

Now that you understand the primary factors that can harm your brain, let's examine the steps you need to take to prevent or reverse such damage.

Diet: The first, and in many respects the most important, step is to adopt a brain-healthy diet. This involves eating foods that do not trigger inflammation and blood sugar spikes, eliminating gluten foods, eliminating foods to which you have sensitivities, and eating meals that have an alkalizing, instead of an acidifying effect, on your body after they are consumed. Chapter 7 provides the guidelines you need to follow for eliminating food sensitivities and for creating alkalizing meals.

The primary dietary key to preventing inflammation and blood sugar spikes is to limit your consumption of carbohydrate foods, and to only consume complex, slow-digesting carbohydrates. Carbohydrates that should be eliminated from your diet begin with all sugars, sweeteners, and simple (white) carbohydrates. Other foods that can cause inflammation and blood sugar spikes include high-glycemic fruits, especially canned and dried fruits, dates, grapes, mango, pineapple, raisins, and watermelon; corn, rice, oats, and other grains; soy and soy products;

all canned and processed foods; alcohol; gluten foods (wheat and wheat products such as bread and pasta, wheat flour, barley, oats, spelt, beer, and various dressings and sauces; you can find a complete list of gluten foods and food products online). For some people, milk and dairy products, as well as eggs and foods that contain eggs, may also need to be eliminated.

The following food categories are your most healthy options: most vegetables, meats and lamb (organically-raised and grass-fed), fermented foods (kimchi, pickles, sauerkraut), and low-glycemic fruits, such as organic apples, apricots, avocados, berries, cherries, peaches, and pears. Various oils are also good for your brain, especially coconut oil (also available as coconut butter, cream, and milk), and organic, extra-virgin olive oil. Drinking plenty of purified, oxygen-rich water and organic herbal teas each day is also important.

Certain fish (those low in mercury and not farm-raised, see Chapter 6) are also excellent "brain foods." This fact was confirmed by a 2014 study in the *American Journal of Preventive Medicine*. In the study, researchers observed 260 healthy adults over a two-year period. They found that both men and women who consumed baked or broiled fish just once a week had increased levels of neuron tissues and up to 14 percent larger brain volumes in the regions responsible for memory and cognitive function. Other studies have confirmed that regularly eating fish at least once a week can reduce the risk of dementia, as well as reducing the risk of brain inflammation and damaged brain tissue. (If you are worried about toxicity from fish, take five chlorella tablets before eating fish, as chlorella will help neutralize any toxins that may be present, especially mercury.)

Another way that you can improve and maintain the health of your brain is to use various spices in your meals. Among the most beneficial spices for doing so are saffron, which has been found to enhance learning and to help prevent depression; turmeric, which has been shown to reduce the incidence of plaque buildup in the brain associated with Alzheimer's and dementia; cinnamon, which helps to balance blood sugar levels and can enhance memory and attention span; cloves, which also help to prevent inflammation; and ginger, another potent anti-inflammatory spice that also helps reduce oxidative stress associated with premature brain cell death and neurodegeneration. You can easily obtain the benefits of these spices simply by adding them to meals. For best results, choose certified organic brands.

Nutritional and Herbal Supplements: A variety of nutrients and herbal supplements can also be very helpful for maintaining the health of your brain. Given the link between the brain-gut axis, I typically recommend that my patients support their gut health by using probiotic supplements, along with GI-protecting supplements such as aloe vera leaf extract, L-glutamine, chamomile, licorice, marshmallow extract. B vitamins are also essential, especially methyl B12 and methyl folate. Used in conjunction with a healthy diet and the strategies for leaky gut that you learned about in Chapter 7, these nutrients can be quite effective.

For helping to control blood sugar and insulin resistance helpful supplements include alpha lipoic acid, chromium, Co-Q10, L-carnitine, vitamin E (tocopherols), magnesium, pectin, vanadium, and zinc, along with the B vitamins biotin, inositol, and niacin.

To help manage and prevent brain damage caused by stress, I recommend the mind/body strategies I shared in chapters 5 and 8, along with supplementation with phosphatidylserine, along with the herbs, holy basil extract, ashwagandha, rhodiola, and Siberian ginseng. These herbs act as adaptogens that aid the hypothalamic-pituitary-adrenal axis, thus protecting the stress pathways of the brain. They can be used individually, but best results are usually achieved when they are used in combination with each other.

To increase blood flow to and oxygenation of the brain, useful supplements include butcher's broom extract, feverfew extract, gingko biloba, huperzine A, vinpocetine, and xanthinol niacinate. Of these, huperzine A, vinpocetine, and xanthinol niacinate, along with acetyl L-carnitine, also support nitric oxide signaling (in the form of eNOS) in the brain and nervous system, as well as in the immune and cardiovascular systems.

In addition to the dietary measures above, to address brain inflammation I often recommend flavonoid supplements, such as apigenin, catechin, luteolin, resveratrol, and rutin. Curcumin, the principal ingredient of turmeric, is also very helpful in this regard.

Other useful supplements for protecting your brain include bacopa monnieri, cordyceps, the essential fatty acid compounds DHA and EPA, glutathione, gotu kola, milk thistle, vitamin D, ginger, boron, and carnosine. Intravenous therapies with glutathione and phosphatidylcholine can be extremely helpful, as well.

Neurotransmitter Support: In order for your brain to function properly its neurons must be able to communicate effectively with each other via chemical messengers known as neurotransmitters. Poor diet, nutritional deficiencies, blood sugar and hormone imbalances, and brain inflammation can all damage and interfere with neurotransmitter function. Addressing these and other factors is therefore vitally important.

The primary neurotransmitters that are usually in need of most attention are acetylcholine, dopamine, GABA, and serotonin.

Symptoms of low acetylcholine levels include comprehension and memory problems (especially memory related to verbalization and visual images), diminished creativity, difficulty with math skills, difficulty comprehending directions and spatial orientation, and difficulty recognizing faces and objects.

Symptoms of low dopamine usually manifest as a lack of self-motivation, inability to start or complete tasks, feelings of despair (hopelessness, unworthiness, etc.), inability to manage anger and stress, feelings of apathy (including towards family and friends), and a desire for isolation from others.

Imbalanced levels of GABA include feelings of anxiety and panic, feeling overwhelmed for no reason, feeling restless or tense, difficulty relaxing, scattered attention, and unexplained worries about issues that normally do not concern you.

Symptoms of imbalanced serotonin levels include lack of joy and contentment, lack of interest in and pleasure from hobbies and interests, depression, unexplained anger, susceptibility to seasonal affective disorder (SAD), inability to achieve restful sleep, and an inability to enjoy meaningful relationships with family and friends.

Both diet and nutritional supplementation can often result in significant improvements in neurotransmitter levels and function. Acetylcholine levels can often be improved by a diet rich in the amino acid choline, such as beef, liver and organ meats, egg yolk, and nuts. Supplementing with huperzine A, acetyl-l- carnitine, GPC (glyceryl-phosphoryl-choline), ashwaganda, DMAE, and pantothenic acid (vitaminB5) can also help.

Most people in America do not develop a lack of dopamine as a result of their diets. More often, it is other factors that cause dopamine imbalances. Nutrients that help support dopamine activity include alpha lipoic acid, beta-phenylethylamine (PEA), D,L-phenylalanine (DLPA), N-acetyl L-tyrosine, vitamin B6 in the form of pyridoxal-5'-phosphate (P5P), and the herb, mucuna pruriens. Eating blueberries on a regular basis can also help. Addressing blood sugar and hormonal imbalances are also important.

As with dopamine, one of the most effective ways to boost and balance GABA activity is through the use of nutritional supplements. These include lithium orotate, magnesium, manganese, P5P, taurine, and zinc. The herbs passion flower and valerian root can also help. The primary dietary intervention is to eliminate all sources of gluten foods and food products because gluten can trigger an autoimmune reaction against an enzyme known as GAD, which is responsible for the body's manufacture of GABA. This is one more reason why I strongly advise against eating gluten foods. For women, progesterone will also increase GABA, which is why it is effective in women with PMS.

With the exception of vegetarians and people who subsist on the standard American diet, most Americans obtain enough serotonin-precursor proteins in their diet. The bigger issues that primarily result in serotonin deficiencies are stress, blood sugar imbalances, and overall impaired brain function. Low estrogen levels can also cause an inadequate supply of serotonin in the brain. Helpful nutrients for supporting serotonin production and activity include folic acid, magnesium (especially magnesium citrate), methyl B12, niacinamide, P5P, SAMe, L-tryptophan, and 5-HTP. The herb St. John's wort can also be useful.

There are also two very effective brain stimulation acupoints. One is gall bladder 14, which is located on the forehead, directly above the pupil, half an inch above the midpoint of the eyebrow. The other is called triple warmer 21. It is located in front of the ear in the depression caused by opening the jaw. These points can also be stimulated by acupressure, where the point is rubbed clockwise for 30 seconds twice a day, on both sides of the face.

Improving Brain Plasticity Through New Learning and New Experiences: Brain, or neuro-, plasticity refers to the brain's ability to adapt and change throughout life in response to new experiences, challenges and what we learn. The first instances of brain plasticity in your life occurred after you were born, when your infant brain began organizing itself in response to all that you were exposed to as you interacted with your new environment outside the womb. The process of brain plasticity continues throughout the rest of our lives. However, as we get older and more set and comfortable in our habits, too many of us stop actively seeking out and engaging in new experiences and life challenges. As a result, the plasticity of brain becomes less active and eventually can decline. Yet, just as the brain can compensate for and create new neural pathways in cases of brain injury in order to regain ability and functions caused by such injuries, so too can its levels of plasticity be enhanced when we purposely undertake new experiences and challenges.

Researchers are continuing to discover how doing so can keep our brains resilient and youthful, constantly forming new neural networks. This is exciting news, considering that until recently neurologists and other brain experts believed that, as we grow older, the brain's neural networks and connections became fixed. Scientists have now discovered that that brain is designed to never stop changing and creating new neural networks, as well as changing and improving the internal structure of existing networks and their synapses. The key is to keep the brain stimulated with new experiences. It is interesting to note that at autopsy, Einstein's brain was 10 percent smaller than the average brain; his genius was attributed to the increased connections between his neurons (neuroplasticity).

There are a number of effective, and enjoyable, ways that you can enhance your brain's plasticity. One of them is to learn and master new skills, such as learning a new language or computer program, learning how to dance, or learning how to play a musical instrument. Learning how to juggle is another fun and very effective way to improve brain plasticity because juggling well involves the activation of both the left and right brain hemispheres, enhancing whole brain learning. Essentially, studying any sort of new information and learning to master it can improve neuroplasticity. Each time you learn something new or master a new skill, your brain structure physically changes, a fact that has been proven by researchers using MRI scans.

Other methods for enhancing brain plasticity include meditation, practicing focused attention (listening attentively to others, noticing your environment as you walk or drive, etc.), seeking out and engaging in stimulating relationships and conversations, taking up a new hobby, traveling to new places, and consciously seeking to do things differently than your normal routine.

As an example of doing things differently, experiment with brushing your teeth or opening doors with your non-dominant hand. Or try eating your meals with your eyes closed, relying on your other senses to experience what you are eating and to determine where your food and plate is. Your brain is designed to develop in response to play and novelty. In fact, neurologists now believe that more than 90 percent of all the learning we experience during the course of our entire lives, including how to walk and speak and recognize other elements of our environment, occurs within the first two to three years of our lives. Nearly all of that learning is self-directed out of a sense of curiosity and play. There is no reason why this same sense of playfulness and curiosity should not be part of our entire lives.

By consciously adopting at least some of the suggestions above, not only will you be helping to keep your brain young and "plastic," you will also very likely soon find you are enjoying yourself more, and gaining fulfillment and satisfaction from the new skills you start to master.

Other Helpful Approaches: In addition to a healthy diet, appropriate nutritional and herbal supplementation, and addressing neurotransmitter function and imbalances, as you learned above, to maintain a healthy, ageless brain, you need to keep your brain stimulated, avoid the use of pharmaceutical drugs, manage stress, get enough restful sleep, and ensure your brain is getting enough oxygen each day (see the sections on stress, sleep, exercise and breathing in Chapter 8 for how to do so), as well as address your body's overall hormone status (see Chapter 10). Regularly practicing the drainage and detoxification measures that you learned in Chapter 6 is also essential. All of these steps, when made part of an ongoing healthy lifestyle can keep your brain sharp and resilient for many years to come.

Key Points To Remember

One of the most important keys to achieving and maintaining ageless vitality now is to optimize the health of your brain. Despite the widespread prevalence of brain diseases such as Alzheimer's and dementia, you can protect yourself and your brain by taking action now.

Growing older, of itself, is *not* the cause of diminished brain health and mental capacity. Rather, the cause is due to a variety of interrelated factors. Some of these factors, such as poor diet and nutritional deficiencies and imbalances, environmental toxins, and chronic stress, are well-known. Others, such as blood sugar imbalances, brain inflammation, lack of oxygen, thyroid and other hormonal imbalances, gluten sensitivity and impaired gut health and related gastrointestinal problems, and the overuse of pharmaceutical drugs, are only now coming to be understood.

Dealing with all of the above factors is essential to protecting your brain and keeping it healthy and youthful.

One of the most significant "brain poisons" is gluten, which can negatively affect the brain even more than it impairs gastrointestinal health. A healthy, gluten-free diet is therefore most important, especially because of the relationship that exists between the brain and the GI tract via the "brain-gut axis."

In addition to proper diet, preventing and reversing brain inflammation, blood sugar imbalances, and keeping the brain properly supplied with oxygen are also important.

Managing hormone levels and keeping the brain's neurotransmitters healthy is also essential, as is getting adequate levels of restful sleep, and regularly participating in activities that enhance your brain's plasticity (its ability to adapt and change throughout life in response to new experiences, challenges and what you learn).

CHAPTER 12

Heal Your Heart;
Hold the Sugar

Heart disease remains our nation's most prevalent health issue, with heart attack alone continuing to be our nation's number one killer, and death by stroke ranking third. These facts are proof that everything we, as a nation and within our medical system, have been doing to combat and prevent heart disease is not working. In this chapter, I will explain why, and then provide you with the information you need to prevent heart disease, as well as high blood pressure. You will also learn how to protect yourself from insulin resistance, an important risk factor for heart disease, as well as cancer, diabetes, and other serious health conditions, and what you can do to prevent unhealthy weight gain and obesity.

What We've Been Told About Heart Disease Is Wrong

For many people, including physicians, the first step in improving and maintaining the health of the heart and overall cardiovascular system is to set aside the erroneous assumptions that have been accepted as fact since the late 1950s. Since that time, we have all been told—by the medical establishment, the American Heart Association, drugs companies, and government health agencies alike—that the primary cause of heart disease is due to elevated cholesterol levels (especially LDL, the so-called "bad" cholesterol). Other risk factors, such as high blood pressure, poor lifestyle choices (especially smoking), and pre-existing disease conditions like diabetes and obesity, have also long been warned against. In addition, during this time, the health of the arteries, not the heart itself, was considered to be most important when it came to the development of heart disease.

Today's mainstream treatment approaches to prevent heart disease are all based on the above factors and assumptions. That being so, why is it that, despite an annual expenditure of over $440 billion in the United States alone to prevent and treat heart disease (according to the Centers for Disease Control and Prevention, or CDC), heart disease remains our nation's number one killer, and affects one out of every three adult Americans? Just as importantly, why is it that approximately 50 percent of all people who develop heart disease do so despite having normal, seemingly healthy levels of the above risk factors? The answer is because the assumptions about what causes heart disease that have guided how physicians work to treat and prevent it are, if not entirely wrong, definitely incomplete. This is particularly true with regard to cholesterol.

Cholesterol, Of Itself, Is Not the Problem and Statin Drugs Are Not the Answer

Also known as the "lipid hypothesis" and the "diet-heart theory", the high cholesterol model of heart disease is based on the belief that heart disease, especially heart attack and stroke, is caused by elevated cholesterol levels that cause arteries to become hardened and blocked (atherosclerosis), which in turn cuts off the supply of blood and the oxygen it contains to heart tissues (ischemia). Based on this theory, physicians screen their patients to monitor their HDL, LDL and HDL/LDL ratio (total cholesterol) levels. These levels are used as markers for heart disease risk. HDL is considered "good" cholesterol, while LDL is considered "bad" cholesterol. When LDL and total cholesterol levels are high, or elevated, and HDL levels are low, patients are considered to be at high risk for developing heart disease. To reduce that risk, they will often be prescribed cholesterol-lowering drugs (statins).

Because of the blame placed on cholesterol today, statins continue to be the most widely prescribed class of medications in the US. Yet, despite their widespread use, statin use has done very little to combat heart disease. In fact, a meta-analysis of more than 65,000 patients without a pre-existing condition of heart disease who were prescribed and used statin drugs for a period of five years found that the drugs provided no benefit whatsoever in 98 percent of patients. Moreover, the drugs only reduced the incidence of heart attack and stroke by 1.6 percent and 0.4 percent respectively.

The benefits of statin drugs for people with a pre-existing condition of heart disease are not that much better. Studies of patients with a known history of heart disease, as well as of patients who have previously suffered a stroke, reveal that only 4 percent of patients derive any benefit from the use of statin drugs after five years of use, and that statins prevented a recurrence of heart attack or stroke by only 2.6 percent and 0.8 percent respectively.

In addition to their overall ineffectiveness, statin drugs also pose serious health risks. For example, in 2014 the Food and Drug Administration declared that the warning label for statin drugs be upgraded to warn of a heightened risk of type 2 diabetes and elevated blood sugar levels, both of which, ironically, are associated with an increased risk of heart disease. Statins also deplete the body of essential nutrients, including CoQ10, which is very important for maintaining a healthy heart and helping heart cells produce energy. Research has also determined that statin use can increase the risk of other disease conditions, as well, including cancer, kidney failure, cataracts, and, in men, erectile dysfunction. Statins can also cause a type of serious memory loss known as transient global amnesia (TGA), a condition in which memory is nearly completely wiped out, sometimes for days. As I mentioned, in the section on brain health above, the widespread use of statins over the past decades may be another factor in the rising incidence of Alzheimer's disease and dementia.

Statins have also been implicated as a cause of diastolic dysfunction, in which the filling phase of each heart beat is altered. In addition, statins have been found to cause a depletion of an immune enhancer called TNF alpha, which some researchers believe can result in cancer, especially when statin drugs are taken for more than ten years.

The results of these and other studies about statins raises this question: Is cholesterol truly the villain in the story of heart disease?

In a word, no.

In fact, you would not be alive were it not for cholesterol. The proof of that statement is provided by your body itself, which, primarily in your liver, manufactures between 80 to 90 percent of all the cholesterol in your system. It has to, because cholesterol is essential for many of the functions that keep you alive and healthy. It is a major structural component of every cell in your body and plays an especially important role in maintaining the integrity of the cell membrane which encloses and protects the cells themselves. Cholesterol is also needed by your body to manufacture various hormones, including adrenal hormones, estrogen and testosterone, as well as vitamin D from the sun (vitamin D acts far more like a hormone than it does a vitamin). Your body also needs cholesterol to produce fat-soluble vitamins, as well as the bile salts that your body requires for the proper absorption of fats.

Cholesterol also acts as a natural anti-inflammatory agent. When inflammation is present in the body, cholesterol levels automatically rise as the body attempts to cope with the inflammation. This is especially true when unhealthy, acidifying and inflammation-causing foods and beverages are consumed. Stress will also result in increased cholesterol levels on a blood test. It is known that professional race car drivers, for instance, will have a spike of 100 mg in their blood cholesterol levels one hour after a race, due to the stress involved in race car driving.

While it is true that certain foods high in saturated fats, such as dairy products, eggs, and meats, also contain cholesterol, the diet of the average American today only contains between 250 to 350 mg of cholesterol. In comparison, each and every day, your liver produces around 1000 mg of cholesterol. Moreover, studies have shown that when people eliminate or restrict their intake of cholesterol-rich foods, liver production of cholesterol increases by as much as an additional 500 mg. Given that the human body is designed to keep itself alive through a continuous repair and adjustment process known as *homeostasis,* why would it produce so much cholesterol if cholesterol poses a threat to its health?

Proponents of the high cholesterol theory of heart disease answer this question by pointing to the two kinds of cholesterol mentioned above, "good" HDL (high density lipoprotein) cholesterol and "bad" LDL (low-density lipoprotein) cholesterol. But the distinction between HDL and LDL cholesterol is not as clear cut as it is commonly believed to be.

What *is* important to note is the role that HDL and LDL play in your body. HDL acts to return cholesterol from your body's tissues back to the liver, while LDL acts to transport cholesterol from the liver out to the rest of your body. To better understand this point, imagine two lines of workers in a factory, carrying materials to and from a machine shop. Would you characterize the workers who returned the materials to the machine shop as any better than the workers who carried the materials away from the shop if those duties were precisely what the workers were hired to do? No, of course you wouldn't.

Similarly, it makes just as little sense to characterize LDL as bad cholesterol when it is simply carrying out the tasks it was designed to do, just as HDL is doing. But LDL is still branded "bad" because of its link to heart disease when it becomes oxidized ("rusts"). And while it is true that there is a *correlation* between oxidized LDL and heart disease, that does not mean heart disease is *caused* by it. Correlations and causes are not the same thing. Just because you were at the scene of the crime, doesn't mean that you caused the crime. This is a very important point to understand.

In addition, a 2014 study published in the *Journal of Lipid Research* further challenges the assumption that even oxidized LDL cholesterol is bad. The truth now appears to be just the opposite: *oxidized LDL cholesterol may in fact be a potential lifesaver.* In this study, researchers reexamined the role that oxidized LDL cholesterol plays in the development of plaque inside the arteries. Previously it was thought that oxidized LDL cholesterol moved rapidly into the arterial walls where it was converted into plaque, causing blockages in the arteries and, in worst case scenarios, rupturing to send clots into the bloodstream, causing heart attacks and stroke. Based on the results of this new study, however, preliminary indications are that oxidized LDL cholesterol may actually be a "good guy," according to one of the studies leader authors, Jason Meyer, an MD, PhD candidate at the University of Kentucky.

In the study, researchers examined the pathway of cholesterol transport known as "selective lipid (fat) uptake." "Based on our analysis," Meyer says, "we were surprised to find that instead of increasing the amount of cholesterol uptake and accumulation in the macrophage foam cells, mildly oxidized LDL almost completely prevents increases in cholesterol." Macrophage foam cells are a specific type of fat-laden immune cells considered to be an indication of arterial plaque buildup. If Meyer and his fellow researchers are correct in their analysis, the demonization of oxidized LDL cholesterol as a major villain in the heart disease story may finally be put to rest.

Blocked Arteries and Unstable Plaque Aren't the Real Problem Either

From the time it was first theorized, the high cholesterol model of heart disease has been tied to the blocked artery model, which holds that plaque buildup in the arteries is another cause of heart disease. More recently, both the high cholesterol and blocked artery models have given way to a focus on unstable plaque. As it turns out, neither blocked arteries nor unstable plaque are the actual causes of heart disease, either.

The blocked artery model of heart disease is something you are probably already familiar with. It holds that the cause of most heart attacks is due to blockages in, and calcification (hardening) of, the arteries due to the progressive buildup of plaque caused by elevated cholesterol. Eventually, the combination of blockages and calcification inside the artery (specifically the lumen, the space through which blood flows) diminishes the blood supply to parts of the heart. As this occurs, the lack of oxygen in that area of the heart due to decreased blood flow triggers sensations of pain (angina). If unaddressed, this, in turn, can cause a heart attack.

The primary treatment options employed by conventional medicine to treat blocked arteries are either angioplasty or stenting. If either of those options is not possible, then coronary bypass surgery is often used. Angioplasty involves the insertion of a deflated balloon on a guide wire known as a balloon catheter into the area of the artery that is blocked. Once there, the balloon is then inflated using water pressure, forcing the expansion of the plaque deposits and surrounding arterial wall to enable improved blood flow. The balloon is then deflated and withdrawn. If necessary, an open tube called a stent is then inserted into the artery to keep the area from narrowing again.

Bypass surgery (coronary artery bypass grafting, or CABG) is a procedure in which a blood vessel is removed, or redirected, from one area of the body and placed around the area or areas of narrowing in the coronary arteries in order to "bypass" the blockages and restore blood flow to the heart muscle. The blood vessel is called a graft. Grafts can come from patients' chest, legs, or arms. Bypass surgery is one of the most commonly performed surgeries in the United States.

While all of these surgical procedures can save lives during acute emergencies, research has shown that their overall benefits are minimal. Recent findings help to explain why. First, studies have found that a significant percentage of heart attacks occur in the areas of the heart where blood flow is not diminished by blocked arteries. Additionally, other research, including a large 2003 study conducted by the Mayo Clinic that evaluated the effectiveness of angioplasty, stenosis, and CABG, found that, although the procedures can relieve symptoms of heart disease, they do not prevent further heart attacks and that only high-risk patients(specifically patients with blockage of the left main coronary artery) whose lives are in acute danger receive any benefit from bypass surgery in terms of their improved chances of survival.

Of greater significance, however, is the discovery by researchers that large arterial blockages (those that block at least 90 percent of an artery) are frequently and effectively dealt with by the body on its own through the development of its own "bypass" network of blood vessels that keep blood flowing to the heart. This extensive network of small blood vessels, which are called **collateral** vessels, actually begins to be formed shortly after birth, and compensates for diminished blood flow in any of the body's major blood vessels, including the heart's four major coronary arteries. (Exercise also stimulates collateral blood vessel formation.) This fact was first proven by experiments conducted by Giorgio Baroldi, MD, PhD of Italy. Dr. Baroldi injected diseased and blocked hearts with plastic so that he could make molds of the blockages that we considered the cause of death. Much to his surprise, he discovered, and definitively proved, how collateral blood vessels work to maintain blood flow to the heart

Based on Dr. Baroldi's research, we now know that the human cardiovascular system, whenever it senses a problem in the heart's "plumbing" (arteries), sets about constructing an alternative pathway of arteries *de novo* (from scratch) to compensate for arterial blockages and keep blood flowing as nature intended. Dr. Baroldi subsequently co-authored a clinical paper with his colleague, Malcolm Silver, MD, PhD, in which they explained that, both clinically and scientifically, the blocked artery theory of heart disease does not hold up.

What the findings of Dr. Baroldi and other researchers mean is that, in the vast majority of cases, angioplasty, stenosis, and CABG may not even be necessary to restore blood flow to the heart, since the body, via its collateral vessels, has already done so. It is primarily for this reason that studies continue to find that none of these three procedures provide much benefit to many patients with heart disease despite how commonly they are performed.

As a result of these findings, a growing number of cardiologists and other physicians have switched their focus away from the blocked artery model to what is known as vulnerable, or unstable, plaque model. The focus on vulnerable plaque first began following the publication of a monograph in 1998 by the American Heart Association (AHA) that was edited by its president, Valentin Fuster, M.D., Ph.D., Director of the Cardiovascular Institute at Mount Sinai School of Medicine, in New York City. The monograph stated that 85 percent of all heart attacks and strokes were due to vulnerable plaque, a "soft" form of cholesterol, proteins, and blood cells that builds up within the arterial wall.

The findings of the monograph were widely reported in both conventional medical journals and the mainstream media and debunked the belief that heart disease is primarily due to hard arterial plaque that obstructs the artery (the high cholesterol and blocked artery models). Given the fact that Dr. Fuster is the only cardiologist to receive four major research awards from the world's top four cardiovascular organizations (the AHA, the American College of Cardiology, the European Society of Cardiology, and the Inter-American Society of Cardiology), the monograph proved quite influential.

Vulnerable plaque primarily consists of soft cholesterol and clotting proteins that are different than the type of obstructing plaque common in atherosclerosis, and which is contained by a fibrous cap that is thinner and weaker than obstructing plaque, and more easily ruptured. As a result of a stressful event, whether it be physical or emotional, the body reacts to vulnerable plaque in much the same way that it deals with infection, releasing blood cells to attack and inflame the fibrous cap. This attack and the subsequent inflammation that results from it can cause the cap to break, spilling the powerful coagulants found in its interior into any artery where they can form a clot that impedes blood flow. If this occurs in a coronary artery, it is called coronary thrombosis, which is commonly believed to be the cause of most cases of heart attack.

Yet, it now appears this isn't true, either, as evidenced by pathology studies, which are the most accurate way to determine the causes of disease and how they occurred. The first major pathology study to examine how often thrombosis occurred in cases of heart attack was published by German researchers in 1974. It found that thrombosis severe enough to cause a heart attack occurred in only 20 percent of cases. Other studies, including a larger one conducted by Dr. Baroldi, increased that figure to 41 percent, yet that still means that nearly 60 percent of people who experience a heart attack, do so without clotting being the cause. Moreover, other research indicates that thrombosis is often a *consequence* of heart attack, *not* its cause. Clearly, then, the three primary models used to explain heart disease are incomplete.

What Really Causes Heart Disease

As research into heart disease continues to progress, it appears the underlying causes of heart disease, including heart attacks can be traced to the autonomic nervous system (ANS), which you first learned about in Chapter 3. Understanding the link between the ANS and heart disease is leading to a revolution in the ways more and more doctors will eventually work to treat and prevent heart disease. My goal in this section is to provide you with the information you need so that you don't have to wait for this revolution to come to pass.

As we discussed in Chapter 3, the ANS controls all of your automatic functions (those functions which do not require your conscious attention, such as blood pressure, respiration, and pulse rate) of your body's organs, including your heart. It is composed of two branches, the sympathetic and parasympathetic systems. The sympathetic nervous system regulates energy production and your body's stress coping mechanisms, as well as the "fight or flight responses" and immune stimulation triggered by emergency situations, while the parasympathetic system is responsible for regulating energy recovery, repair, regeneration, and relaxation.

It is the parasympathetic branch of the ANS that is of particular importance when it comes to reversing and, especially, preventing heart disease. One reason this is so is because the primary nerve of the parasympathetic system responsible for nerve impulses to the heart is the vagus nerve, which you learned about in the brain section above. The vagus nerve, under the direction of the parasympathetic nervous system, slows and relaxes the heart. By contrast, the sympathetic nervous system, especially when it activates the body's "fight or flight" response, causes the heart to beat faster. According to Thomas Cowan, MD, who has spent years researching the link between diminished parasympathetic activity and heart disease, "It is the imbalance of these two branches [sympathetic and parasympathetic] that is responsible for the vast majority of heart disease."

My own experience as a physician confirms this. Using a diagnostic technique called heart rate variability (HRV), which accurately measures both sympathetic and parasympathetic activity in real time (you will learn more about HRV in Chapter 14), researchers have conducted studies showing that patients with ischemic heart disease have a reduction in their bodies' parasympathetic activity of at least 33 percent or more. Ischemia is characterized by restricted blood flow to the heart and its tissues, causing a loss of oxygen and reduced energy supply. The studies also show that the lower parasympathetic activity is, the greater the degree of ischemia that exists. "Furthermore," Dr. Cowan states, "about 80 percent of ischemic events have been shown to be preceded by significant, often drastic reductions in parasympathetic activity related to physical activity, emotional upset, or other causes." My own use of HRV testing also shows this to be true.

By contrast, other studies have shown that people with healthy parasympathetic activity who experience spikes in their sympathetic activity due to physical or emotional shocks, never suffer from ischemia. What this research shows is that increased activation of the sympathetic nervous system does not cause heart attack and other types of heart disease unless such activation is preceded by decreased parasympathetic activity. As Dr. Cowan explains, "We are meant to have times of excess sympathetic activity; that is normal life. What's dangerous to our health is the ongoing, persistent decrease in our parasympathetic, or life-restoring, activity."

Based on this new understanding of heart disease, researchers are now beginning to understand that heart attack and other types of heart disease, in the vast majority of cases, will not occur unless there is first a decrease in parasympathetic activity. Typically, this decrease is followed by an increase in sympathetic activity, most usually due to the "fight or flight" response in reaction to physical, emotional, or other stressors. This combination of events results in heart cells dramatically increasing their production of lactic acid, something which occurs in virtually 100 percent of heart attack events, whether or not the coronary arteries are negatively impacted. Due to the increased acidity in the heart, the heart cell walls become rigid, making them less able to contract, and leading to edema and impaired function of the heart muscle itself, as well as heart cell death, all of which are involved in causing heart attacks. In addition, the swelling (edema) of heart tissue results in changes in pressure of the arteries that run through the affected area of the heart. This increase in pressure, in turn, is what causes vulnerable plaque in the arteries to rupture, further blocking the arteries involved, and/or creating dangerous clots.

What is most important to remember about this process is that *none of it happens unless and until parasympathetic activity is first decreased.* "Only this explanation accounts for all of the observable phenomena associated with heart disease," Dr. Cowan says. "The true origin of heart disease could not be more clear."

Directly related to this process of decreased parasympathetic activity and the cascade of events that can follow it, is what occurs in the endothelium, the very thin layer of cells that line your body's arteries. A healthy endothelium is necessary for proper blood flow and overall cardiovascular function, especially in relation to the smooth vascular muscle that makes up most of the blood vessel walls. The events described above that are associated with decreased parasympathetic activity can all negatively impact the endothelium, resulting in one or more of three possible responses: inflammation, oxidative stress (increased level of free radicals), and vascular autoimmune dysfunction (your body mistakenly attacks your blood vessels with an antibody), all of which are linked to heart disease.

Compounding this problem is the fact that, each time blood vessels and the endothelium are negatively affected, a type of "memory" is created within them so that subsequent harm to blood vessels and the endothelium can trigger a heightened reaction by way of the three endothelial responses mentioned above. This is true even if the subsequent harm is seemingly of little consequence. Research has shown, for instance, that even short-term exposure to an inflammatory agent such as sugar can lead to a long-term inflammatory response.

However, again, it is important to stress that problems within the heart and overall cardiovascular system most often occur only if there is first a decrease in parasympathetic activity. For example, although atherosclerosis is a result of endothelial dysfunction and has long been viewed as a significant risk factor for heart disease, the presence of atherosclerosis of itself does not mean that angina, heart attack, or other types of heart disease will occur. So long as parasympathetic activity is healthy, the autonomic functions will override atherosclerosis, aided by the collateral blood vessels you learned about earlier in this chapter.

This does not mean that you can, or should, ignore atherosclerosis if it is present, any more than you should ignore any other risk factors that have been linked to heart disease. All such factors need to be addressed. But it is the activity of your parasympathetic nervous system that is of paramount importance when it comes to protecting your heart.

Heart Disease Is Different For Women

Heart disease has traditionally been considered a disease that most commonly affects men. Most people also assume that cancer, not heart disease, is the number one killer of women in the United States. Both of these assumptions are no longer true, and can be dangerous if believed. In actuality, 10 percent of all American women between the ages of 45 and 64 are now living with some form of heart disease, and over 40 percent of all deaths among women in the US are caused by heart disease (approximately 500,000 deaths each year), with heart attacks killing six times as many women each year as breast cancer.

Women who suffer a heart attack also have lower survival rates compared to men (38 percent to 25 percent), and are more likely to suffer from another heart attack within six years (35 percent to 18 percent). Female heart attack survivors are also more than twice as likely to be disabled due to heart failure within six years compared to men (46 percent to 22 percent), and nearly twice as many women as men die after bypass surgery. Making matters worse, most of the research conducted on heart disease today is focused on men, with women comprising only 25 percent of all participants in medical studies related to heart disease.

Compounding matters is the fact that women often do not experience symptoms of heart disease in the same way that men do, and therefore are more likely to not recognize what the symptoms mean, or to ignore them altogether. For example, while chest pain is the most common symptom of a pending heart attack, **women are far more likely than men to not experience chest pain before a heart attack strikes**. Women are also less apt to experience other common warning signs of heart disease, such as pain in the left arm and shortness of breath.

Instead of experiencing the most common male warning signs of heart disease, women are more likely to experience what are known as "atypical warning signs". Such symptoms include pain in the back, neck or jaw; nausea; vomiting; indigestion; weakness; unexplained fatigue; dizziness or lightheadedness; and sleep disturbances. Research has shown that 95 percent of women who suffered heart attacks first experienced one or more of these atypical symptoms rather than common warning signs. In the majority of cases, they did not recognize the symptoms for what they were. Had they done so, the majority of them might have avoided heart attacks by receiving medical attention in time.

Physicians, too, can fail to detect heart disease in women. One reason this is so is because women aren't as likely to have fatty plaque buildup in their arteries compared to men. This is especially true among younger women. In addition, women typically develop heart disease an average of 10 to 15 years later than men do. Researchers attribute this delay to two factors: menstruation, which helps to thin blood, making it easier for the heart to pump it; and the rich supply of female hormones that are produced prior to menopause, which have heart-protecting properties. Once menopause sets in, however, women who previously exhibited no signs of heart disease might quickly develop them, but because of their health history their doctors might fail to screen for them.

All of the above facts make it essential that women become proactive when it comes to heart disease. This means knowing the different and atypical warning signs of heart disease that most commonly affect women, and making sure to request a thorough screening for heart disease from their doctors, especially once they enter into menopause.

Managing High Blood Pressure (Hypertension)

High blood pressure, or hypertension, is a serious health condition that can lead to other health problems, including heart attack and stroke. According to the American Heart Association, approximately one-third of all American adults have high blood pressure, including many people in their early 20s, and another third of all Americans suffer from pre-hypertension, meaning their blood pressure levels are higher than normal. In addition, all too often high blood pressure is also undiagnosed. over 20 percent of people with high blood pressure not being aware of their condition.

Here are some simple yet powerful steps you can do to prevent high blood pressure from developing, and to reduce it if it already has developed.

See Your Doctor and Get Tested: The first step is to consult with your doctor and have him or her measure your blood pressure. Doing so is a quick and easy procedure. Today, you can also find blood pressure monitors at your local drug store. Most of these devices are inexpensive and reasonably accurate, allowing you to check your blood pressure level on a regular basis without the need to see your doctor. However, if you currently do not know your blood pressure level, I recommend that you initially see your doctor so that he or she can work with you to create an optimal healthy lifestyle.

Unfortunately, just as physicians continue to focus on the less essential risk factors for heart disease, so too are they ignoring the most effective way for evaluating their patients' blood pressure levels. The majority of physicians rely on traditional one time office blood pressure measurements. A far better approach is to measure mean blood pressure levels over the course of 24 hours. This is accomplished using what is known as ambulatory 24-hour blood pressure measurements in which a patient's blood pressure is measured throughout the day and night. (The use of home blood pressure tests can make accomplishing this task easier.)

24-hour blood pressure monitoring also helps to determine if a patient is what is known as a "dipper" or "non-dipper". Blood pressure tends to drop when we sleep. This is called "dipping". Some people with high blood pressure do not "dip" when sleeping, putting them at risk for a stroke. These people can benefit from taking small doses of melatonin before bed, which will result in dipping.

I, along with many other heart specialists, also find that nighttime blood pressure readings are typically more important than day blood pressure levels. Although high blood pressure is not a disease, it is a valuable marker for heart disease, and therefore it is crucial that it is correctly identified. When measuring blood pressure levels, you and your doctor should consider the following facts:

Blood pressure readings of 120/80 mmHg are considered normal. The number 120 is called the systolic blood pressure, which is the pressure in the artery when the heart pumps. The number 80 is called the diastolic blood pressure, which is the pressure in the artery when the heart relaxes (fills).

Each blood pressure increase of 20/10 mmHg can double the risk of heart disease.

Before age 50, the diastolic blood pressure is the best predictor of heart disease risk; after age 50, the systolic blood pressure is a better indicator of risk.

When measuring blood pressure, it is best to use arm cuffs, not wrist or finger monitors.

If your doctor finds that your blood pressure is high, be advised that he or she may recommend blood pressure medication. In cases of dangerously high blood pressure levels, such drugs can literally be lifesavers. However, although such drugs may relieve the symptoms of high blood pressure, they do little or nothing to resolve its underlying causes. Additionally many of these drugs can cause unhealthy side effects. Therefore, if you have high blood pressure, ask your doctor to help you determine whatever factors may be contributing to your condition. Then, if your blood pressure level isn't at a dangerous level, take a few months implementing the following self-care measures below. Should you still require blood pressure medications after this time frame, bear in mind that all blood pressure medications (except diuretics) should be taken at night, because they will have a 25 to 50 percent increased effectiveness, at the same dose, compared to when they are taken during the day.

Diet: A healthy diet is one of the most important factors in preventing and reducing high blood pressure. The best diet is one that is low in unhealthy fats, sugar, and salt, and rich in foods containing potassium, calcium, and magnesium. Fiber-rich foods are also important. Overall, try to eat meals that contain plentiful supplies of fresh, organic vegetables, along with free-range lean meats and poultry and wild caught fish. Try to also limit your intake of carbohydrate foods.

In at least one meal each day, be sure to also include garlic and/or onions, both of which have been shown to reduce both systolic and diastolic pressure levels. Also be sure to eliminate all refined and simple carbohydrate foods, processed foods, and beverages while drinking lots of pure, filtered water throughout the day.

Nutritional Supplements: There are a number of nutrients that can help keep blood pressure levels under control. Some of the most beneficial are fish oils, vitamins B3 and B6 along with a complete B-complex supplement, vitamin C, vitamin D, omega-3 fatty acids, lycopene, magnesium, potassium, selenium, and zinc. CoQ10, and the amino acids cysteine, and taurine can also be helpful.

Herbal Remedies: One of the best herbal remedies for preventing and reducing high blood pressure is hawthorne. Hawthorne is well known for its ability to strengthen and protect the cardiovascular system, so it's not surprising that it is beneficial for helping to manage blood pressure levels too. Other helpful herbs include celery seed extract, which acts as a natural calcium channel blocker, and olive leaf extract, which acts as a natural inhibitor of angiotensin converting enzyme (ACE), which can harm blood vessels and cause them to constrict, thus increasing the risk of hypertension.

Lifestyle: A healthy lifestyle is another significant factor for maintaining healthy blood pressure levels. Healthy life style choices include limiting your daily alcohol and caffeine intake, as well as not smoking and avoiding exposure to secondhand smoke. If you are overweight, seek help so that you can get to within ten pounds or less of your ideal weight, as healthy weight loss can dramatically reduce high blood pressure. (For more on weight loss, see below.)

Managing stress is also very important, as chronic stress is one of the primary causes of high blood pressure. Meditation can be particularly effective in this regard, so much so in fact that in 1984 the National Institutes of Health (NIH) recommended meditation over prescription drugs as a treatment for mild cases of high blood pressure. Regular exercise is also important. Exercise not only helps to lower high blood pressure, it is also excellent for reducing stress.

Social Health: In addition to the above steps, be honest with yourself and evaluate your relationships, both at work and at home. Try to avoid spending time with people who are habitually negative or who cause you stress in other ways. In addition, if you need help with your personal relationships, consider counseling or receiving some other type of guidance. Just as importantly, try not to spend too much time alone. Numerous scientific studies show that people with strong and supportive social ties on average are healthier, have better blood pressure levels, and usually live longer than people who tend to be "loners."

Screening For Heart Disease

One of the main reasons why heart disease continues to be our nation's number one killer has to do with how most physicians today screen for it. For the most part, they are only concerned with monitoring their patients HDL, LDL, and total cholesterol levels, along with their blood pressure and triglyceride levels. All of these markers have their place, but if you want to truly know how healthy your heart and cardiovascular system is, your doctor needs to go much further in his or her testing. For me, this starts with a heart rate variability screening at every patient checkup.

As I mentioned earlier, HRV testing provides a real-time, accurate and completely noninvasive measurement of both sympathetic and parasympathetic activity in real time, letting me know how well my patients' autonomic nervous system is functioning, and alerting me to any signs of diminished parasympathetic activity, and increased sympathetic activity. In conjunction with HRV testing, I also recommend hormone testing, in order to screen for imbalanced levels of hormones associated with both the sympathetic and parasympathetic nervous systems. Should these tests show diminished parasympathetic activity, I will immediately start patients on a program to restore parasympathetic function to optimal levels (see below).

In addition to the tests mentioned above, I also recommend an advanced lipid profile test. The comprehensive test goes far beyond measuring HDL, LDL and total cholesterol alone. In addition, I recommend you ask to have your C-reactive protein (CRP) tested. CRP is a marker for inflammation. Elevated blood homocysteine is also a risk factor for vascular disease. A fasting blood sugar test is also advisable. High blood sugar also increases the risk of endothelial dysfunction. (**Note:** Many physicians today consider a fasting blood sugar level of 100 mg to be normal. For my patients, I aim for levels between 75 to 85 mg.) Regular monitoring of your blood pressure is also important, as is monitoring your blood hemoglobin A1 C for signs of insulin resistance.

I also order a fasting serum insulin level for my patients. The ideal level for this test is 5; 7-9 is good; while a serum insulin level greater than 10 equates to a 600 percent greater risk of having a heart attack. You can also look at a ratio of triglycerides/HDL to determine cardio-vascular health. The ideal ratio is 1:1, or a reading of 1 (triglycerides level divided by HDL level). A reading of 2 is good. The average American has a reading of 3.5. If your triglycerides/HDL reading is greater than 4, you will most likely be diabetic or pre-diabetic.

Strategies To Keep Your Heart Healthy

In the Bible (Proverbs 4:23), it is written, "Above all else, guard your heart, for everything you do flows from it." The following guidelines can help you do just that.

Maintaining Healthy Parasympathetic Activity: Now that you understand how diminished parasympathetic activity is always associated with heart disease, you also realize how important it is to keep the parasympathetic nervous system functioning optimally. I shared a number of ways for how you can do so in Chapter 3, but they bear repeating. Such measures include:

- Eating potassium-rich foods (avocado, bananas, dark leafy greens, legumes, wild caught salmon) and using potassium supplements.
- Consuming warm drinks and avoiding cold drinks and drinks that have been sweetened.
- Drinking peppermint, lavender, and linden (tilia) teas.
- Taking time throughout the day to perform deep breathing exercises.
- Gargling (this stimulates and tones the vagus nerve).
- Singing loudly (this also stimulates and tones the vagus nerve).
- Stimulating your gag reflex (this stimulates and tones the vagus nerve, as well).
- Practicing yoga.
- Meditating.

Another exercise that is also effective is to take a deep breath in and hold it. As you do so say out loud the vowels A, E, I, O, U. This is an additional way for you to stimulate the vagus nerve.

In addition, regularly seek out experiences that that promote relaxation, calm, and feelings of peace, and that also rekindle your sense of vitality and enthusiasm for life. This includes making it a habit to spend time each week in nature. Ideally, try to do so barefoot whenever possible, for the energizing and anti-inflammatory grounding ("earthing") benefits this provides. Also spend time creating and reconnecting to positive, supportive relationships in your life.

If you are married or in a relationship with a significant other, you can also sustain optimal parasympathetic activity by frequent love-making. Not just the act of sex itself, but also taking time to cuddle, hug, kiss, etc. Doing so releases oxytocin, a powerful hormone that acts as a neurotransmitter in the brain, and which increases feelings of trust, emotional security, and empathy for, and a deeper sense of connectivity to, others. All of these positive emotions are extremely beneficial to the health of your heart.

Diet: Given the interrelationship that the heart and the brain have, it is not surprising that the dietary recommendations I shared with you in the brain section above are also important for maintaining a healthy heart and protecting overall cardiovascular function. For the most part, you want to follow a low-carbohydrate, alkalizing diet that provides you with a plentiful supply of fresh, ideally organic, vegetables and organic meats, poultry, lamb, and wild-caught, healthy fish.

In addition, don't be afraid of healthy, saturated fats, despite how long they have been demonized as a cause of heart disease. Like your brain, your heart requires a certain amount of saturated fat in order to optimally function. You can help ensure that you obtain enough healthy fats by regularly consuming one or two eggs from free-range chickens during each week. Other healthy fat food sources include avocado, grass-fed meats, fatty fish (such as lake herring, lake trout, mackerel, salmon, sardines), butter, and nuts. For cooking, you can also use coconut oil and extra virgin, organic olive oil, which can also be used on salads.

Certain nutritional compounds found in food are also highly beneficial for your heart, and for protecting the health and integrity of the endothelium. These include luteolin, which is found in carrots, celery, green peppers, olives, and oranges; quercetin, which is found in apples, capers, onions, and tomatoes; and sulforaphane, which is found in broccoli, Brussels sprouts, cabbage, cauliflower, collard greens, and kale. Resveratrol, which is found in grapes and red wine, epigallocatechin-gallate (EGCG), which is found in green tea, and pomegranate, are also heart-healthy, endothelium-protecting nutrients. Garlic is particularly important for cardiovascular health, as it helps to keep the blood thin. Other natural blood thinners are gingko, vitamin E (tocopherols), nattokinase, and fish oils. You want your blood to flow like red wine, not like ketchup.

Finally, certain spices can also protect your heart. These include black pepper, cinnamon, coriander, curcumin (turmeric), garlic, ginger, and oregano. As they can do for your brain, spices can not only aid your heart, but also make your meals more delicious and flavorful.

Nutritional and Herbal Supplements: Heart-healthy nutritional supplements include alpha lipoic acid (ALA), betaine, bromelain, carnitine, CoQ10, L-arginine, omega 3 fish oils, vitamin C, vitamin E (tocopherols), niacin (vitamin B3), vitamin B6, grapeseed extract, lycopene, magnesium, potassium, taurine, zinc, nattokinase, proteolytic enzymes, serrapeptase, lysine, proline, and trimethylglycine (TMG).

Helpful herbs include bilberry, ouabain (which is especially useful for helping to maintain optimal parasympathetic nervous system function), Boswellia serrata, cayenne, gingko biloba, guggul, and hawthorne berry.

Exercise: Ideally, you should try to get at least 30 minutes of exercise each and every day. The benefits of regular exercise for preventing heart disease have long been verified by medical research. This fact was again confirmed in a meta-analysis study published in *Mayo Clinic Proceedings in September 2014.* In the study, researchers analyzed 10 previously published studies that examined over 42,000 elite athletes. They discovered that the athletes not only lived longer, compared to the general population, but that their risk of dying from heart disease was reduced by 27 percent. (They also had a 40 percent less risk of dying from cancer.)

If you don't already exercise, be sure to consult with your doctor so that the two of you can work together to create an exercise program that is most appropriate for your specific needs. For more about exercise, see Chapter 8. (**Note:** People who have previously experienced a heart attack should not overexert themselves with exercise, and should limit their total exercise activities to no more than 30 minutes per day. Recent research has shown that overexertion and prolonged exercise in heart attack patients not only offers diminishing returns, but can increase the risk of further problems. One reason this is so may be because of how prolonged exercise and overexertion can diminish parasympathetic activity.)

Lifestyle: If you are overweight, work with your doctor, who can help you devise a program for losing excess weight. If you smoke, seek help so that you can quit. It is also important that you get a good night's sleep for at least 7 to 8 hours.

Stress Management: Given how closely linked chronic stress is to heart disease, it's important that you take time each day to "de-stress" yourself. Useful ways for doing so are meditation, deep breathing exercises, regularly engaging in hobbies and other enjoyable activities, and spending time with loved ones. If stress continues to be a problem in your life, consider working with a health professional who specializes in stress relief. For more on effective ways to manage stress, see Chapters 5 and 8.

The bottom line, when it comes to heart disease is this: For the vast majority of people, heart disease is largely the result of long-standing unhealthy habits. By following the above recommendations, you can go a long way toward preventing and reversing heart disease, both on your own and, if necessary, by working with your doctor. The most important key is to get started now.

Insulin Resistance and Obesity

Before ending this chapter, I want to briefly discuss insulin resistance and our nation's increasing problem of obesity. Today, more than half of all Americans are overweight or obese, and the segment of our population in which obesity rates are greatest is among children and teenagers. Of all children born in the USA today, one-third will develop diabetes, and half will become obese. What this means is that the youth of today, if this dangerous trend is not reversed, will experience rates of Alzheimer's and dementia, heart disease, and many other serious degenerative diseases, including cancer and diabetes, that will likely far surpass current rates, most of which are already at an all-time high.

The sad irony about this pending disaster is that insulin resistance is primarily a "lifestyle disease," meaning it is mostly the result of everyday lifestyle choices people make, such as eating poorly, forgoing exercise, and engaging in various other unhealthy activities. But individuals alone are not solely to blame. Other culprits include the food industry and our own government, which for decades encouraged people to follow the dietary guidelines of the USDA's Food Pyramid, which, it turns out, was primarily created at the behest of special interest organizations and other industry groups and their lobbyists. Shortly after the USDA issued its recommendations, starting in the 1980s, our nation began experiencing a steady and inexorable rise in degenerative diseases, nearly all of which are due primarily to insulin resistance and obesity.

Following the creation of the USDA Food Pyramid, food manufacturers swapped out fats from most food products and replaced them with sugar in various forms, especially fructose, dextrose, high fructose corn syrup, and other sugars, as well as low-calorie artificial sweeteners. Plain and simple, *sugar, in all of its forms, except as it naturally occurs in fruit, is the enemy to your health, and artificial sweeteners are no better!*

One of the leading voices warning of the dangers of sugar, especially with regard to our nation's children, belongs to Robert H. Lustig, MD, a pediatric endocrinologist and professor of clinical pediatrics as the University of California, San Francisco. After nearly two decades spent researching the effects of sugar, especially on children, Dr. Lustig has found that the more we eat sugar, the more sugar creates an appetite in the body and brain for more sugar. It does this, he states, via hormone activities that are triggered by sugar consumption, especially on the part of cortisol.

"When cortisol floods the bloodstream, it raises blood pressure [and] increases the blood glucose level, which can precipitate diabetes," he points out. "Human research shows that cortisol specifically increases caloric intake of 'comfort foods'." Based on his research, he adds, "The problem in obesity is not excess weight. The problem with obesity is that the brain is not seeing the excess weight."

According to Dr. Lustig, the brain doesn't recognize excess weight because appetite is determined by a dual system known as *anorexigenesis*, which is characterized by feelings of not being hungry and ready to "burn energy", and *orexigenesis*, which triggers sensations of hunger and the body's need to store energy in the form of calories. This dual system is mediated by leptin, the hormone that regulates body fat. But leptin is unable to do its job when insulin levels rise, because too much insulin blocks the leptin signal, thus preventing the brain from recognizing when it is no longer necessary to keep eating. This process of leptin dysfunction and insulin resistance is primarily caused by excess consumptions of sugars and carbohydrate foods (including too many complex, healthy carbohydrates) and a lack of healthy fats in the diet.

The mechanisms by which sugar tricks the brain into desiring even more sugar is very much related to the overall mechanisms of addiction. In this case, instead of an addiction to alcohol, cigarettes, or drugs (both legal or illegal), the addiction is to food. And the foods that are most likely to cause addiction fall within the sugar and carbohydrate family.

Thus, as a nation, we are becomingly increasingly addicted to the very foods and food ingredients (sugars and sweeteners) that cause insulin resistance and the many diseases that are in turn caused by it.

Moreover, a growing body of addiction research demonstrates that the risk of alcohol and drug addiction is significantly increased among children and teens with a "sweet tooth." That's because consumption of sugar and excess carbohydrates create similar receptor sites in the brain that are created from the use of alcohol and drugs. These receptor sites multiply each time the addicting substance is used or consumed, which is why addiction can often prove so difficult to recover from.

In addition to sugar, excess carbohydrate consumption, lack of healthy fats, and food addictions, a number of other factors can also contribute to insulin resistance and obesity. These include lack of exercise, lack of fiber in the diet, low thyroid function, environmental toxins, and unresolved psychological issues.

The link between lack of exercise and both insulin resistance and unhealthy weight gain is well-established. Failing to exercise regularly results in a slower metabolism, worsens insulin spikes after eating insulin-raising foods, and impairs the body's ability to burn calories and keep blood sugar levels balanced.

Lack of fiber makes it more difficult for your body to eliminate wastes products and toxins, and can also cause blood sugar spikes, promoting insulin resistance.

Low thyroid function, or hypothyroidism can also trigger insulin resistance, and can lead to a slower metabolism and sluggish digestion. Diminished thyroid function also causes the body to retain fluids, which in turn can cause sugar to bind with fluids, triggering swelling and weight gain. In addition, low thyroid levels interfere with the body's ability to burn fat (thermogenesis).

Environmental toxins can also trigger insulin resistance and is virtually always present in cases of unhealthy weight gain and obesity. One of the primary reasons for this is that the body uses fat cells to trap and store toxins it cannot otherwise eliminate. The more toxins you are exposed to, the more fatty tissues that are built up in your body.

Unresolved psychological issues can also play a role in unhealthy weight gain and obesity. Such issues usually manifest as overeating and cravings for so-called "comfort foods," even when a person knows they are unhealthy. Emotional eating and consumption of unhealthy foods can serve as a temporary way to "stuff down" painful emotions and/or to deal with stress.

Preventing and Reversing Insulin Resistance

The good news about insulin resistance and the diseases it can cause, including brain diseases, heart disease, and obesity, is that, since it *is* largely a condition caused by one's lifestyle choices, there is much you can do on your own to significantly reduce your risk of developing it, and to reverse it if you are already experiencing it. For the most part, that means following the recommendations I shared above for keeping your brain and heart healthy and ageless.

Those same dietary and lifestyle recommendations will also go a long way to preventing and eliminating insulin resistance, and towards helping you lose weight if you need to. You can also improve your results by supplementing with the nutrients alpha lipoic acid, biotin, chromium, CoQ10, magnesium, and vanadium, all of which are proven to help manage insulin resistance. In addition, be sure to regularly employ the drainage and detoxification measures I shared in Chapter 6. And, if psychological issues are playing a role in your unhealthy eating habits, please refer back to the information and techniques I shared in Chapter 5, and consider working with a trained counselor to help you heal painful emotions.

By following all of the recommendations I have shared with you in this chapter, you now have the tools you need to keep both your heart healthy, and to protect yourself from insulin resistance and the tendency toward unhealthy weight gain. By adhering to these recommendations you will soon find that your heart markers are improving, that you feel more rested and energized due to maintaining the health of your autonomic nervous system, and that, if you need to lose weight, not only will you be doing so, you will also find that you can keep it off without having to resort to faddish, quick-fix diets that don't work in the long run. In short, you will become healthier and leaner, and a fit example of what it means to create outstanding health now.

Key Points To Remember

To properly maintain the health of your heart, you need to set aside the erroneous assumptions that have been accepted as fact, and which have guided cardiologists and other physicians since the late 1950s. Chief among these assumptions are the beliefs that heart attack and other types of heart disease are caused by high cholesterol levels, blocked arteries, and vulnerable plaque. While each of these factors can certainly be involved in heart disease, they are *not* the causes.

It is the parasympathetic branch of your body's autonomic nervous system that is of particular importance when it comes to reversing and, especially, preventing heart disease. Diminished parasympathetic activity is a key factor in heart disease. Even when other risk factors for heart disease are present, it will not occur unless parasympathetic activity is first diminished.

Stress of any kind is the single most important factor that diminishes parasympathetic activity. Chronic stress and its corresponding depletion of parasympathetic activity, accompanied by a sudden increase in sympathetic activity, causes heart cells and tissues to become acidic, thereby depleting the flow of nutrients and oxygen to the heart and causing heart cell death that trigger heart attack and other cardiovascular events.

As parasympathetic activity declines, the cascade of events that can follow it harms the endothelium, the very thin layer of cells that line your body's arteries. In response, the endothelium reacts in one of three possible ways, triggering inflammation, oxidative stress (too many free radicals), or vascular autoimmune dysfunction, all of which are linked to heart disease.

Heart disease in women is often different than it is in men, presenting different symptoms that can often go unrecognized by doctors and female patients alike.

Conventional screening tests for heart disease are also inadequate. Proper screening includes heart rate variability testing to determine the health of both the parasympathetic and sympathetic nervous systems in real time, hormone testing, comprehensive lipid profile screening, fasting blood sugar testing, and screening for markers of inflammation by testing blood levels of C-reactive protein and homocysteine.

Regular and proper screening of your blood pressure level is another important step you need to take in order to screen for, and prevent heart disease.

The traditional single blood pressure measurement most doctors typically reply upon is far less effective than 24-hour ambulatory blood pressure screening. Determining whether a patient is a "dipper" or "non-dipper" is also important.

Should blood pressure medications be needed to help you control your blood pressure levels, keep in mind that, with the exception of diuretic drugs, taking your medications at night can increase their effectiveness by 25 to 50 percent, compared to taking them during the day

To maintain the health of your heart, you need to ensure that your parasympathetic nervous system continues to function at optimal levels. Keys to doing so include eating potassium-rich foods, consuming warm drinks and avoiding cold drinks and drinks that have been sweetened, drinking peppermint, lavender, and linden (tilia) teas, and regularly performing deep breathing exercises during the day. Other helpful measures include gargling, singing, and stimulating your gag reflex, all of which stimulate and tone the vagus nerve. Yoga and meditation can also help, as can regularly spending time outdoors in nature, and making love with a loved one.

A healthy, low-carbohydrate, organic diet containing healthy, fatty foods and a plentiful supply of vegetables is also essential for protecting your heart, as are various nutritional supplements, herbal remedies, regular exercise, and proper management of stress.

Many of the same factors that protect against heart disease, such as a healthy diet, proper supplementation with nutritional supplements and herbs, managing stress, and exercising regularly, can all help to prevent and reverse high blood pressure. Socializing with people whose company you enjoy is also important, rather than being a "loner" or spending time in relationships with people who do not support your mental and emotional well-being.

To protect your heart, it is also vital that you prevent or reverse insulin resistance and corresponding unhealthy weight gain.

CHAPTER 13

Radiant Skin

Your skin is one of your most important, yet most often over-looked, organs in your body, and its condition can be a significant indicator of your overall health. Your skin also performs many essential functions, including regulating your body temperature, protecting underlying body tissues, synthesizing vitamin D from sunlight, and aiding in immunity via specialized skin cells. Skin also excretes water, salts, various organic compounds and toxins via sweat, and is the interface between you and the stimuli of your external environment.

One of skin's most important roles is as an organ of detoxification. Because of the vital role it plays in this area, it is sometimes called the body's "third kidney," since many of its functions having to do with fluids and electrolyte balance are similar to those that the kidneys perform. During times of chronic toxicity, which is far too common today, all the key organs of drainage, such as the liver, lymph, and kidney become overloaded, making the role the skin plays in drainage all the more important. When these internal organs cannot clear the toxic load, toxins will be pushed out through the skin resulting in skin eruptions, odors, discolorations, blemishes, and rashes. These conditions will usually resolve and disappear as the body becomes purified.

It is possible to quickly assess the relative efficiency of elimination through the skin by looking at a person's iris (the colored portion of the eye). The skin is represented by the outermost part of the iris. If it is very dark and dense, this is an indication that the skin is relatively blocked as an organ of elimination. To open it up, skin brushing before a shower (see Chapter 6) and vigorous use of a loofah sponge in the shower are recommended.

In addition to the many important roles skin plays in helping to maintain your body's overall health, it, of course, greatly contributes to your outer appearance. A clean, "glowing" complexion is both a sign of good health and something that makes us more attractive and confident. Conversely, poor skin conditions are signs of other health issues, and can lead to feelings of insecurity and unattractiveness. The rest of this chapter shares the most effective ways that you can achieve healthier, more attractive skin.

Factors That Can Affect Skin Health

There are a number of factors that can affect the health of your skin, ranging from poor hygiene and poor diet to impaired gut health, hormonal imbalances, chronic low-grade dehydration, smoking, exposure to ultraviolet (UV) radiation, stress, and lack of sleep and one's sleep positions.

Poor Hygiene: Proper hygiene is essential for healthy skin. Poor hygiene habits, on the other hand, expose your skin to the buildup of unhealthy bacteria, dirt and grime, and environmental toxins and harmful chemicals.

Poor Diet: It should be no surprise that poor diet can cause unhealthy skin, given how important your diet is to your overall health. When it comes to your skin, the biggest dietary culprits are dietary habits characterized by the regular consumption of processed foods, sugar and artificial sweeteners, excess proteins, unhealthy fats, wheat and other gluten foods, and foods to which you are allergic or sensitive.

Impaired Gut Health: You learned about the relationship between the skin and the gut in Chapter 7. To briefly recap here, impaired gut health leads to a buildup of toxins, pathogens, and undigested protein particles, all of which create burdens on your body's internal organs of detoxification. The more these organs are overwhelmed by such factors, the less able they are at performing their tasks, forcing the skin to have to aid in excreting them. As I mentioned above, this, in turn, can lead to a variety of unhealthy skin conditions.

Hormonal Imbalances: Just as they do to the rest of your body's organs, hormonal imbalances can significantly impair the health of your skin. When hormones become imbalanced, the skin's thickness, pH levels, and ability to repair and regenerate itself are all diminished. This is particularly true of thyroid hormones. Low or imbalanced thyroid hormone levels are a common cause of unhealthy, dry skin, for example. Excess levels of testosterone and DHEA can result in both oily skin and acne.

Dehydration: The health of the skin depends on an adequate daily intake of pure, filtered water. Lack of water can lead to dry skin, wrinkling, and other skin disorders.

Smoking and Exposure to Secondhand Smoke: It should be self-evident to all health-conscious people that smoking and exposure to secondhand smoke is not good for you. Smoking and exposures to cigarette smoke causes a reduction of blood supply to the skin, depriving the skin of vital nutrients and oxygen. As a consequence, skin can become dry or take on an unhealthy pallor, and prematurely start to wrinkle.

UV Radiation: Ultraviolet radiation, not only from the sun, but from other sources, such as tanning booths, black lights, halogen lights, and fluorescent and incandescent light bulbs, can cause a variety of harmful effects on the skin, including skin cancer, as well as premature wrinkling, pigmentation problems, and dry skin.

Stress: Stress can harm healthy skin because of how it depletes the body of various essential nutrients, impairs gut health, and interferes with the body's normal processes of detoxification.

Lack of Sleep: Like the body itself, during sleep, skin repairs itself. You are doubtless familiar with the expression "beauty sleep." It turns out it contains a lot of truth. Regular, healthy sleep improves skin health, while lack of sleep can impair it. As you learned earlier in this book, when you fail to get enough sleep, your body produces more of the stress hormone cortisol. Elevated levels of cortisol can lead to increased stress and inflammation, harming the overall quality of your skin, and resulting in bags and dark circles under the eyes. Lack of sleep and its resulting increase in cortisol and other stress hormones can also exacerbate existing skin conditions, such as acne and eczema, while a good night's sleep can help improve such conditions. Lack of sleep can also cause a breakdown of collagen and hyaluronic acid, which are what gives skin its glow and translucency.

Self-Care Tips for Healthier Skin

Addressing each of the factors above that can harm your skin, or cause it to become unhealthy, is the first and, in many ways, most vital step along the road to a more vibrant complexion. Fortunately, doing so is both easy, and something you can do on your own.

Healthy Hygiene: Proper skin care starts with proper hygiene. This means washing your skin (both face and body) on a daily basis. Castile or other pure soaps should be used, but minimal amounts, since heavy soaping can wash away valuable skin oils, and can cause the skin to overproduce oil in order to compensate. You should also shampoo your hair frequently with a non-chemical soap or shampoo, which can be found in most health food stores.

Regular showers and baths are also important. At the end of a shower, turn the water to cool, and then to warm. As you become accustomed to the temperature change, you may go from hot to cold and back several times. This exercises the tiny muscles in the skin, which control dilation and contraction of the pores. As pores become stronger, they can better respond to the various exposures skin is subjected to on a daily basis.

For added benefit, after showering, sit in a tub of water to which a cup of apple cider vinegar has been added. Doing so can help restore and strengthen the acid mantle layer that sits on top of the skin. Afterward, dry and rub your body briskly with a towel until a warm glow is felt. Epsom salt baths can also be used to help draw toxins out of the skin. These baths are especially beneficial during times when you are also using internal drainage and detoxification methods (see Chapter 6). Such a bath works best after skin brushing (see below) and use of a loofah sponge. Fill your tub with warm to hot water and four or more cups of Epsom salt, letting the salt dissolve. This bath is quite relaxing and good for tense, sore muscles, and may be taken as often as needed.

Diet: To keep your skin healthy, follow the dietary guidelines in Chapter 7, emphasizing plentiful amounts of fresh, raw or lightly steamed vegetables, especially dark leafy greens and cruciferous foods, such as broccoli, cabbage, and cauliflower. Bragg's Liquid Amino Acid can also be added to meals to enliven taste and to help make your skin luminous.

In addition, to improve your body's GI function, add more fermented foods to your diet, such as sauerkraut, miso, or kimchi. You also need to remove sugar from your diet, and eliminate all low-nutrition, processed foods, all of which can cause inflammation, blood sugar spikes, and insulin resistance (see Chapter 12), causing harm to skin cells and tissues. Wheat and other gluten foods should also be avoided for the same reason.

You also want to be sure to keep your body supplied with healthy oils, which help maintain the integrity of the skin, keeping it moisturized and supple. Good sources of healthy dietary fats include organic coconut oil, organic olive oil (extra-virgin), chia and other seeds, nuts, and hemp oil. Avoid polyunsaturated foods, which are quick to go rancid, and are commonly used in processed foods. In cases of excess estrogen production, you also need to avoid soy and all soy foods and drinks, because soy stimulates estrogen production.

Another rich source of healthy fats, as well as vitamin D and vitamin K, are eggs, organic yogurt, butter, and cheeses. Be sure to choose foods from this group that are obtained from pasture raised (grass-fed) animals, as animals raised on grains are lacking in nutritional value, and are also usually laden with antibiotics, growth factors, and other harmful additives.

Finally, to protect against dry, itchy, or flaking skin, you need to keep your body supplied with enough iodine. Iodine-rich foods include kelp and other seaweeds, wild caught fish, cranberries, organic cranberries and strawberries, organic potatoes, and various legumes (beans), such as navy beans. Adding iodized sea salt can also be helpful.

Proper Hydration: To optimize the health of your skin be sure to keep your body hydrated by drinking adequate amounts of pure, filtered water each and every day. "When it comes to skin health, it is important to focus on hydration, specifically consumption, lymphatic drainage, and air humidity," states skin care specialist and esthetician Melanie Simon, of Jackson Hole, Wyoming and Santa Barbara, California. "I recommend that people drink water with minerals, and to avoid chlorinated and fluoridated water whenever possible. Also avoid water filtered through reverse osmosis, which strips out both good and bad minerals, unless you add mineral drops to it. Half your body weight in fluid ounces of healthy water is a good place to start when looking for ideal consumption amounts. But drinking enough water of itself is not enough. It is also critical to move the water and stimulate the lymphatic fluid. This can be accomplished with regular exercise and deep breathing. Our bodies are composed primarily of water, and it is amazing how you can change the appearance of your skin if you properly manipulate the fluids in your body."

In addition to healthy water, adding fresh-squeezed, organic vegetable juices to your daily diet can also be helpful, as can drinking organic herbal teas. You can also drink almond milk mixed with coconut water and a sprinkle of cinnamon. Not only is this drink delicious, it is also good for your skin.

"You must also consider air humidity," Melanie adds. "If your air is very dry, make sure to run a humidifier in your room at night. This really makes a difference if you are exposed to dry air all day long. Also, in the winter when the heat comes on, I also recommend the use of a humidifier. In the long run, this will make a big difference in the appearance of your skin."

Nutritional Supplements: Various nutritional supplements can also help maintain the health of your skin. Among the most essential are vitamin A, B complex vitamins, vitamin C, vitamin E (tocopherols), vitamin D3, vitamin K2, omega-3 oils, magnesium, chlorella, selenium, silica, and zinc. Fulvic acid taken internally once a day with freshly squeezed organic juice is also helpful. Fulvic acid powder can also be applied topically (mixed with water) to heal skin irritations and cuts and burns. Probiotic supplements, and both digestive and proteolytic enzymes (taken away from meals), can also be beneficial because of their ability to improve and maintain proper GI function, as can oxygen-release powder supplements.

Homeopathic Remedies: To help maintain skin health a class of homeopathic remedies known as cell salts can be especially helpful. Cell salts are homeopathic preparations of 12 vital minerals that act as building blocks in the body, including the skin. Because they are diluted and potentiated, only small biochemical amounts of the mineral salts are taken up by the body's cells and tissues. This allows for their better absorption, enabling them to more effectively fortify and energize living tissue. The effectiveness of cell salts for protecting and repairing the skin, has been proven for over 200 years, as has the effectiveness of homeopathy itself.

"Like minerals themselves, cell salts are the foundation needed by your body to carry out its many enzyme-based activities, and act as the catalysts in your body's energy cycles and other functions, including keeping cells, tissues, and organs properly nourished," Jeannette Baer says. "Cell salts also facilitate the cells basic functions, including water balance, removal of toxins, cellular elasticity, oxygenation, and sodium-potassium balance. By maintaining and improving such function, cell salts provide multiple positive benefits for the skin, including preventing and eliminating acne, dark circles under the eyes, enlarged pores, brown and liver spots on the skin, skin redness and rashes, sagging skin, and broken capillaries."

Cell salt remedies are of particular importance today because of many decades of destructive farming practices, which has left crop soil around the world denatured and demineralized. There are 12 basic cell salts, grouped by their overall mineral class. Calcium cell salts are *Calcium fluoride, Calcium phosphate,* and *Calcium sulphate.* Potassium cells salts are *Kali muriaticum, Kali phosphate,* and *Kali sulfur,* while the three cell salts in the sodium group are Nat Muriaticum, Nat Phosphate, and Nat Sulfur. The remaining three are *Ferrum phosphate (iron), Magnesia phosphate (magnesium),* and *Silicea (silica).*

Cell salts, which typically are sold in a potency of 6X and are available at most health food stores, are an excellent way to restore and rebuild the body and its organs, including the skin, because of how they address biochemical and bioenergetic imbalances, rather than suppressing or covering up symptoms. They are safe to use for all ages and can be taken on a regular basis. They can be taken on an individual basis, or as a combination formula containing all 12 cell salts. Two combination cell salt formulas I recommend are Bioplasma, manufactured by Hyland's, and Cell Salts Complex, by Apex Energetics. The Hyland's formula can usually be found at local health foods store. To learn more about Cell Salts and other Apex products, visit www.apexenergetics.com.

Herbal Remedies: Herbal remedies have been used to improve and maintain the skin for centuries. Among the most effective herbal remedies are alma, which is rich in vitamin C; astragalus, which can be mixed with sesame oil and applied topically, and is especially useful for healing skin burns and benign tumors; holy basil, which can improve skin elasticity and help prevent and reverse wrinkles; licorice root, which helps combat inflammation and, when applied topically as a paste, can speed healing of skin irritations, including eczema and psoriasis; and shatavari root, an Ayurvedic remedy that has been used for centuries to treat skin conditions. Other herbs include Saponaria, Fumaria, and Viola Tricolor.

Skin Brushing: Although I already covered skin brushing in Chapter 6, I want to emphasize its benefits for healthy skin in this chapter, as well. This simple and invigorating ritual before baths and showers is an excellent way to exfoliate your skin, ridding it of dead skin cells, while also supporting the overall health of your body's immune system because of how it stimulates the lymphatic system and improves circulation. Skin brushing can also enhance your body's endocrine (hormone) function.

To perform skin brushing you will need a long-handled natural bristle brush, which you can find at some health stores, bath and beauty boutiques, and online. Prior to bathing or showering, gently, yet firmly, brush your skin, starting with your hands and arms, then progressing to your upper torso, and finally your legs and feet. Always remember to brush toward your heart.

For added benefit, you can use high quality essential oils when skin brushing. To do so, place a single drop of essential oil on your palm, then rub the dry brush tips onto the oil. Good essential oil choices for skin brushing include cypress, eucalyptus, laurel, rosemary, and yarrow. With or without the use of essential oils, I recommend you get in the habit of dry skin brushing for about five minutes each day before you shower or bathe.

Lifestyle: Important lifestyle measures include avoiding smoking (seek professional assistance if you currently smoke and need to quit), avoiding exposures to secondhand smoke, harmful exhaust and other chemicals and toxins, getting enough sleep, managing stress (see Chapter 8), and exercising to induce sweating, which helps rid the skin of toxins, and improves blood flow and muscle and skin tone, while also helping to keep blood pressure and hormone levels normalized. Regular, moderate exercise is best, as over-exertion places excess stress on the body and can counteract the health benefits of moderate exercise.

Also, avoid frowns, squinting, and other facial motions that can cause wrinkling because such motions weaken elastin, diminishing the skin's ability to spring back to its previous smooth state.

Protecting Yourself From Ultraviolet (UV) Light: Avoiding, or at least minimizing exposure to ultraviolet light is also important, including from the sun. In addition to being linked to basal cell and squamous cell skin cancer, UV light can cause wrinkles by damaging the production of collagen in the layer of the skin known as the dermis.

When you are out in the sun, it is best wear a hat or other head covering, and to use a sun block, or screening lotion, with minimal chemicals. As my friend Jeannette Baer, PA-C, cofounder of "Aesthetics Montecito" in Montecito, California, explains, "Sun blocks that contain parabens and other chemical components are harmful because these ingredients literally can get 'cooked" into the skin during sunlight exposure. Sunlight also causes these chemicals to become denatured and change their structure, making them even more toxic and dangerous as they are heated by the sun and absorbed into the skin. Zinc and titanium dioxide are safe alternatives to chemical sun blocks. Vitamin C products are also recommended because of their ability to protect against free radical damage, both externally and internally." If you need a quick and healthy tan, you can apply a natural vegetable oil called Sun FX to your skin.

Peptides, a specific class of proteins, can also be very helpful for creating, maintaining, and protecting ageless skin from ultraviolet light and other harmful exposures. "These proteins are important for skin care because of how they can trigger cells, including skin cells, to behave like younger, healthier cells," Jeannette states. She also recommends retinoid creams. "Originally used in products that treat acne, retinoids are compounds related to vitamin A. They help protect the skin by encouraging cellular turnover. As we get older, it takes longer and longer for our new skin cells to push off the old cells that affect our skin's appearance, whereas, by contrast, the skin of children turns over every 28 days or so, which is why healthy children have such luminescent skin."

I would like to add that several of my patients have been able to heal their basal cell skin cancers with a topical cream called BEC5 (Curaderm). BEC5 is an extract derived from eggplant. It is applied twice a day to the affected area, and covered with a Band-Aid. It takes one month for it to resolve.

Sleep: As I mentioned above, getting enough restful sleep each night is also vital for healthy, youthful skin. "I would say that sleep deprivation, by far, is the quickest way to accelerate the aging of skin," Melanie Simon says. "I have seen this consistently with insomniacs and, in contrast, the clients I have worked with who have made sleep a priority are the ones that have spectacular skin."

To improve the quality of your sleep, follow the recommendations I shared in Chapter 8. Jeannette Baer also recommends avoiding sleeping with your face pressed against your pillow. "Regardless of pillow softness," she says, "sleeping in this fashion puts pressure on your face, and can result in the appearance of lines on your chin, cheeks, or forehead."

Face Cleansing Tips: In addition to practicing good daily hygiene, here are some other useful tips for cleansing your face. Melanie Simon recommends that you begin by using your hands to massage the lymph nodes along your neck in a small, circular motion, starting at the base of your neckline and moving up to the jaw line and the front of your ears. Doing this gently pumps lymph, helping it to move instead of clumping. "The lymph nodes in your neck are responsible for most of the fluid that drains out of your face, so it's important to give them some attention when you are cleansing your skin."

Once you are done massaging your neck, move to your mouth and cheek area and massage those areas in the same manner, followed by the area around your eye sockets. "I like to circle the eyes and, with my thumbs, guide the lymph down the sides of the nose. The fluid in the face drains out only if the lymph nodes have been cleared. That is why it is important to start at the base of the neck and then work upward to move lymph out of the face. For best results, I have my clients look up a

picture of the lymph nodes in the neck and face to more accurately perform this daily ritual." Melanie adds that you can also use skin care massage devices to perform this lymphatic massage. In her practice, she will
often use the Foreo Luna™. (For more information, see www.foreo.
com.) There are a variety of similar products on the market, as well.

Once you complete your neck and facial lymphatic massage you are
ready to begin cleansing your face. Melanie recommends a five-step
routine for optimal results. "I begin by cleansing the forehead, and then
progress all along the rest of the face and neck line," she says. "I start
with a gentle, non-chemical cleanser that cleans the skin without stripping it. Look for gentle, non-foaming cleansers that feel almost like
moisturizers when they are applied, such as the CIRC-CELL clay oil
cleanser. Such cleansers remove dirt from the skin while leaving the oils
of the skin intact."

The next step in Melanie's approach is the use of a skin toner. "I
know this scares many people," she says, "but I would never skip a toner." She recommends avoiding alcohol-based products because of how
they can cause skin to dry out. "A good toner is meant to prep the skin's
pH," she explains. "Look for products that include lactic acid and witch
hazel. This is a nice combination that will leave your skin looking and
feeling moisturized, as opposed to parched. I prefer skin toners with a
pH that is slightly acidic, with a pH of about 5.5. You can buy pH strips
at your local drugstore to test different toners to be sure they are within
the correct range."

Melanie recommends applying toners with gauze, pressing it into
your face and neck firmly, and holding it in place on each section for at
least five seconds. Once you finish, allow the toner to set up. "You don't
want to instantly add a serum and alter the toner and its ability to affect
your skin's pH," she says. "You have to give it a minute or so to do its job."

After this step, it is time to apply a skin serum to add protective,
health-enhancing compounds to your skin. "A serum should be primarily comprised of a water weight formulation that soaks into the skin immediately as it is applied," Melanie says. "Look for a serum that contains

high concentrations of at least one of the following ingredients: amino acids, elastin, or placenta extract."

The fourth step is the application of a skin moisturizer or creme. "Such products should contain lipids or have a butter-like consistency to keep your skin protected," Melanie advises. "If you are dealing with acne, look for a creme that also contains ingredients like arnica and sulfur. Alternately, if you are lacking in hormones, look for cremes that contain non-GMO soy or wild yam." Such cremes and moisturizers both protect skin and feed its tissues.

Melanie then recommends that you complete this cleansing process with a finishing fluid or spray, applying it to both your face and neck to lock in all of the above benefits, and to keep your skin moisturized and protected against dehydration.

Professional Skin Care Options

In cases of persistent skin problems, such as acne, eczema, psoriasis, or rash, I recommend that you work with your physician in conjunction with a dermatologist. If your skin problems are due to hormone imbalances, I also recommend that you consult with an integrative physician who specializes in anti-aging medicine and bio-identical hormone therapy. Ideally, he or she will also practice Energy Medicine in order to detect any previously unsuspected factors that may be involved.

In addition to the need for possible medical assistance, you can also benefit from working with a professional esthetician, such as Jeannette and Melanie, who take a non-toxic, holistic approach to skin care. Two valuable skin care methods such estheticians provide are Microneedle rolling and the photofacial.

Microneedle Rolling: Microneedle rolling helps to stimulate your skin to produce more collagen. "Insufficient collagen is the common factor in skin conditions such as wrinkles, scars, and stretch marks, "Jeannette Baer explains. "If your skin would manufacture more collagen then you wouldn't develop these conditions. Frequent use of the Microneedle Roller provides nature with a helping hand by triggering collagen production, which can be very effective in reversing and preventing such conditions."

The Microneedle Roller is a hand-held tool that can be used by both men and women. In addition to stimulating collagen production, it also stimulates production of elastin, and offers several other beneficial effects, including helping to reverse scars (including acne scars, stretchmarks, wrinkles, cellulite, and hyper-pigmentations. It can also help prevent hair loss in some cases.

"Microneedling has equivalent results to chemical peels, laser treatment, and dermabrasion, but it is much less invasive and safer, and is available at only a small fraction of the cost of these other treatments," Jeannette explains. "As you roll the Microneedle Roller across your skin, it makes pinpoint punctures into the dermis, the majority of which are simply temporarily opening your pores. Your skin perceives this as damage, though it really isn't, which causes the release of growth factors that trigger the production of elastin and collagen. Your skin reacts to any damage or injury by initiating the healing process, but in general it will only heal as far as it has to in order to keep you in good health. By frequently initiating this healing process using the Microneedle Roller, you stimulate your skin to keep repairing until the process is complete."

In addition to triggering greater collagen and elastin production, the resulting micro channels that the Microneedle opens results in greater penetration of topical skin cleansers, lotions, moisturizers, and cremes, signficantly increasing their overall effects. "Clinical studies in the US, as well as in Europe and South Korea, have proven that the absorption of topical skin care products is increased by as much as 1,000 times when they are applied following Microneedling," Jeannette says.

Photofacial: The photofacial is a cosmetic procedure designed to produce younger, healthier skin. It is a 30-minute procedure in which intense pulses of light (IPL) therapy are used to penetrate deep into the skin. "The IPL photofacial then causes collagen and blood vessels below the epidermis to constrict, reducing redness and age lines," Melanie Simon explains. "The procedure involves only minimal discomfort, such as minor redness and swelling that can sometimes occur after treatment and then quickly disappear. Pigmented spots and areas of redness selectively absorb the intense pulsed light delivered by photofacials, resulting in significant improvements in the appearance of skin without peeling or burning. The IPL photofacial process leaves skin with a clear, glowing, youthful complexion, making it one of the most popular procedures requested by my clients."

According to Melanie, a variety of skin conditions, such as red complexion, rosacea, fine lines and wrinkles, large pores, freckles, and pigmented spots, respond well to IPL photofacial treatments. Other skin conditions for which IPL photofacial treatments offer benefit include broken capillaries on the skin, mild acne scars, dull complexion, sun and smoke damage, and liver spots.

Key Points To Remember

Your skin, though often overlooked, is one of your body's most overlooked organs and a key indicator of your overall health.

Among the many important functions your skin performs are regulating body temperature, protecting underlying body tissues, synthesizing vitamin D from sunlight, and aiding in immunity via specialized skin cells. Skin also excretes water, salts, various organic compounds and toxins via sweat.

Because of the important roles it plays as a major organ of detoxification, skin is sometimes called the body's "third kidney," since many of its functions are similar to those the kidneys perform.

Various factors can affect the health of your skin, especially poor hygiene, poor diet, impaired gut health, hormonal imbalances, chronic low-grade dehydration, smoking, exposure to ultraviolet (UV) radiation, stress, and lack of sleep.

To maintain the health of your skin and reverse skin conditions it is essential that you practice good hygiene daily, eat nutritious meals, drink plenty of pure, filtered water, and make healthy lifestyle choices, such as getting enough sleep, regularly engaging in moderate exercise, not smoking, and avoiding exposures to secondhand smoke, harmful exhaust, and other toxins and chemicals. Avoiding excessive exposure to ultraviolet light is also important.

Various nutritional supplements, herbal remedies, and homeopathic formulas can also help maintain healthy skin. Homeopathic formulas known as cell salts can be of particular benefit because of their ability to provide vital minerals to skin cells and tissues in a highly absorbable way.

Managing stress, getting adequate sleep each night, avoiding sleeping with your face pressed into your pillow, and avoiding frowning, squinting, and other facial motions, are all also important.

And excellent daily ritual to improve skin health is to dry brush your entire body for at least five minutes in the morning before you bathe or shower.

Properly cleansing your neck and face is also important. This starts with gently massaging the lymph nodes from the base of your neck up to your jaw line, and then over your face, in order to move fluids and prevent lymphatic congestion. Following such a massage, and the five-step process of cleansing your face and neck can make a significant difference in your appearance. This process begins with using a gentle face and neck cleanser, followed by the application of a skin toner, a protective skin serum, a skin creme or moisturizer, and a finishing fluid or spray.

For persistent skin problems, working with an integrative, anti-aging physician is advised. In some cases, a dermatologist may also be necessary.

Two innovative, professional skin care therapies that can also make a healthy difference in your appearance are Microneedle Rolling and the IPL photo facial.

CHAPTER 14

Medicine's Exciting Future

Although the main purpose of this book is to empower you to immediately begin your journey towards ageless vitality on your own by incorporating the many proven self-care techniques and guidelines I have shared with you, I would be remiss if I did not also inform you of a number of very exciting professional care therapies that have the potential to completely revolutionize modern medicine as they become more well-known and utilized. All of the therapies outlined below have been personally investigated by me, and I have used many of them for my own health, and in treating my patients. It is my hope that they will soon become adopted by more doctors and other health care specialists across the country. Your awareness of them, and demand for them, can help make that happen. What follows is a brief overview and explanation of each of them.

Cold Laser Therapy

Cold laser therapy, also known as soft, or low-level laser therapy, has been used as a treatment for various health conditions for the past few decades, but it was not until 2001 that the Food and Drug Administration (FDA) approved cold lasers as a medical device. Since that time, a number of cold laser devices have come to market, including models designed for home use.

Cold laser therapy can be used to either target and activate acupuncture points, thus acting like acupuncture without the needles, making it an ideal alternative for patients who have a phobia about needles, or to provide a beam of low intensity laser, or photon, light to initiate a series of bioenergetic reactions in the body that stimulate the body's overall healing mechanisms at the cellular level. The therapy is completely noninvasive and has now been approved by the FDA as a treatment for a variety of health conditions, including acute and chronic pain (including back, neck, and shoulder pain), arthritis, bursitis, carpal tunnel syndrome, fibromyalgia, ligament sprains, muscle strain and tension, tendonitis, and tennis elbow. Cold lasers are also used in conventional medicine for cosmetic surgery, eye surgery, heart surgery and various other conditions.

In addition, research has shown that cold laser therapy provides a number of important overall physiological benefits. These include:

- Increased cell growth and reproduction
- Increased metabolic activity
- Increased cellular energy (by stimulating production of the mitochondria to produce more adenosine triphosphate (ATP)
- Increased blood flow and overall circulatory function
- Reduced formation of scar tissue
- Improved nerve function
- Faster wound healing.

During cold laser therapy, photon light is emitted at specific wavelengths and at various levels of penetration into the body. Low levels of penetration are all that is necessary for conditions such as surface scarring and lymphatic congestion, while deeper penetration (up to four to five inches into the body) may be necessary to effectively treat joint pain.

In my practice I use the TerraQuant Quantum Low Level Laser. The TerraQuant System has added features for clinical use that other laser systems lack, and is covered by many health insurance plans. TerraQuant is one of the few medical devices available today in the world that provides a unique combination of super pulsed laser with infrared, visible red light, and magnetic field therapy based on Low Level Quantum Therapy. TerraQuant provides preset treatment protocols, as well as a custom treatment mode, providing a low-intensity, noninvasive, safe treatment to transform cells from an unstable state into a stable healthy state. For more information, please contact Apex Energetics @ (800) 736-4381.

Overall, cold laser therapy is easy to apply, very safe, free of side effects, cost effective for both the practitioner and patient, and a superior treatment option compared to pain medications and other drugs that are incapable of going beyond managing symptoms. Cold laser therapy may eliminate the need for surgery, has a high success rate, and can be an excellent synergistic treatment with other therapies. I regard cold laser therapy to be an important addition to other medical treatments, and with the recent development of low-cost professional cold lasers, I expect the use of cold laser therapy will be a rapidly growing medical treatment option.

The CVAC™ Process

The CVAC process, while still little known to the public at large, got a boost of recognition a few years ago when it was revealed by the *Wall Street Journal* that Novak Djokovic, one of the world's elite professional tennis players, attributed his number 1 ranking in the world, in part, to CVAC. Djokovic, like many other elite athletes, is known for his interest in the latest research in health, including cutting edge therapies. Prior to discovering CVAC he had already adopted a gluten-free diet to enhance his athletic performance, which he stated helped improve his strength and endurance on the tennis court. CVAC stands for Cyclic Variations in Adaptive Conditioning□.

CVAC treatments consists of reclining in an egg-shaped pressure chamber, or CVAC pod. Once inside, the device delivers from 200 to 400+ patterned cycles of low pressure. A proprietary proportioning system assures that only filtered fresh air is allowed into the pod. A high performance regenerative vacuum blower suctions air out of the pod, while the proportioning system continuously vents fresh air back into it. At no time is air allowed to recirculate or become stale.

The temperature naturally changes in the pod in concert with the changes in pressure. As the pressure lowers, so does the temperature; as the pressure increases, it gets warmer. This is continuously changing during every session.

There are three basic stressors that create a system of exercise in every CVAC session. They are temperature, air density and pressure. The body naturally adapts to these stressors, which then enhance the body's ability to adapt and thrive in a variety of conditions. Even though users do nothing more than sit inside the pod as a treatment session unfolds, the CVAC sessions produce many of the same benefits that may be acquired from intense aerobic and anaerobic (strength training) exercise. CVAC sessions also help improve the body's ability to absorb oxygen more effectively. This is a natural outcome derived from the body's adaptation to the three stressors (temperature, air density, and pressure).

During each CVAC session the body's exertion and recovery phases occur in sequence, with the body's cellular energy systems benefiting from the pressure changes inside the pod, and the lymphatic system is "massaged," or stimulated, to enhance its ability to eliminate cellular waste matter. The many changes in air pressure during a session creates a greater than normal stress on the body, which, over time, allows for greater physiological adaptation to take place.

A number of studies have validated the CVAC processes' ability to improve fitness levels to a degree similar to regular periods of physical exercise. One such study conducted at Stanford University involving a group of insulin-resistant sedentary, middle-aged men demonstrated that as little as 120 minutes of CVAC therapy each week for a total of 10 weeks was enough to dramatically lower the men's blood-fasting glucose level, thus decreasing their risk of diabetes, as well as cancer and heart disease. By contrast, the control group which was given sham (placebo) sessions, continued to decline toward diabetes. Another study involving student athletes showed significant improvements in their blood's capacity for carrying oxygen. When I first tried the CVAC process for myself I was pleasantly surprised with the improvement in my energy level after a 15 minute session, and a feeling of well-being that persisted for about 24 hours.

Though the CVAC process can be effective for improving physical conditioning and overall fitness levels, it is important to note that it is not intended as a replacement for regular exercise, nor is it a method for diagnosing, treating, or managing any type of health condition. And, as with exercise itself, before trying CVAC therapy, I recommend that you first consult with your physician.

For more information about CVAC therapy, visit www.cvacsystems.com.

EECP Therapy

EECP stands for Enhanced External Counterpulsation Therapy. Though EECP has been in use for many years in the U.S. (and even longer in other countries), and is approved by the Food and Drug Administration and covered by Medicare and most private health insurance, many doctors still do not use or recommend it to their patients. This is very short-sighted on their part, in my opinion, given EECP's proven effectiveness for helping with the symptoms associated with heart disease, especially chest pain and symptoms of coronary heart disease. Despite this, currently less than 20 percent of our nation's cardiology clinics offer or even recommend EECP treatments.

During EECP treatments, cuffs similar to those used to measure blood pressure are applied to the body at the calves, thighs, and buttocks, and then mechanically inflated, starting at the calves. This inflation sequence forces blood back into the heart during its diastolic phase (filling between heartbeats). The arteries that supply the heart with blood are called the coronary arteries. These arteries deliver blood to the heart while the heart is filling. The squeezing of the cuffs during the filling phase of the heart cycle increases blood flow to the heart. The cuffs are quickly deflated before the next heart beat, which increases blood flow to the lower extremities, and simultaneously reduces the workload of the heart. Additionally EECP has been found to stimulate VEGF (vascular endothelial growth factor), which results in the formation of new blood vessels throughout the body, thus increasing the delivery of oxygen and glucose to all the organs.

Research from nearly 200 clinical studies has shown that EECP is effective for increasing both the strength and overall health of the heart because of the increased oxygenated blood it supplies the heart, especially to parts of the heart muscle that may have reduced blood flow. Studies on EECP have found that it can significantly improve a patient's quality of life, reduce the risk of heart failure, and reduce the frequency and intensity of angina attacks, as well as the need for angina medication. Moreover, heart patients who receive EECP typically become better able to exercise and engage in other physical activities for longer periods of time without experiencing chest pain. EECP has also been shown to provide improvements in patients suffering from other types of cardiovascular disease, including stroke and peripheral artery disease, or PAD.

Outside of the U.S., EECP is used for a wider range of conditions than it is used for here, including Alzheimer's and dementia (to increase the flow of blood and oxygen to the brain), diabetes, erectile dysfunction (ED), macular degeneration, and Parkinson's disease. In addition to a reduction and elimination of chest pain, heart palpitations, and leg pain caused by heart disease, as well as a reduced need for heart medications, the overall benefits of EECP include increased energy, improved brain function and mental alertness, improved eye health, improved lung capacity and respiration, improved kidney and liver function, and improved sexual function in men. EECP therapy has also been shown to have a better than 80 percent success rate.

My Los Angeles patients receive EECP at a facility, owned by Sara Soulati, that can be located by going to www.globalcardiocare.com. To locate other clinics or hospitals that offers EECP, visit www.eecp-therapy.com/find-an-eecp-treatment-facility.

Gene Diagnostics

Gene diagnostics, or gene testing, is a means of testing patients for the presence of genetic disease, gene mutations, and genetic predispositions for a variety of health conditions and other physiological issues for which they may be more at risk because they carry genes linked to such conditions. Testing involves analyzing chromosomes, DNA and various proteins found in blood, hair, skin, or samples from inside of the cheeks obtained from a mouth swap. Advances in gene diagnostics continue to unfold, largely due to the discoveries of the Human Genome Project. Currently there are over 1,200 genetic diagnostic tests available.

While gene diagnostics offer many benefits to physicians and patients when it comes to health, it is important to state that gene tests for medical reasons remain controversial. The primary reasons for this controversy have to do with the fears the results of such tests can trigger, as well as privacy concerns about the results, and how the results might impact a person's employment and health insurance premiums. Medical privacy and other laws help to minimize these latter concerns, but the issue of fears related to gene testing results remains a very real problem.

An example that highlights the seriousness of the fears that can arise from gene diagnostics is that of women who, upon learning that their gene tests found they carry genes for breast or ovarian cancer, elect to have both of their breasts and/or ovaries removed despite their current state of good health. In a number of cases, such drastic procedures are undertaken with the encouragement and full support of their physicians.

I am vigorously opposed to such drastic measures for three reasons. First, because they rarely are necessary; second, because of the immense toll such surgical procedures place on the body, diverting energy and other resources away from its many other normal, health-protecting functions; and finally because, as the saying goes, *your genes are not your destiny*. Just because you may have a genetic predisposition for a particular disease, including cancer, in no way means you will develop it (genes are like recipes; they don't tell you what's for dinner). As the growing and exciting field called *epigenetics* (the study of the processes involved in the development, activation and deactivations of genes) is increasingly making clear, it is not whether or not you carry a gene linked to a disease that is important, *it is whether or not that gene is ever activated to trigger that disease.* The understanding of this latter fact is what makes gene diagnostics an important new tool in helping doctors guide their patients to achieving and maintaining optimal health.

Here's an example of how I put gene diagnostic results to work in my practice. Suppose one of my female patients is found to carry one or more of the cancer genes that have been linked to breast cancer. Compounding this issue, let's say that there is also a history of breast cancer in her family (mother, sister, grandmother, aunt, etc.). Such a family history can understandably create fear that she too will develop breast cancer one day, and that fear is likely to rise when she learns of her gene test results.

As a caring physician, it is my responsibility to take her fears and concerns seriously, not dismiss or make light of them. At the same time, it is also my duty and responsibility *not to feed her fears.* Instead, my goal is to first help her fortify her mind and beliefs, using the methods I shared in Chapter 5, and then do all that I can to help ensure that she and I work together to do everything else that is necessary to reduce her breast cancer risk and keep her cancer-free. It is because of this proactive, preventive, comprehensive approach that the incidence of breast cancer among my patients, as well as all other serious disease conditions, as I mentioned in Chapter 6, is nearly nonexistent, whereas the incidence of such conditions continues to skyrocket among patients of most other physicians today.

Gene diagnostics can be a very helpful aid for fine-tuning the proactive, preventive, and comprehensive approach that characterizes my medical practice, and can be the same for you, as well. By using it to determine what, if any, genetic predispositions for illness you may have, you will be better informed and empowered to address those genetic "weaknesses" so that the genes involved are not activated or expressed. In the process, you will also be improving all other aspects of your health, as well. And, instead of fearing future outcomes, you will achieve greater confidence and optimism about your health, knowing that you are doing all you can to stay healthy.

In the years ahead, I expect more doctors to begin incorporating gene diagnostics into their practice. For now, if you are interested in obtaining a medical gene test for yourself or a loved one, I recommend that you only work with doctors who are not only familiar with, and already using, this new technology, but who also take a similar approach to my own when it comes to interpreting and acting on the test results.

Intravenous Vitamin Therapy

When I was an ER doctor, my colleagues and I all knew of the beneficial effects of intravenous fluids and intravenous medications, because of how they work fast to save lives. Intravenous nutrients are very powerful because they facilitate the excretion of toxins and can rejuvenate organs such as the liver and the brain. Intravenous vitamin therapy, or IVT, has been used for decades by a small, yet growing, number of nutritionally-oriented physicians, including me. It involves using IV's to administer certain vitamins, minerals and amino acids, directly into the bloodstream.

This approach offers a number of advantages compared to oral nutritional supplementation. First, IVT allows for nutrients to quickly reach the body's cells without having to first pass through the digestive tract and liver to be metabolized. Moreover, IVT enables physicians to administer high doses of nutrients safely and effectively without the typical side effects, such as stomach cramping or loose bowels, that can be caused when high doses of nutrients are taken orally. This is especially true of nutrients like vitamin C and magnesium.

In addition, the highest doses of nutrients that can be safely administered intravenously would be impossible to consume orally. And even if that were not the case, because of how the digestive process breaks down oral supplements, a good percentage of them is often excreted by the body without being utilized by cells, tissues, and organs, unlike what happens with IVT.

Another important benefit that IVT provides is its ability to administer more effective therapeutic doses of nutrients. This is important, because research has established that, for certain nutrients, high blood or tissue concentrations must be achieved in order for them to be most active and effective. Vitamin C is a good example of this.

Numerous studies show that high concentrations of vitamin C in the bloodstream and intracellular fluids are necessary before it can achieve its beneficial effects. Large doses of vitamin C administered via IVT can stimulate the immune system, help the liver work better, and strengthen and improve the functioning of the adrenal glands, as well as other organs that are not functioning efficiently. Using intravenous vitamin C, I can dramatically help many patients. Some of my patients, for example, are receiving chemotherapy for cancer at three- to four-week intervals. In between these chemotherapy sessions, they receive 25,000 mg of intra-venous vitamin C from me on a weekly basis, in order to reduce toxicity from the chemotherapy. This protocol in no way interferes with the action of chemotherapy, and can improve its effectiveness.

Besides vitamin C, the nutrients most commonly administered via IVT include phosphatidylcholine (for its liver and brain effects), glutathione (for its ability to detoxify), trace minerals, and alpha lipoic acid (ALA). A very popular IV is a combination of vitamin C, various B vitamins, calcium, and magnesium known as the Myers Cocktail, which is named after John Myers, MD, the physician who invented it in the 1970s, and which has proven to be an effective treatment for a range of conditions including acute and chronic asthma, cold and flu, chronic fatigue (CFS), Epstein-Barr virus, fibromyalgia, headache and migraine, and for managing the withdrawal symptoms of drug addiction.

Intravenous vitamin C and glutathione can be very helpful to help your body get rid of the effects of general anesthesia. This can be done one week after surgery, and followed with an additional IV one week later. If you are in need of surgery, ask your integrative doctor to make sure that he uses IVT in his practice.

All IVT treatments are first custom-tailored to each patient's specific needs and can be administered either quickly, as an IV "push" (over 10-15 minutes), or as a standard IVT treatment, which usually lasts between 30 to 90 minutes while the patients sits comfortably, and is able to listen to music, read a book, or simply relax. IVT has been an essential component of my overall treatment protocol for many of my patients, and both they and I can personally attest to its effectiveness.

If you are interested in exploring IVT for yourself, contact a physician who is trained in its use. You can find such physicians in your area by contacting the American College for Advancement in Medicine (ACAM). To learn more, visit www.acam.org.

Ionized Oxygen Therapy

Ionized Oxygen Therapy (IOT) has been utilized and researched since the 1920's, with most of the research being performed in Germany, where it was first developed. IOT is both a very basic (simple to administer) and highly effective therapy, with far-reaching benefits. It affects every aspect of the body's health, and can be used as a treatment for any health condition, either by itself or as a complement to other therapies.

IOT involves the use of medical grade oxygen that has first been treated to produce either a negative or positive charge on the oxygen. The patient simply inhales the treated oxygen, through an oxygen mask. In general, negative ions have a relaxing effect(parasympathetic) and positive ions have a stimulating effect(sympathetic). I use the negative ions much more often with my patients. Both types of ions produce a profound regulatory effect on the body's nervous, immune, gastrointestinal, intercellular matrix, and inflammatory systems, and also act to change the body's "biological terrain", a term primarily used to refer to the physical characteristics of the body's fluids. These characteristics help determine what types of illnesses and infections a person is susceptible to. Changing these characteristics via IOT helps to eliminate these susceptibilities and improve overall health.

As with IVT, the benefits of IOT are many. They include increased mood and mental/cognitive functioning, increased energy and endurance, decreased healing time, decreased susceptibility to infections and illness, improved gut health and function (including normalizing the ecosystem of the gut microbiome), and improved cellular function. Some of the health conditions for which IOT has been proven to be especially effective are allergy, arthritis, difficulty concentrating and other cognitive problems, dizziness, fatigue, both high and low blood pressure, heart disease and circulatory conditions, migraine, dizziness, all respiratory conditions, and stress.

Another useful application of IOT is its use to create oxygen-rich, ionized water. Like IOT itself, ionized water provides energy directly to the body's organs of the body. For general health purposes, between half to one liter of ionized water is consumed per day. For most conditions, negatively ionized water is drunk for three days, followed by the use of positive water for one day, with this cycle continuing for three to four weeks. After that, no ionized water is drunk for between three to four weeks, and then the cycle is repeated. Energy deficiency is not only caused by the lack of nutrition, vitamins, and minerals, but also by the lack of oxygen and water. Ionized oxygen energizes the respiratory air, the drinking water, and the body water.

Note: In recent years a number of home ionizing water units have become popular, both in the U.S. and abroad. These units cannot provide the same degree of benefits as those from IOT administered by a physician. Although there are an estimated 3,000 or more physicians who use IOT worldwide, the majority of them live and work outside the U.S. Hopefully, more U.S. physicians will join their ranks in the coming years

Light and Sound Therapies (Sensory Resonance)

The origins of both light and sound therapy date back to ancient times. Ancient healers from all healing traditions recognized the importance of sunlight for health and well-being, and I'm sure you have often experienced the benefits of "sunlight therapy" for yourself each time you stepped out into a bright, sunny day and felt your mood improve as a result. As you learned in Chapter 5, the experience of positive emotions also produces numerous physiological benefits within your body.

The earliest forms of sound therapy include chanting and verbal prayers, as well as drumming and other forms of music. Such methods continue to be used today, and their benefits continue to be verified by modern science. Each time your mood lifts when you hear a favorite song or piece of music you, too, are verifying the effectiveness of sound as a healing tool.

Light Therapy: Since the 20th century a number of exciting developments have occurred within the field of light and sound therapies. In the field of light therapy, one such development is the cold laser therapy we discussed above. Another, increasingly popular, therapy in this field is full-spectrum light therapy, which involves the use of light boxes, lamps, and wall units comprised of full-spectrum lights that mimic the light of the early morning sun.

Full-spectrum light therapy is especially well-known for its ability to prevent and reverse the effects of seasonal affective disorder (SAD), which is caused by a lack of sunlight exposure, especially during winter months, and is characterized by depression, lack of energy, excessive eating and sleeping, mood swings, and a lowered sex drive. Because of how full-spectrum light treatments have been shown to help people with SAD, today full-spectrum light bulbs can be found at most hardware stores. Other conditions for which full-spectrum light therapy has been shown to have benefit include high blood pressure, hyperactivity (especially in children and teens), insomnia, migraine, and PMS.

Other useful types of light therapy include UV light therapy, which involves the use of ultraviolet light applied either directly to the skin or to irradiate drawn blood that is then reintroduced to the body; colored light therapy (one form is called syntonics), which involves the use of various colored lights to treat disease; and photodynamic therapy, which is used to treat tumors via the application of dyes or medications that absorb light and which are in turn absorbed by the tumors. The tumors are then exposed to specific types of light, causing cancer cells to die without harming healthy cells.

A type of light therapy that I am particularly interested in, and which I use in my medical practice, is called Biophoton therapy. Biophoton therapy involves the application of light to particular areas of the skin for healing purposes. It is via Biophotons that cells communicate and transfer information, in other words, using light particles as the primary carriers of information in the body. The light, or photons, that are emitted by Biophoton diodes are absorbed by the skin's photoreceptors and then travel throughout the body, where they help regulate what is referred to as human bioenergy. By stimulating certain areas of the body with specific quantities of light, Biophoton therapy can help reduce pain, as well as aid in various healing processes throughout the body. The theory behind Biophoton therapy is based on the work of F.A. Popp, who theorized that light can affect the electromagnetic waves of the body and regulate enzyme activity. Through the use of Biophoton therapy, human bioenergy can be rebalanced and strengthened, thus alleviating and improving numerous health conditions.

Since body and mind are connected through this energy, I find that I am not only able to improve my patient's physical conditions, but can also aid them in achieving a greater state of mental and emotional health. Initially, Biophoton therapy was used primarily for cosmetic, skin care, and scalp conditions. It was only much later that its effectiveness was discovered for treating chronic pain and a variety of other health conditions. Even when cells die, energy is produced because the cell emits photons(light) at the time of its death to its living neighbors (like passing on an inheritance).

Sound Therapy: There are many types of sound therapy approaches, such as auditory integration, or Tomatis, therapy, developed by Alfred Tomatis, MD; BioAcoustics™, developed by Sharry Edwards, director of the Sound Health Institute in Ohio; cymatic therapy, developed by the Swiss researcher Hans Jenny; and various forms of music therapy, such as those popularized by Don Campbell and Steven Halpern. A full explanation of these and other sound therapies goes beyond the scope of this book. Suffice it to say that, like light therapy techniques, the benefits of sound therapy are wide ranging. Such benefits include improvements in ADD/ADHD, autism, cognitive dysfunctions, headache, high blood pressure, insomnia, mental and emotional problems, and pain (including pain caused by medical and dental surgeries).

The VibraSound[(R)]:VibraSound® is a proprietary technology that enables people to feel music in every cell of their body. It was developed by my friend and pioneering researcher Don Estes. According to Don, music is meant to be seen and felt, as well as heard, and the key to health and happiness is the ability to *experience* life as much as to *analyze* it. Too much analysis leaves one short of experience. Experience actualizes in human consciousness as either pleasure or pain. The VibraSound system can help bring about a state of pleasurable experience, what Don has termed *sensory resonance.* This type of healthy pleasure has applications in just about every field of medicine, psychiatry, stress management, recreation, and entertainment.

Sensory resonance is a state of mind that occurs when one is extremely excited, challenged or relaxed in a pleasurable experience. It cannot be achieved under conditions of boredom, threat, or pain. VibraSound was designed to help users relax and become inspired at the same time by synchronizing their senses of sight, sound, and vibration with a unique form of music therapy that allows them to simultaneously see, hear, and feel harmonic, health-inducing vibrations. Being relaxed and stimulated at the same time can bolster one's health by helping to balance the autonomic nervous system.

VibraSound® consists of four main parts:

1. Vibrotactile mattress that sends music as vibration to the body.
2. Visual display that sends music as light pulsations to the eyes.
3. Immersion headphones that send music as sounds to the ears.
4. Sensorium™ LSV, an interface that synchronizes the sound, light and vibration with the music.

VibraSound is a state of the art neurotechnology that blends almost every aspect of Sensory Resonance. It synchronizes light, sound, color, intent, aroma, breath, and intense vibration with music so beautiful that it can send chills of pleasure up your spine. The internal massage performed by the music leaves your body feeling relaxed, refreshed, and invigorated at the same time. By synchronizing all of the body's main sensory input channels, it transforms the mind into a state that can result in a Peak Experience. Beyond the benefits already discussed, this Regenerative Innertainment can assist in stress management, creativity, emotional release, self-discovery, and spiritual evolution.

To learn more about the VibraSound and Don's work, visit www.vibrasound.com.

Nutrigenomics

Nutrigenomics is another exciting new field that explores how the interaction between one's diet and nutritional status and one's genetics affects health. More importantly, it helps physicians to more effectively and accurately create a personalized dietary and nutritional plan to improve and maintain optimal health for their patients.

As you learned early on in this book, each of us has a unique *biochemical individuality*, as well as a specific metabolic type and key hormonal gland. Recognizing and working with each of these factors is a hallmark of the holistic, individualized, patient-centered approach I take as a physician. With the help of nutrigenomics testing, I can take this approach to the next level, significantly improving my patients' outcomes and further ensuring the likelihood that the ageless vitality they achieve by working with me will be theirs for many more decades to come.

Nutrigenomics testing works in much the same way as gene diagnostics does, with testing usually conducted using a saliva or inner cheek swab sample. From such samples, physicians can learn the specific nutrients their patients need, as well as what dosage levels they need, which foods are optimal for their health, and which foods they should avoid, as well as a variety of other important health information, such as how patients metabolize alcohol, caffeine, carbohydrates, proteins, and fats; how they metabolize nutrients, including vitamin D; how their bodies regulate insulin; their bodies' detoxification status; and their risk factors for various disease conditions, including heart disease, diabetes, and osteoporosis. Nutrigenomics testing can even determine which types of exercise (aerobic or anaerobic) are most optimal for each patient, and improve their ability to lose weight and keep it off, usually simply from adopting a dietary and nutritional program that "is right for their DNA," thus eliminating the need for dieting, which is rarely effective long-term. Thanks to nutrigenomics testing, physicians such as myself are now better able than ever before to determine our patients' unique nutritional and metabolic needs, and to create the most effective overall health program tailored to those needs.

Although there are a number of companies that allow you to order home-testing nutrigenomic kits, I recommend that you not do so. Instead, work with a physician who is knowledgeable about such tests, and who can then work with you to tailor the most appropriate treatment program based upon your test results.

PEMF

PEMF stands for Pulsed ElectroMagnetic Field therapy. In recent years, a number of scientists and inventors, recognizing the importance of the earth's natural pulsed magnetic field, as well as the frequencies of what is known as the Schumann Resonance of the earth's ionosphere, to human health, and the fact that, since the early 20th century, the earth's magnetic field has started weakening, have developed a number of PEMF devices to introduce these frequencies to the body. As the frequencies are introduced, the body's flow of energy is stimulated and balanced, bringing the body into a more harmonious, energized state.

There are a variety of PEMF devices today, all of which utilize the principles of Energy Medicine. PEMF therapy is approved by the FDA for certain applications, including for stimulating bone growth, heal bone fractures, and as a complementary therapy to cervical fusion therapy. According to William Pawluk, MD, MSc, one of the world's leading experts on PEMF devices and PEMF therapy, other health benefits of PEMF therapy include increased circulation, improved immune function, enhanced energy levels, enhanced muscle function and relief of muscle tension, enhanced oxygenation of blood and cells, reduced inflammation, improved nerve and liver function, improved detoxification, improved sleep, improved assimilation of nutrients, and overall stress relief.

In my practice, I use the Ondamed, a battery-powered biofeedback device that enables me with the help of the Autonomic Nervous System to determine which frequencies of pulsed electromagnetic fields will cause the best therapeutic response, and more importantly, where the dysfunctional areas are located on the body, which are potentially responsible for the patient's symptoms.

Invented over 20 years ago by the German engineer, Rolf Binder, the Ondamed continues to offer the most advanced biomedical technology using a personalized approach to fine tune the therapy that is needed for the patient. This unique PEMF therapy has been further developed by The Binder Institute for Personalized Medicine in Germany, by founders Rolf Binder and his wife, Sylvia Binder, ND, PhD.

Ondamed stimulation induces subtle current impulses in the body's fluids, organs, tissue, cells, and connective tissue, (also known as "the matrix," which practitioners of energy medicine consider to be the body's largest organ in the body, connecting all cells, tissues, and organs). Temporary stimulation with Ondamed-focused frequencies promotes relaxation, muscle re-education, and increased flow of electrons, that returns the body to its former state of wellness.

Although there are a number of PEMF devices designed for home use, when first exploring PEMF I recommend you first work with a physician or other health care expert trained in its use. To learn more about PEMF and the types of devices available, visit Dr. Pawluk's website, www.drpawluk.com. For more information about Ondamed, go to www.ondamed.net.

Stem Cell Therapy

Stem cell therapy has the potential to revolutionize nearly all aspects of medicine. Even though the practical applications of stem cell therapy are currently limited in scope, if the theoretical applications bear fruit we may soon see stems cells used to treat everything from heart disease and cancer to spinal cord injuries, Parkinson's disease, and Alzheimer's, to even baldness and blindness.

Stem cells are considered the "mother cells" of all other cells in the body because they are undifferentiated cells that can differentiate, or turn, into specialized cells, and also divide (through a process known as *mitosis*) to produce additional stem cells. There are two primary types of stem cells in humans and other mammals: embryonic stem cells and adult stem cells. In the developing fetus, embryonic stem cells differentiate into specialized cells that form and regenerate all of the organs and tissues of the body. Adult stem cells are found in bone marrow and fat, as well as other tissues and organs of the body. These cells have a natural ability to repair damaged tissue, although their ability to do so declines as we age.

The best known and most widely used form of stem cell therapy to date is the bone marrow transplant, which has been used for more than 30 years as a treatment for certain types of cancers, especially leukemia and lymphomas. In this procedure, a donor's healthy bone marrow re-introduces stem cells to replace the cells lost in the recipient's body as a result of chemotherapy treatment, which kills both cancer and healthy cells indiscriminately. The transplanted stem cells also trigger an immune response that helps to kill off cancer cells. Also, a patient's bone marrow can be removed prior to cancer chemotherapy, and then is re-introduced into the body after chemotherapy is completed.

In 2012, a proprietary stem cell drug known as Prochymal[R] was granted limited approval by the Canadian government for the management of acute graft-versus-host disease in children who fail to respond to steroid treatments. Stem cell therapy is also gaining interest within the field of orthopedic and sports medicine (along with PRP or platelet rich plasma), where it is showing promise as a treatment for injuries or defects affecting bone, cartilage, ligaments, and tendons in animals.

Aside from the above uses for stem cell therapy, all other stem cell approaches are experimental and in the early stages of research and development. Much of this research is focused on *autologous* stem cell therapy, meaning treatment involving stem cells harvested from a person's own body. There are three sources of autologous adult stem cells in humans: bone marrow, extracting stem cells from pelvic bone; adipose tissue (fat cells), which involves harvesting of stem cells via liposuction; and blood, which involves drawing blood and then harvesting stem cells through a process called *apheresis*. During apheresis the drawn blood passes through a machine that extracts stem cells and returns the rest of the blood back to the donor's body. Stem cells can also be harvested from umbilical cord blood following birth, and then banked for future use.

Until recently, embryonic stem cells were considered to have the most promising wide-scale applications because of their ability to differentiate into specific organ and tissue cells. Because embryonic stem cells are typically harvested from aborted fetuses, however, research into their use remains controversial, and opposed by certain religious groups, including the Catholic Church.

Fortunately, recent advances in adult stem cell research may make the controversy moot. Today, researchers are discovering new methods to cause adult stem cells to differentiate into various cell types, potentially opening the door for their use as a method to regenerate a wide range of organs in the body, as well as for treating and reversing a broad range of diseases. Given the ongoing developments in the field of stem cell therapy, it is highly likely that it will soon move out of the realm of theoretical application to play an important and practical role as a primary treatment modality for many of today's most difficult to treat diseases.

Telomeres

Another recent and exciting development in the field of longevity medicine is the research into telomeres and telomerase, the enzyme that activates and controls them. Telomeres are specialized cap-like structures at the end of chromosomes. They resemble the plastic tips at the end of shoelaces.

Telomeres protect chromosomes from degradation, and from becoming fused together. They also preserve the integrity of chromosomes, as well as genes, by ensuring the complete replication of the ends of chromosomal DNA each time that the cells divide. In addition, telomeres facilitate the correct positioning of chromosomes within the nucleus of cells during the process of replication.

Each time DNA replicates, however, telomere loss and shortening naturally occurs because the ends of the telomeres themselves are not replicated. As this occurs, their tips can also become frayed and the telomeres shorten, to the point where they can no longer protect the gene-carrying portion of the chromosomes. This results in chromosomal instability and loss of cell viability, which, in turn, leads to accelerated aging, altered or loss of normal gene functions, and impaired immunity, and can contribute to various chronic, degenerative diseases, including cancer.

Most cells in your body can only divide between 30 and 50 times before the telomeres they contain become too short and are no longer able to function properly. When they get too short, cells can no longer make fresh, healthy copies of themselves. This is precisely what happens as we grow older, as the tissues and organ systems that depend on continued healthy cell replication begin to falter. The average number of telomeres that are lost each year varies, depending upon both genetic and environmental factors. Telomere loss can also be hastened by a sedentary lifestyle, oxidative stress caused by free radicals, and insulin resistance.

Telomerase regulates telomere activity and ensures that it is carried out properly. Research dating as far back as the 1980s has demonstrated the importance of telomerase for maintaining telomere integrity, and therefore the prevention of premature aging and disease. Beginning in the 1990s, a team of researchers led by William Andrews, PhD, showed that when telomerase was added to normal cells, they could continue dividing healthfully well past their normal limit of healthy cell division. Based on his research findings, Dr. Andrews equates the known underlying causes of aging to sticks of dynamite, with shortened telomeres having the shortest fuse. "I believe there's a really good chance that if we defuse that stick," he stated in an article about him published in *Popular Science* in 2011, "and the person doesn't smoke and doesn't get obese, it wouldn't be surprising if they lived to be 150 years old."

The key to such longevity, Dr. Andrews and other scientists believe, lies in activating telomerase so that it can in turn slow, and possibly reverse, the natural shortening process of telomeres as cells replicate. Thus far, researchers has found that the herb astragalus, long used by practitioners of traditional Chinese medicine as an adaptogenic remedy (adaptogenic herbs increase resistance and resilience to stress and also support adrenal function), contains a telomerase-activating compound. Based on this finding, a company called T.A. Sciences (TA stands for telomerase-activation) introduced TA-65[R] in 2007 as the world's first specific formula for telomerase-activating in the marketplace. (TA-65 contains the compound found in astragalus.) According to Garry Gordon, MD,DO, the herb Pueraria Mirifica, which is indigenous to Thailand, may also activate telomerase. No doubt we will soon see other such products in the near future.

For now, however, the most practical value to come out of telomere research involves telomere testing so that patients and their doctors can have a better idea of their overall telomere status. One such company that offers telomere testing is Life Length in Madrid, Spain. The test consists of an analysis of blood and tissue samples to measure the percentage of short telomeres in individuals. For more information, visit www.lifelength.com. Given the role that telomeres play in our health, I foresee a day soon when telomere testing will be an essential component of regular patient testing.

UVLrx Station®

We have all read about the negative effects that toxins have upon the body, producing harmful free radicals, that need to be neutralized by antioxidants. But there is a different type of therapy available, called oxidative therapy, which has been shown to be effective in killing bacteria, viruses, and fungus. Examples of oxidative therapy include intravenous ozone, intravenous hydrogen peroxide, and ultraviolet blood irradiation (UBI). These therapies are much more popular in countries like Germany, Russia, and Cuba than they are in the United States. They have been studied in major medical research centers throughout the world, including Baylor University, Yale University, UCLA, and Harvard, as well as medical schools and laboratories in Great Britain, Germany, Italy, Russia, Canada, Japan, and Cuba.

During the 1960's, researchers at Baylor University discovered that IV hydrogen peroxide had an energizing effect on heart muscle, and that it could remove arterial plaque efficiently. These studies were largely ignored by the medical establishment. Currently, the legal status of these oxidative therapies is unclear in this country. If a practitioner wishes to use these therapies, he must be part of a research study that is registered with the FDA, and is called an Institutional Review Board (IRB).

Ultraviolet Blood Irradiation (UBI) has been used in this country since the early 1900's, but became less popular after the advent of antibiotics. The book *Into The Light* by William Campbell Douglas, MD, describes the early use of UV blood treatments. UV irradiation is used to sterilize surgical instruments and surgical operating rooms. A company called Therakos has developed an effective machine that utilizes UV light therapy in the treatment of certain blood cancers.

A new and innovative technology, the UVLrx Station®, offers a significant improvement on ultraviolet blood irradiation (UBI). Traditional UBI has been shown to be an effective therapeutic solution for the treatment of numerous medical conditions. Until now, UBI has been administered via an extracorporeal technique, which involves the extraction, irradiation, and return of approximately five percent of a patient's total blood volume. The blood, once drawn, is then irradiated with a single wavelength within the ultraviolet light spectrum, and then returned to the patient's body. The absorbed light energy oxygenates the blood, which, as it flows back into the body, then carries oxygen and healing light energies to the body's cells and tissues. The therapeutic benefits of this approach have been well documented, and include the elimination of harmful microorganisms (bacteria, fungal, and viral infections), cellular detoxification, improved immune function, and enhanced overall biochemical balance. Conditions that have benefited from UBI include arthritis, asthma, infections, chronic hepatitis, and HIV.

The UVLrx Station® significantly improves upon traditional UBI methods in a number of ways. First, it eliminates the need for blood to be drawn before it can be irradiated with ultraviolet light. Instead, it makes use of a ground-breaking intravenous delivery system that delivers UV light directly into the patient's vein, without the need for tubes, pumps, or cuvettes (small glass tubes)filled with circulating blood. To receive treatment, patients sit comfortably in a chair while an IV is started. A thin fiber optic cable is attached to a small, plastic hub, called a Dry Light Adapter® (DLA) that integrates an IV saline drip with a fiber optic delivery mechanism. From a single catheter, the patient receives the light therapy together with a normal saline infusion. The patient can rest, read, watch TV, or simply relax during the 60-minute treatment cycle. When the cycle is complete, the catheter and DLA are removed and disposed of and a small bandage is placed on the site. The patient experiences no more discomfort than from a vitamin infusion or donating a pint of blood.

An additional advantage of the UVLrx Station® is that there is no need for patients to first receive blood thinning medications before their treatments begin, which is often used with traditional UBI treatments. This greatly reduces the risk of complications. Moreover, patients avoid having to watch their blood be physically extracted from their body. Many people have an innate fear when it comes to needles and seeing their own blood, and traditional UBI methods subject a patient to both of these experiences.

The biggest advantages of the UVLrx Station®, however, go far beyond the ease and convenience it provides compared to other UBI methods. During treatment,100 percent of a patients' total blood volume receives light therapy, in contrast to the 5 percent total blood volume that is treated using traditional UBI. Additionally, the UVLrx Station® delivers three specific wavelengths of light tailored to achieve a desired clinical effect. Use of these different wavelengths improves and expands the therapeutic potential of the UVLrx Station®. Each wavelength targets natural photoreceptors in targeted cells. When stimulated with light, the photoreceptors activate key biochemical pathways, generating the therapeutic effect. The multi-wavelength (multi-light) protocol is designed to help maximize the desired clinical effects, and each of the three wavelengths has been chosen for both their safety and therapeutic benefit.

All UBI systems use the same mechanism of action, namely deactivation of pathogens. What this really means is that the UV light breaks up strands of DNA in the pathogen's cells. This causes the cells to deform and deflate and, more importantly, prohibits the pathogen from reproducing. Once a pathogen is deactivated in the body, the body will then filter it through the liver, lymph, and kidney drainage systems, and then excrete it into the stool or urine.

The UVLrx Treatment System with its multi-wavelength protocol possesses the capability to stimulate another natural process in the bloodstream called *phagocytosis*. This process occurs when white blood cells are activated and target pathogens, and then consume and digest the pathogens. This mechanism helps to clear the body's viral load. Having this mechanism integrated into the UVLrx Treatment System allows patients to be treated two to three times a week, enabling the physician to treat conditions more aggressively when the conditions justify it.

Finally, the UVLrx Treatment System administers UVA light, as opposed to other UV systems that use UVC light. Research has shown that UVA light is effective at low doses and is safe to administer over extended periods of time, if necessary. UVA light has also been shown to increase cellular ATP production.

Overall, the UVLrx Treatment System represents a breakthrough therapeutic approach that not only improves upon the benefits already established by traditional UBI approaches, but which will likely also expand access to treatment so that many more people can gain those benefits.

In the future, the UVLrx Treatment System may help optimize organ transplants, especially bone marrow and stem cell transplants, because it may help reduce the risk of graft versus host disease (GVHD) that often follows such procedures. Indications are that the UVLrx Treatment System may also help optimize stem cell therapy in the future, as well as possibly potentiating standard pharmaceutical drug treatments through its ability to photo-activate and more effectively catalyze the delivery mechanism of such drugs once they enter the bloodstream. In short, the UVLrx Treatment System represents a substantial new treatment approach for doctors to use, and patients to benefit from, and I am very excited about the solutions it may soon provide to our nation's health-care crisis. Physicians wishing to participate in this technology would need to join an IRB and register with the FDA.

Key Point to Remember

The key point to remember from this chapter is that medicine and medical science are not static. Just like you and your body, it continues to grow and adapt. New discoveries, innovations, and improvements to our understanding and the practice of medicine occur far more frequently than most people realize, even if it can sometimes take decades or more before such discoveries, and the therapies and techniques they can result in, become widely accepted.

That is why, many years ago, I chose to explore and investigate so-called "alternative" therapies and treatments that could potentially be of benefit to me, my family and friends, and my patients. Had I not chosen to do so, it is very likely that I would only be offering the drugs and surgery approach to medicine that I was trained in during the years of my formal medical education. Thankfully, that is not the case, because if it were I know I would not have been able to have achieved the consistently high success rates for the wide range of conditions my patients present with.

In sharing the above techniques with you, I want to both inform you of their existence and benefits, and to open your eyes to new possibilities that can positively impact your own health needs. Expanding your horizons of knowledge and understanding in this way has been a primary goal of mine throughout this book. Despite all of the burdens and obstacles we as a nation face when it comes to health care, I remain confident that the future is very bright, and that we will continue to see the introduction of new, highly effective and innovative approaches for not only preventing and reversing illness, but also for significantly expanding the human lifespan while simultaneously increasing our ability to achieve and maintain outstanding health. I hope that you share my sense of optimism, and that you will seek out at least some of the therapies you learned about in this chapter.

May you stay forever young.

Dancing Your Way to 120 and Beyond

"Time is the only coin of your life.
It is the only coin you have,
And only you can determine how it will be spent.
Be careful lest you let other people spend it for you."

~ Carl Sandburg

C ongratulations! By reading this book, you now know more about how to go about creating outstanding health than most doctors today. More importantly, you now have the information you need to begin putting what you've learned into action.

This new knowledge empowers you to take control of your health in ways that might once have seemed impossible to you. As you work with the **Six** Essential Keys that I've shared with you, and conscientiously apply the self-care tools I've outlined for each of them, I can promise you that you will soon begin to notice positive changes in the way you look and feel, and in your attitudes and beliefs about your life. In the process, you will come to a deeper understanding of yourself as first and foremost a "being of energy." This is not something you will simply come to believe; it is something you will increasingly begin to experience and prove for yourself.

The key to all of the above, of course, depends on whether or not you *take action*. I raise this point because, sadly, it is a fact that as many as 80 percent or more of all people who buy and read books about health never actually apply what they learn. This is similar to people who purchase gym membership. Industry data show that year after year only about 20 percent of those who do so make regular use of their gym membership. The rest either quit within a few weeks or never set foot in the gym at all. If you expect to improve your health and overall well-being, and attain the ultimate goal of this book—dancing your way to 120 and beyond—you must get started now.

There is a saying I like that has relevance here: Time means nothing, but *timing means everything.* To me, the first part of the saying relates to age; it's just a number and really doesn't matter. In the course of my medical career I have met countless people who were old in their 20s, 30s, and 40s who are now vibrantly healthy and youthful decades later because the timing was right for them to discover what they didn't know, yet needed to do, to dramatically improve their health. Having found and read this book, the timing is now right for you to do the same, and start your own journey to new levels of wellness.

This is especially true and important given the abject failure of our current medical system to effectively meet our nation's massively growing health care problems, all of which are being made even worse each day by the amount of stress, environmental toxins, and other health and hormone disruptors all of us are exposed to. Simply put: *In order to not only survive, but also thrive, in today's stress-filled, toxic world, you have to be willing to take charge of your health and the health of your loved ones, becoming your own personal health expert and seeking out physicians like me whose practice of medicine rests upon a whole person, energy-based foundation.* I wrote this book so that you could best be able to do so.

As you learned, the path to outstanding health starting now rests on addressing all of the following:

Cleansing and fortifying your mind, including your attitudes, beliefs, and habitual life patterns.

Cleansing your body using the drainage and detoxification techniques you learned about in Chapter 6.

Following a health-supporting, alkalizing, energizing diet.

Creating a naturally energizing lifestyle.

Using Energy Medicine to evaluate your current health status and to detect and address energetic imbalances as soon as possible in order to prevent them from progressing to full-blown disease.

And keeping your endocrine glands and the hormones they produce in a state of optimal balance.

Initially, working with all of these six essential keys may seem overwhelming, and also unfamiliar to you. If so, that's okay. Just as it is important to start slow when you are beginning an exercise program, so too is it vital for you to not overdo things as you begin to apply all that you've learned in this book. Go slow at first, and then continue to add other elements to your wellness lifestyle as you progress. Initially, I recommend that you focus on the first essential key to program your mind for success. Doing so will go a long way towards ensuring your success with the other essential keys, as well as in all other areas of your life.

While you begin to create your successful mindset, I also encourage you to adopt the dietary guidelines I've shared with you, along with an appropriate exercise program and regular breathing exercises. Then add in some of the drainage measures I taught you for a few more weeks. After that, if necessary, progress onto the detoxification steps (ideally, by this time, working with an integrative, energy medicine physician experienced in detoxification therapies). You can also make use of the specific homeopathic and herbal formulas I've developed to assist the organs of detoxification. (See the Resources section for more information.) Finally, make use of Energy Medicine and any appropriate hormone therapies to further maximize the healthy benefits of my Outstanding Health program.

No doubt some of the information I've shared with you in this book is new to you. Perhaps you are even skeptical about it. If so, I encourage you to set aside your skepticism until you have tried out my recommendations for at least one month. For most people, that is ample time for them to prove to themselves that my recommendations work.

In addition, let me stress that *everything I have shared with you in this book in no way is intended to mean that I am opposed to conventional medicine, or that you should stop seeing your conventional doctor or using pharmaceutical drugs if they have been prescribed for you.* Not at all! My intention is to *add* to the benefits you may already be receiving from conventional medicine, and to provide you with other options you can use in conjunction with it. This is the approach a number of my patients take with me, seeing me because of what I can offer them (what you learned in this book), while continuing to see their conventional MDs, as well. This best-of-both-worlds approach works well for them. And, over time, as they continue with my treatments, they often find that their need for drugs is reduced, and even eliminated.

I also want to point out that, even after you start to experience success by following what I've taught you, at times you may still find yourself backsliding. If so, know that this is normal, too. No journey of value ever follows a straight, even line. There are always twists and turns, and ups and downs. As they occur in your life, recognize them for what they are, and don't let them discourage you. Change, even when it is for the better, is rarely easy, yet the more that you commit yourself to continue on your path to renewed and lasting health, the easier and more satisfying your journey will become.

It is said that most people who fail or give up on their dreams do so when they are only inches away from attaining them. So, when it comes to your health, never give up.

With that in mind, I want to share this story from my own life. As I mentioned previously in this book, my medical career began in Los Angeles as a Board Certified Emergency Room Physician. During that time I participated in many "Code Blues" (cardiac arrests). By the time the patient got to the ER, it was often too late. We continued CPR, but after 20 minutes, we ended the resuscitation.

Then in 1991, at a self-improvement seminar led my friend and personal transformation expert Tony Robbins on the Big Island of Hawaii, my beliefs about life and death were radically changed. I had just climbed to the top of a 50 foot pole (the ropes course), leaped to catch the trapeze, and missed. I was extremely dismayed as I was slowly being brought down. I began to walk away from my group of 60 people. As I did so I noticed that one of the people in my group was crying because he had also missed the trapeze. Realizing by the law of contrast that my emotional state was far better than his, I rejoined my group and began cheering for my fellow teammates.

One of my teammates, Howard, had just missed the trapeze, and as he was lowered to the ground, he was smiling to all. But as his feet gently landed on the ground, 15 feet directly in front of me, he went into cardiac arrest. I immediately began CPR, and had two teammates massage the inner aspect of his little fingers (the heart meridian in acupuncture), while calling for the paramedics.

It took 30 minutes for the paramedics to arrive. Once they did, we started the IV, put a tube in Howard's trachea, gave him all of the appropriate cardiac drugs, and defibrillated him with the paddles, all to no avail. He had flat-lined.

I continued to work on Howard as he was transferred to the ambulance. As I moved to board the ambulance, the paramedics thanked me for my help, and informed me that my services were no longer needed (it was now their turf). I looked them straight in the eye and said "No way, I'm not leaving now." We took a 30 minute ride to the hospital (it turned out to be an urgent care center), during which time the defibrillator stopped working. By this time I had been administering CPR on Howard for an hour, and I was exhausted. Howard was purple and gray, and it didn't look good.

We were five minutes from the hospital, when the paramedic smacked the defibrillator, like you would do to an old TV set to get it to work, and suddenly a heart rhythm magically appeared on the monitor.

Five minutes later, as we pulled up to the hospital, Howard had a blood pressure of 100, and five minutes later, he woke up. He went on to make a complete recovery, after being without a heart beat for one hour. For the next seven years I received the most beautiful cards from Howard, thanking me for saving his life.

I was taught in medical school that the brain can only survive for five minutes without oxygen before irreversible changes and damage occur, but Howard's body and spirit didn't agree with that theory. The lesson I learned from this experience is "Never say Never," and don't fall into the trap of using old beliefs to guide your present actions and behaviors.

It is old and outdated beliefs and behaviors that are guiding our current, mainstream medical paradigm. This is why it is such a failure when it comes to managing our nation's ever-mounting health crisis, and why it is also resisting Energy Medicine and many of the other solutions I have shared with you, all of which my patients' long-term health successes prove *do* work. Even so, I know that Energy Medicine will definitely succeed and become mainstream in the years ahead, despite the possible continued hostile attitude of some in the medical profession.

I wrote this book so that you don't have to wait for such a paradigm shift to occur. I want you to benefit from the "medicine of the future" right now. It is my sincere desire that the ideas, information and tools contained in this book will help you to create the same level of health that my patients and I enjoy, and which I know is truly possible for all of us.

May you spend the "coin of your life"—your time—doing what most fulfills you. And may your life journey be long and vibrantly healthy!

Resources and Recommended Reading

Dr. Michael Galitzer

Dr. Galitzer regularly consults with patients in person at his offices in Los Angeles, California. He also offers Skype consultations with patients across the United States and all around the world. If you would like to schedule a consultation with Dr. Galitzer or learn more about the services he offers, visit:

www.DrGalitzer.com
12381 Wilshire Boulevard, Suite #102
Los Angeles, CA 90025
Phone: (310) 820-6042

Other Websites for Dr. Galitzer

www.outstandinghealthbook.com
*The official website for the book, **Outstanding Health**, along with its companion free, online newsletter **The Outstanding Health Bulletin**. (Visit the website to sign up to receive it.)*

www.ahealth.com
*The official website for **The American Health Institute**, founded by Dr. Galitzer's wife, Dr. Janet Hranicky, who is also its president. (Dr. Galitzer serves as the Institute's medical director.)*

Organizations

The following physician-based organizations can help you locate doctors in your area who offer many of the services employed by Dr. Galitzer that are mentioned in this book.

American Academy of Anti-Aging Medicine (A4M)
1801 N. Military Trail
Suite 200
Boca Raton, FL 33431
(888) 997-0112
www.A4M.com

American College for Advancement in Medicine (ACAM)
380 Ice Center Lane, Suite C
Bozeman, MT 59718
(800) 532-3688
www.acam.org
info@acam.org

American Board of Integrative Holistic Medicine (ABIHM)
5313 Colorado St.
Duluth, MN 55804
(218) 525-5651
www.abihm.org
www.holisticboard.org
admin@abihm.org

American Holistic Medical Association (AHMA)
27629 Chagrin Blvd.
Suite 206
Woodmere, Ohio 44122
(216) 292-6644
www.holisticmedicine.org
info@holisticmedicine.org

Acupuncture

American Academy of Medical Acupuncture (AAMA)
1970 E. Grand Avenue
Suite 330
El Segundo, CA 90245
(310) 364-0193
www.medicalacupuncture.org

Applied Kinesiology

International College of Applied Kinesiology (ICAK)
ICAK-USA Central Office
6405 Metcalf Ave., Suite 503
Shawnee Mission, KS 66202
(913) 384-5336
www.icakusa.com
www.icak.com (outside of the USA)

Biological/Holistic Dentists

Biological dentists are trained in the proper removal and replacement of dental amalgams containing mercury. The following organizations can help you locate biological dentist near you.

International Academy of Biological Dentistry and Medicine (IABDM)
19122 Camellia Bend Circle
Spring, Texas 77379
(281) 651-1745
www.iabdm.org

International Academy of Oral Medicine and Toxicology (IAOMT)
8297 ChampionsGate Blvd, #193
ChampionsGate, FL 33896

(863) 420-6373
www.iaomt.org
info@iaomt.org

Holistic Dental Association
1825 Ponce de Leon Blvd. #148
Coral Gables, FL 33134
(305) 356-7338
www.holisticdental.org

Mercury Free Dentists
439 East Thompson
PO Box 154
Amity, AR 71921
(252) 288-1541
www.mercuryfreedentists.com

Energy Medicine

Occidental Institute Research Foundation (OIRF)
2002 West Bench Drive
Penticton, British Columbia V2A 8Z3
Canada
(800) 663-8342
www.oirf.com
support@oirf.com

International Society for the Study of Subtle Energies and Energy Medicine (ISSSEEM)
P.O. Box 297
Bolivar, Missouri 65613 USA
(888) 272-6109
www.issseem.org
www.issseemblog.org/
info@issseem.org

Energy Psychology

Emotional Freedom Technique (EFT)

> www.emofree.com (Official website of Gary Craig, founder of EFT)

Eye Movement Desensitization and Reprogramming (EMDR)

> www.emdr.com (Official website of EMDR Institute, Inc.)

Tapas Acupressure Technique (TAT)

> www.tatlife.com

Thought Field Therapy (TFT, also known as Callahan Techniques)

> www.tftpractitioners.net

Environmental Medicine

American Academy of Environmental Medicine (AAEM)

> 6505 E. Central Avenue, #296
> Wichita, KS 67206
> (316) 684-5500
> www.aaemonline.org
> administrator@aaemonline.org

Academy of Comprehensive Integrative Medicine (ACIM)

> www.acimconnect.com
> info@acimconnect.com

Homeopathy

The American Institute of Homeopathy

> 10418 Whitehead St.
> Fairfax, VA 22030
> (888) 445-9988
> www.homeopathyusa.org
> admin@homeopathyusa.org

National Center for Homeopathy
7918 Jones Branch Drive, Suite 300
McLean VA, 22102
(703) 506-7667
www.homeopathycenter.org

North American Society of Homeopaths (NASH)
PO Box 115
Troy, ME 04987
(206) 720-7000
www.homeopathy.org
www.americanhomeopath.com
nashinfo@homeopathy.org

Lab Testing

Cyrex Laboratories
www.cyrexlabs.com
www.cyrexlabs.com/CyrexTestsArrays/tabid/136/Default.aspx

Diagnos-Techs
19110 66th Ave S, Bldg G
Kent, WA 98032
(800) 878-3787
www.diagnostechs.com
diagnos@diagnostechs.com

Forever Health (Suzanne Somers)
(800) 333-2650
www.foreverhealth.com/blood-tests
customerservice@foreverhealth.com

Life Extension Foundation for Longer Life (LEF)
P.O. Box 407198
Fort Lauderdale, FL 33340

(800) 226-2370

www.lef.org

www.lef.org/Vitamins-Supplements/Blood-Tests/Blood-Tests

customerservice@lef.org

Sabre Sciences

2233 Faraday Avenue

Suite K

Carlsbad, CA 92008

(760) 448-2750

(888) 490-7300

www.sabresciences.com

info@sabresciences.com

ZRT Labs

8605 SW Creekside Place

Beaverton, OR 97008

(866) 600-1636

www.zrtlab.com

info@zrtlab.com

Nutritional Supplements

Apex Energetics

16592 Hale Ave.

Irvine, CA 92606

(800) 736-4381

(949) 251-0152

www.ApexEnergetics.com

info@ApexEnergetics.com

Forever Health (Suzanne Somers)

(800) 333-2650

www.foreverhealth.com/products

customerservice@foreverhealth.com

Life Extension Foundation for Longer Life (LEF)
> P.O. Box 407198
> Fort Lauderdale, FL 33340
> (800) 226-2370
> www.lef.org
> www.lef.org/Vitamins-Supplements
> customerservice@lef.org

Personalized Stress Management Consultations

Dr. Janet Hranicky
> www.DrHranicky.com

Metabolic Typing

Healthexcel
> www.healthexcel.com
> info@healthexcel.com

Future of Medicine Therapies and Devices

Cold Laser Therapy TerraQuant
Apex Energetics
> 16592 Hale Ave.
> Irvine, CA 92606
> (800) 736-4381
> (949) 251-0152
> www.ApexEnergetics.com
> info@ApexEnergetics.com

CVAC™Process
CVAC Systems, Inc.
> 43397 Business Park Dr.
> Suite D2

Temecula, CA 92590-3686

(866) 753-2822

www.cvacsystems.com

EECP
Sara Soulati

11860 Wilshire Blvd

Los Angeles, CA 90025

(310) 473-3030

633 Aerick Street

Inglewood, CA 90301

(310) 412-8181

www.globalcardiocare.com

EECP Therapy

www.eecp-therapy.com/find-an-eecp-treatment-facility

Heart Rate Variability (HRV)
Intellewave, Inc.

238 Rockaway Ave, 2nd Floor

Valley Stream, NY 11580

(516) 341-0307, (917) 586-8498

www.intellewave.net

www.nervexpress.com

info@intellewave.net

Intravenous Vitamin Therapy
American College for Advancement in Medicine (ACAM)

380 Ice Center Lane, Suite C

Bozeman, MT 59718

(800) 532-3688

www.acam.org

info@acam.org

Ondamed
Ondamed Inc.
>   2570 Route 9W
>   Cornwall, NY 12518
>   (845) 534-0456, ext. 115
>   www.ondamed.net
>   support@ondamed.net
>
>   Ondamed GmbH
>   Kürzeller Strasse 18
>   77963 Schwanau
>   +49-7824-6466-0
>   www.ondamed.de
>   kontakt@ondamed.de

PEMF Devices
Dr. William Pawluk
>   (866) 455-7688
>   www.drpawluk.com
>   info@drpawluk.com

Telomere Testing
Life Length
>   c/ Miguel Angel 11, 2nd floor
>   Madrid, Spain 28010
>   +(34) 91 737 1298
>   www.lifelength.com
>   info@lifelength.com

UVLrx Therapeutics
>   www.UVLrx.com
>   (844) 885-7979
>   info@UVLrx.com

Vibrasound/Don Estes
InnerSense, Inc.

2118 Wilshire Blvd
Suite 730
Santa Monica, California 90403
(310) 261-1128
www.vibrasound.com
www.harmonicresolution.com
info@vibrasound.com

Skin Care

Aesthetics Montecito (Jeannette Baer, PA-C)

Four Seasons, The Biltmore
1260 Channel Drive
Montecito, CA 93108
(805) 565-8480
www.aestheticsmontecito.com

Melanie Simon

1805 E. Cabrillo Boulevard
Suite B
Santa Barbara CA 93108
(805) 403-6056

Cornelia Spa at The Surrey
20 East 76th Street
New York, NY 10021
(646) 385-3600
For appointments in Jackson Hole, WY, call (805) 708-8656
(Both spa and home treatments available.)
www.MelanieSimon.com
melanie@circcell.com

Suzanne Organics (Suzanne Somers)
(800) 333-2650

> www.foreverhealth.com/suzanne-organics
> customerservice@foreverhealth.com

CircCell

> (855) 372-2355
> www.circcell.com
> info@circcell.com

Other Websites of Interest

Don Estes
Founding Director and President
Psiometric Science, LLC.
Psiometric Science, Inc.
InnerSense, Inc.

> www.psimetricscience.com
> www.theportacle.com
> www.psi-fi-sound.com

Datis Kharrazian, DHSc, DC, MS, MNeuroSci

> http://drknews.com
> http://brainhealthbook.com
> http://thyroidbook.com

Tony Robbins

> www.tonyrobbins.com
> www.tonyrobbinstraining.com
> www.business.tonyrobbins.com

Suzanne Somers

> www.suzannesomers.com

JJ Virgin

> www.jjvirgin.com

Recommended Reading

By Larry Trivieri Jr

Alternative Medicine: The Definitive Guide (editor and principal author, with Burton Goldberg), Celestial Arts, 2002. (Dr. Michael Galitzer and his wife Dr. Janet Hranicky were contributors to the 2nd edition of this book.)

Juice Alive: The Ultimate Guide to Juicing Remedies (with Steven Bailey, ND), Square One Publishers, 2010

The Acid-Alkaline Food Guide (with Susan E. Brown, PhD, CNN), Square One Publishers, 2013

The Acid-Alkaline Lifestyle, Square One Publishers, 2015

The American Holistic Medical Association Guide to Holistic Health, John Wiley & Sons, 2001

Health On The Edge: Visionary Views of Healing in the New Millennium, Tarcher/Penguin, 2003

By Suzanne Somers (featuring Dr. Michael Galitzer)

I'm Too Young for This!: The Natural Hormone Solution to Enjoy Perimenopause, Harmony (2014)

Bombshell: Explosive Medical Secrets that Will Redefine Aging, Harmony (2012)

Sexy Forever: How to Fight Fat After Forty, Harmony (2010)

Knockout: Interviews with Doctors Who are Curing Cancer—and How to Prevent Getting It in the First Place, Harmony (2009)

Breakthrough: Eight Steps to Wellness, Harmony (2008)

Ageless: The Naked Truth About Bioidentical Hormones, Harmony (2007)

The Sexy Years: Discover the Hormone Connection: The Secret to Fabulous Sex, Great Health, and Vitality, for Women and Men, Harmony (2004)

By Tony Robbins

MONEY: Master the Game: 7 Simple Steps to Financial Freedom, Simon and Schuster, 2014

Unlimited Power : The New Science Of Personal Achievement, Free Press, 1997

Awaken the Giant Within : How to Take Immediate Control of Your Mental, Emotional, Physical and Financial Destiny!, Free Press, 1992

By JJ Virgin

The Sugar Impact Diet, Grand Central Life and Style, 2014

The Virgin Diet, Harlequin, 2012

The Virgin Diet Cookbook, Grand Central Life and Style, 2014

By Dr. Datis Kharrazian

Why Isn't My Brain Working?, Elephant Press, 2013

Why Do I Still Have Thyroid Symptoms?, Elephant Press, 2010.

By William L. Wolcott

The Metabolic Typing Diet, Doubleday, 2000.

Acknowledgments

To love and be loved is a true gift. And to be blessed by my wife Janet and wonderful children, Hayley, Connor, Grant, and Justin, is more than I can ask for.

My deep gratitude goes to my parents, Hyman and Isabelle, and my sister Gail, who taught me love, and who were always there for me.

It began with Upstate Medical School, which provided me with a great medical education, and then to the ER, where I learned about the art of delivering medical care.

To my teachers in Energy Medicine, Roy Martina M.D. and Helmut Schimmel M.D. who patiently guided me through the door to a whole new world.

My deep respect for Armond Simonian, President of Apex Energetics, who had the courage to create a special type of health company.

To the doctors at ACAM and A4M who bravely teach so many health care practitioners about the New Medicine.

For Dr. Valerie Hunt, whose wisdom and guidance will always be cherished, and never forgotten.

My deep appreciation for Larry Trivieri, whose brilliance as a writing partner is unmatched, and whose friendship is everlasting.

For Vicki St. George who got the ball rolling on this project.

To Suzanne Somers, my friend, who has inspired and empowered so many women to reclaim their health.

I am grateful for having the opportunity to be of service to my patients. You have been some of my greatest teachers. This book is for you.

And to my dear friends, who have laughed with me and stood beside me over the years.

May you all stay forever young.

~ **Michael Galitzer**

I wish to acknowledge both Dr. Michael Galitzer and his wife, Dr. Janet Hranicky for their friendship, support, and the excellent work they are doing as leading experts in their respective fields of medicine and healing. I also want to thank Michael for inviting me to collaborate with him on this project. His integrity and helpfulness throughout the process of this book's creation has made it one of the most fulfilling projects I've ever worked on.

I also want to thank my dear friend and mentor, Burton Goldberg, for the many decades he has spent helping others as the "Voice of Alternative Medicine," for opening the door to my career, and for introducing me to Michael and Janet.

My deepest thanks also go out to the many other pioneering health physicians and health experts it has been my great good fortune to meet and learn from over the course of my career, especially Drs. C. Norman Shealy, Garry Gordon, Lee Cowden, Alan Gaby, Robert A. Anderson, Rob Ivker, and, most especially, the late, great Valerie Hunt, all of whom have influenced me for the better in ways they most likely don't even realize.

A tip of the hat, as well, to Rudy Shur, another very good friend.

As always, my deepest thanks to, and appreciation for, my Mom, brothers and sisters, nieces and nephews and their children, and all of my friends, without whom my life would be far less fun and love-filled.

Finally, and most especially, I wish to thank my father, Lawrence A. Trivieri, who passed away as this book was in production. Everything I am today I owe to him and the example he set me by the way he lived his life. This is for you, Dad. I love you...

~ **Larry Trivieri Jr**

About the Authors

Michael Galitzer, M.D.

Dr. Michael Galitzer is a nationally recognized expert in Energy Medicine, integrative medicine, and bioidentical hormone replacement therapy (BHRT). For more than 40 years Dr. Galitzer has been a leading figure and innovator in the field of longevity, or anti-aging medicine.

Dr. Galitzer graduated from SUNY Upstate Medical School, and in 1973 he moved to Los Angeles, where he practiced Emergency Medicine for 15 years. (He was among the first 100 doctors in the U.S. to become board certified in Emergency Medicine.) Eventually he began studying integrative medicine, including herbs, nutrition, Energy Medicine, and homeopathy, and in 1990 he completed a course in Medical Acupuncture, which he incorporated into the private practice he established in Santa Monica, California, in 1987.

Today, Dr. Galitzer utilizes revolutionary treatments drawn from both traditional and complementary medicine, including sound and light therapy, toxin elimination, and intravenous supplementation, to produce remarkable and rapid improvements in his patients' health and vitality. His patient list includes many top Hollywood, business, and sports figures, as well as people from all across North and South America, Europe, Asia, Africa, and Australia.

Dr. Galitzer has been a member of the American Association of Medical Acupuncture, the American Association of Acupuncture and Bio-Energetic Medicine, the International Oxidative Medical Association, and the American Academy of Anti-Aging Medicine. He was a Board Member of the American College for Advancement in Medicine, a leading organization of physicians in the area of Alternative and Complementary Medicine. He has given lectures all over the world on longevity, alternative, and bioenergetic medicine.

For the past decade, Dr. Galitzer has been a featured contributor to nine bestselling books by actress, author, and health advocate Suzanne Somers, including *I'm Too Young for This!: The Natural Hormone Solution to Enjoy Perimenopause (2014)*, *Bombshell: Explosive Medical Secrets that Will Redefine Aging (2012)*, *Sexy Forever: How to Fight Fat After Forty (2010)*, *Knockout: Interviews with Doctors Who are Curing Cancer—and How to Prevent Getting It in the First Place (2009)*, *Breakthrough: Eight Steps to Wellness (2008)*, *Ageless: The Naked Truth About Bioidentical Hormones (2007)*, and *The Sexy Years: Discover the Hormone Connection: The Secret to Fabulous Sex, Great Health, and Vitality, for Women and Men (2004)*. Dr. Galitzer's own publications include *Re-ignite Your Spark, No Batteries Required*, a chapter on bioidentical hormones in *Alternative Medicine, the Definitive Guide (2002)*, and research papers published in *Explore Magazine* and *The Townsend Letter for Doctors*. His work has also been featured in articles in the *New York Times Magazine*, and *C Magazine* in California.

In addition to his thriving practice in Santa Monica, Dr. Galitzer is the medical director of The American Health Institute in Los Angeles, an organization dedicated to education and research in the areas of Energy Medicine and cancer. He currently resides in Santa Barbara with his wife and four children.

Larry Trivieri Jr

Larry Trivieri Jr is a bestselling author and nationally recognized lay authority on holistic, integrative, and non-drug-based healing methods, with more than 30 years of personal experience in exploring techniques for optimal wellness and human transformation, including acid-alkaline balance. During that time, Trivieri has interviewed and studied with over 400 of the world's top physicians and other health practitioners in over 50 disciplines in the holistic health field.

Trivieri is the author or co-author of 20 books on health, including *The Acid-Alkaline Lifestyle, The Acid-Alkaline Food Guide, Juice Alive, The American Holistic Medical Association Guide to Holistic Health, The Self-Care Guide to Holistic Medicine,* and *Health On The Edge: Visionary Views of Healing in the New Millennium.* He also served as editor and principal writer of both editions of the landmark health encyclopedia, *Alternative Medicine: The Definitive Guide,* and has written over 200 articles for Internet-based health sites, including 1HealthyWorld.com and IntegrativeHealthReview.com. He has also written numerous feature articles for a variety of publications, including *Alternative Medicine,* for which he also served as contributing editor from 1999 through 2002; *Natural Health, Natural Solutions,* and *Yoga Journal.* He has also been written about in a number of national publications, including *The Washington Post.*

Trivieri is dedicated to sharing the wealth of potentially life-saving information he has learned about with as wide an audience as possible in order to help usher in a new era of wellness and health care in the 21st century. To that end, he also lectures about health nationwide, and has been a featured guest on numerous TV and radio shows across the United States.

Made in the USA
Middletown, DE
04 June 2015